Oncogenes

Cancer Treatment and Research

WILLIAM L MCGUIRE, *series editor*

Livingston, RB (ed): Lung Cancer 1. 1981. ISBN 90-247-2394-9.
Humphrey GB, Dehner LP, Grindey GB, Acton, RT (eds): Pediatric Oncology 1. ISBN 90-274-2408-2.
Decosse JJ, Sherlock P (eds): Gastrointestinal Cancer 1. 1981. ISBN 90-247-2461-9.
Bennett JM (ed): Lymphomas 1, including Hodgkin's Disease. 1981. ISBN 90-247-2479-1.
Bloomfield CD (ed): Adult Leukemias 1. 1982. ISBN 90-247-2478-3.
Paulson DF (ed): Genitourinary Cancer 1. 1982. ISBN 90-247-2480-5.
Muggia FM (ed): Cancer Chemotherapy 1. ISBN 90-247-2713-8.
Humphrey GB, Grindey GB (eds): Pancreatic Tumors in Children. 1982. ISBN 90-247-2702-2.
Costanzi JJ (ed): Malignant Melanoma 1. 1983. ISBN 90-247-2706-5.
Griffiths CT, Fuller AF (eds): Gynecologic Oncology. 1983. ISBN 0-89838-555-5.
Greco AF (ed): Biology and Management of Lung Cancer. 1983. ISBN 0-89838-554-7.
Walker MD (ed): Oncology of the Nervous System. 1983. ISBN 0-89838-567-9.
Higby DJ (ed): Supportive Care in Cancer Therapy. 1983. ISBN 0-89838-569-5.
Herberman RB (ed): Basic and Clinical Tumor Immunology. 1983. ISBN 0-89838-579-2.
Baker LH (ed): Soft Tissue Sarcomas. 1983. ISBN 0-89838-584-9.
Bennett JM (ed): Controversies in the Management of Lymphomas. 1983. ISBN 0-89838-586-5.
Humphrey GB, Grindey GB (eds): Adrenal and Endocrine Tumors in Children. 1983. ISBN 0-89838-590-3.
DeCosse JJ, Sherlock P (eds): Clinical Management of Gastrointestinal Cancer. 1983. ISBN 0-89838-601-2.
Catalona WJ, Ratliff, TL (eds): Urologic Oncology. 1983. ISBN 0-89838-628-4.
Santen RJ, Manni A (eds): Diagnosis and Management of Endocrine-Related Tumors. 1984. ISBN 0-89838-636-5.
Costanzi JJ (ed): Clinical Management of Malignant Melanoma. 1984. ISBN 0-89838-656-X.
Wolf GT (ed): Head and Neck Oncology. 1984. ISBN 0-89838-657-8.
Alberts DS, Surwit EA (eds): Ovarian Cancer. 1985. ISBN 0-89838-676-4.
Muggia FM (ed): Experimental and Clinical Progress in Cancer Chemotherapy. 1985. ISBN 0-89838-679-9.
Higby DJ (ed): The Cancer Patient and Supportive Care. 1985. ISBN 0-89838-690-X.
Bloomfield, CD (ed): Chronic and Acute Leukemias in Adults. 1985. ISBN 0-89838-702-7.
Herberman RB (ed): Cancer Immunology: Innovative Approaches to Therapy. 1986. ISBN 0-89838-757-4.
Hansen HH (ed): Lung Cancer: Basic and Clinical Aspects. 1986. ISBN 0-89838-763-9.
Pinedo HM, Verweij J (eds): Clinical Management of Soft Tissue Sarcomas. 1986. ISBN 0-89838-808-2.
Higby DJ (ed): Issues in Supportive Care of Cancer Patients. 1986. ISBN 0-89838-816-3.
Surwit EA, Alberts DS (eds): Cervix Cancer. 1987. ISBN 0-89838-822-8.
Jacobs C (ed): Cancers of the Head and Neck. 1987. ISBN 0-89838-825-2.
MacDonald JS (ed): Gastrointestinal Oncology. 1987. ISBN 0-89838-829-5.
Ratliff TL, Catalona WJ (eds): Genitourinary Cancer. 1987. ISBN 0-89838-830-9.
Nathanson L (ed): Basic and Clinical Aspects of Malignant Melanoma. 1987. ISBN 0-89838-856-2.
Muggia FM (ed): Concepts, Clinical Developments, and Therapeutic Advances in Cancer Chemotherapy. 1987. ISBN 0-89838-879-5.
Frankel AE (ed): Immunotoxins. 1988. ISBN 0-89838-984-4.
Bennett JM, Foon KA (eds): Immunologic Approaches to the Classification and Management of Lymphomas and Leukemias. 1988. ISBN 0-89838-355-2.
Osborne CK (ed): Endocrine Therapies in Breast and Prostate Cancer. 1988. ISBN 0-89838-365-X.
Lippman ME, Dickson R (eds): Breast Cancer: Cellular and Molecular Biology. 1988. ISBN 0-89838-368-4.
Kamps WA, Humphrey GB, Poppema S (eds): Hodgkin's Disease in Children: Controversies and Current Practice. 1988. ISBN 0-89838-372-2.
Muggia FM (ed): Cancer Chemotherapy: Concepts, Clinical Investigations and Therapeutic Advances. 1988. ISBN 0-89838-381-1.
Nathanson L (ed): Malignant Melanoma: Biology, Diagnosis, and Therapy. 1988. ISBN 0-89838-384-6.
Pinedo HM, Verweij J (eds): Treatment of Soft Tissue Sarcomas. 1989. ISBN 0-89838-391-9.
Hansen HH (ed): Basic and Clinical Concepts of Lung Cancer. 1989. ISBN 0-7923-0153-6.
Lepor H, Ratliff TL (eds): Urologic Oncology. 1989. ISBN 0-7923-0161-7.
Benz C, Liu E (eds): Oncogenes. 1989. ISBN 0-7923-0237-0.

Oncogenes

edited by

CHRISTOPHER BENZ
Cancer Research Institute
University of California, San Francisco

and

EDISON LIU
Lineberger Cancer Research Center
The University of North Carolina at Chapel Hill

1989 KLUWER ACADEMIC PUBLISHERS
BOSTON / DORDRECHT / LONDON

Distributors

for North America: Kluwer Academic Publishers, 101 Philip Drive, Assinippi Park, Norwell, Massachusetts 02061 USA
for all other countries: Kluwer Academic Publishers Group, Distribution Centre, Post Office Box 322, 3300 AH Dordrecht, THE NETHERLANDS

Library of Congress Cataloging-in-Publication Data

Oncogenes / edited by Christopher Benz and Edison Liu.
    p. cm.—(Cancer treatment and research)
  Includes bibliographies and index.
  ISBN 0-7923-0237-0
  1. Oncogenes. 2. Oncogenesis. I. Benz, Christopher. II. Liu,
Edison T. III. Series.
  [DNLM: 1. Oncogenes. W1 CA693 / QZ 202 05418]
RC268.42.O525 1989
616.99'4071—dc20
DNLM/DLC
for Library of Congress   89-2717
                                                                                                                CIP

Copyright © 1989 by Kluwer Academic Publishers

All rights reserved. No part of this publication may be reproduced, stored in a retrieval system or transmitted in any form or by any means, mechanical, photocopying, recording, or otherwise, without the prior written permission of the publisher, Kluwer Academic Publishers, 101 Philip Drive, Assinippi Park, Norwell, Massachusetts 02061.

PRINTED IN THE UNITED STATES OF AMERICA

Table of Contents

Foreword to the Series vii

Preface ix

List of Contributors xi

I. Basic Aspects of Oncogenes in Malignant Transformation

1. Oncogenes and proto-oncogenes: General concepts 3
    C. V. DANG

2. Molecular biology: Concepts and techniques 25
    E. LIU AND J.W. LARRICK

3. The *myc* family of nuclear proto-oncogenes 37
    W.M.F. LEE

4. The *ras* family of oncogenes 73
    C.J. DER

5. *src*-related protein tyrosine kinases 121
    A. VEILLETTE AND J.B. BOLEN

6. The epidermal growth factor receptor and its ligands 143
    A. WELLS

7. The platelet-derived growth factor system 169
    S.R. COUGHLIN AND M.T. KEATING

8. Transforming growth factors-α and -β and their potential
    roles in neoplastic transformation 177
    R. DERYNCK

II. Clinical Aspects of Oncogenes in Human Neoplasia

9. Oncogenes in human solid tumors 199
   C.F. ROCHLITZ AND C.C. BENZ

10. Oncogenes in human leukemias and lymphomas 241
    E. LIU

11. Human retrovirus-associated malignancy 267
    M.S. MCGRATH AND V.L. NG

12. The human DNA tumor viruses: Human papilloma virus   285
    and Epstein-Barr virus ....
    N. RAAB-TRAUB

13. Molecular biology of the human retinoblastoma gene 303
    Y.K.T. FUNG, A. T'ANG AND T.L. THOMPSON

14. Therapeutic applications of oncogenes 319
    J.W. LARRICK AND E. LIU

Index 331

Cancer Treatment and Research

Foreword

Where do you begin to look for a recent, authoritative article on the diagnosis or management of a particular malignancy? The few general oncology textbooks are generally out of date. Single papers in specialized journals are informative but seldom comprehensive; these are more often preliminary reports on a very limited number of patients. Certain general journals frequently publish good in-depth reviews of cancer topics, and published symposium lectures are often the best overviews available. Unfortunately, these reviews and supplements appear sporadically, and the reader can never be sure when a topic of special interest will be covered.

Cancer Treatment and Research is a series of authoritative volumes that aim to meet this need. It is an attempt to establish a critical mass of oncology literature covering virtually all oncology topics, revised frequently to keep the coverage up to date, and easily available on a single library shelf or by a single personal subscription.

We have approached the problem in the following fashion: first, by dividing the oncology literature into specific subdivisions such as lung cancer, genitourinary cancer, pediatric oncology, etc.; and second, by asking eminent authorities in each of these areas to edit a volume on the specific topic on an annual or biannual basis. Each topic and tumor type is covered in a volume appearing frequently and predictably, discussing current diagnosis, staging, markers, all forms of treatment modalities, basic biology, and more.

In *Cancer Treatment and Research*, we have an outstanding group of editors, each having made a major commitment to bring to this new series the very best literature in his or her field. Kluwer Academic Publishers has made an equally major commitment to the rapid publication of high-quality books, and to worldwide distribution.

Where can you go to find quickly a recent authoritative article on any major oncology problem? We hope that *Cancer Treatment and Research* provides an answer.

WILLIAM L. MCGUIRE
Series Editor

Preface

Like the other volumes in this series, *Oncogenes* addresses a diverse academic audience, ranging from clinical hematologists and oncologists to basic biochemists and molecular biologists. Clearly, this subject no longer belongs to one clinical or research specialty and is increasingly being accorded chapter status in a variety of comprehensive medical textbooks.

It has been less than two decades since the first oncogene, *src*, was identified in the chicken-infecting Rous sarcoma viral genome, and less than 15 years since J.M. Bishop and H.E. Varmus first discovered that v-*src* has a normal cellular counterpart, the proto-oncogene c-*src*. In this short span of time and with the increasing number of newly identified human proto-oncogenes (now approaching 50), there has been the co-emergence of an entire field of study related to oncogene structure and function; and yet the diversity of their many molecular forms and poorly understood cellular activities still challenges our ability to simply categorize them. The introductory chapter in this volume offers a general overview of oncogenes and proto-oncogenes, their current and historical relationship to tumor viruses, and a system of classification based on the biochemical properties and cellular functions of their encoded products, oncoproteins. The second chapter provides another overview, describing the many different experimental methods that are being applied to the study of oncogenes and oncogenesis; these analytical techniques are repeatedly referred to in the remaining chapters dealing with both basic and clinical aspects of this subject. A comprehensive basic review of all known oncogenes and their role in malignant transformation is well beyond the scope of this text. Instead, in the first part of this volume we have chosen to focus on selected oncogene systems that show promising clinical relevance: the *myc* and *ras* oncogene families, and those encoding growth factors and growth factor receptors with tyrosine kinase activity.

The most timely challenge of this volume, however, is its attempt to assess the clinical relevance of the rapidly accumulating data showing activation and expression of oncogenes in human malignancies. Underlying this worldwide study is the hypothesis that normal cellular proto-oncogenes can be activated to cancer-causing oncogenes by any number of different genetic alterations; this remains an appealing theory that is, no doubt, overly simplistic. Nonetheless, an expanding number of activated oncogenes have been detected in subsets of human leukemias, lymphomas, and solid tumors and are impressive pieces of evidence supporting this oncogene theory. The sum of this clinical evidence is presented in the second part of this volume. Additional chapters in this section provide important illustrations showing how RNA and DNA tumor viruses can directly and indirectly contribute to human tumorigenesis, and also describe the important and newly recognized role of tumor suppressor genes as uncovered in the study of hereditary retinoblastomas. No less important, a final chapter is devoted to novel approaches for anticancer therapies designed to reverse or inactivate oncogene abnormalities. These approaches, though speculative, emphasize the potential of applying oncogene research to clinical targets.

List of Contributors

BENZ, CC, M-1282 Cancer Research Institute, University of California San Francisco, San Francisco, CA 94143-0128

BOLEN, JB, Laboratory of Tumor Virus Biology, Building 41, Room D824, National Cancer Institute, N.I.H., Bethesda, MD 20892

COUGHLIN, SR, Howard Hughes Medical Institute, Box 0724, U412, University of California San Francisco, San Francisco, CA 94143

DANG, CV, Blalock 1063, Johns Hopkins Medical School, 600 North Wolfe Street, Baltimore, MD 21205

DER, CJ, La Jolla Cancer Research Foundation, 10901 North Torrey Pines Road, La Jolla, CA 92037

DERYNCK, R, Genentech, Inc., Department of Developmental Biology, 460 Point San Bruno Boulevard, South San Francisco, CA 94080

FUNG, YKT, Division of Hematology and Oncology, Department of Pediatrics, Microbiology, and Ophthalmology, Children's Hospital of Los Angeles, PO Box 54700, Los Angeles, CA 90054-0700

KEATING, MT, Howard Hughes Medical Institute, Box 0724, U412, University of California San Francisco, San Francisco, CA 94143

LARRICK, JW, Genelabs Inc., 505 Pnobscot Drive, Redwood City, CA 94063

LEE, WMF, Cancer Center, 7 Silverstein, H.U.P., 3400 Spruce Street, Philadelphia, PA 19104

LIU, E, CB#7295, 227 Lineberger Cancer Research Center, University of North Carolina at Chapel Hill, Chapel Hill, NC 27599

MCGRATH, MS, San Francisco General Hospital, WD-84, 1001 Potrero Avenue, San Francisco, CA 94110

NG, VL, San Francisco General Hospital, WD-84, 1001 Potrero Avenue, San Francisco, CA 94110

RAAB-TRAUB, N, Department of Microbiology and Immunology, Lineberger Cancer Research Center, The Medical School, University of North Carolina at Chapel Hill, Chapel Hill, NC 27599-7295

ROCHLITZ, CF, Free University of Berlin, Universite Klinikum Charlottenburg, Spandauer Damm 130, 1000 Berlin 19, West Germany

T'ANG, A, Division of Hematology and Oncology, Department of Pediatrics, Microbiology, and Ophthalmology, Children's Hospital of Los Angeles, PO Box 54700, Los Angeles, CA 90054–0700

THOMPSON, TL, Division of Hematology and Oncology, Department of Pediatrics, Microbiology, and Ophthalmology, Children's Hospital of Los Angeles, PO Box 54700, Los Angeles, CA 90054–0700

VEILLETTE, A, Laboratory of Tumor Virus Biology, Building 41, Room D-824, National Cancer Institute, N.I.H., Bethesda, MD 20892

WELLS, A, Division of Laboratory Medicine, University of California San Diego, Medical Center, San Diego, CA 92103

Basic Aspects of Oncogenes
in Malignant Transformation

1. Oncogenes and proto-oncogenes: General concepts

Chi V. Dang

Theoretically, the cancerous phenotype of cells can result from epigenetic or biochemical regulatory changes without alteration of the genotype. Although epigenetic changes may contribute to neoplasia, overwhelming evidence supports the concept that neoplasia results from heritable changes allowing unrestrained growth of cells that are associated with altered expression of certain 'cancer genes,' or oncogenes [1,2]. The normal cellular counterparts that probably play some role in normal cell proliferation and differentiation are called proto-oncogenes. Genetic alterations (such as proviral insertional mutations, chromosomal translocation, gene amplification, or point mutations) can activate cellular oncogenes that in turn contribute to neoplasia.

In this brief review, the following topics will be discussed: 1) the control of normal cell proliferation and mechanisms of transmembrane and intracellular signal transduction; 2) the concepts of viral oncogenes and cellular oncogenes; and 3) the mechanism of how altered expression or structure of cellular oncogene products contributes to neoplasia. These general concepts will provide the background for detailed discussions of specific oncogenes in the subsequent chapters.

Cell proliferation

The cell cycle

The mechanisms that produce cancer cells are likely to involve processes that control normal eucaryotic cell growth. Although the process of normal cell proliferation is incompletely understood, cells that proliferate in culture appear to progress through a growth cycle or cell cycle (figure 1) [3]. The cell cycle is resolvable into discrete stages: 1) S phase (DNA replication); 2) G_2 phase, which follows S phase; 3) mitosis (M), which follows G_2; and 4) G_1 phase, which precedes the S phase. Cells can withdraw from the cell cycle into a resting G_0 phase or terminally differentiate into nondividing cells.

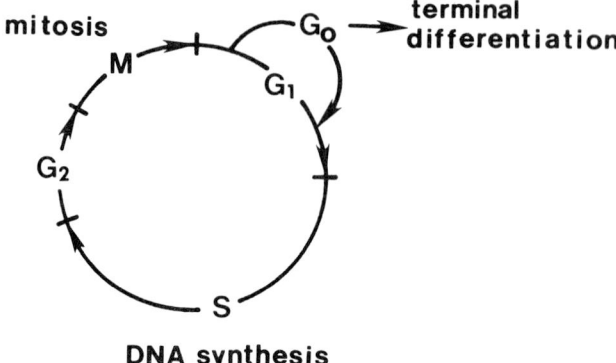

Figure 1. The cell cycle.

For specific cell types, each phase of the cell cycle has a predetermined length. During the S phase, replication of DNA occurs with the synthesis of histone proteins. At the G_2 stage, each cell contains two copies of each of the DNA molecules. The cell then divides in the mitotic (M) phase, when identical copies of DNA are distributed to each daughter cell. The most variable period is the G_1 phase, which can vary from hours to many days. Since control of cell growth involves the flux of cells into and out of the resting G_0 phase, it is critically important to understand the mechanisms that regulate this process.

Growth factors

Cells in culture and presumably those in animals can be stimulated to grow by soluble extracellular growth factor polypeptides, hormones, or mitogens [4]. Extracellular signals can be classified based on the distance over which the signal must act. Endocrine signals are produced by endocrine organs and carried to the target cells by the blood circulation. Paracrine signals produced by signaling cells only affect adjacent target cells. In autocrine signaling, the cells respond to substances that they themselves release.

The mode of cellular stimulation by steroid or thyroid hormone appears to be more direct than the way peptide growth factors act [5]. Steroid or thyroid hormones cross the plasma membrane to bind specific hormone receptors. The hormone receptor–hormone complex can affect gene expression by direct specific interaction with DNA.

Certain growth factors such as epidermal growth factor (EGF) are poor mitogens, but their activities can be potentiated by other factors such as platelet-derived growth factor (PDGF). PDGF and insulinlike growth factors share this property and are so-called competence factors because they can potentiate progression factors, such as EGF. The detailed mechanisms by

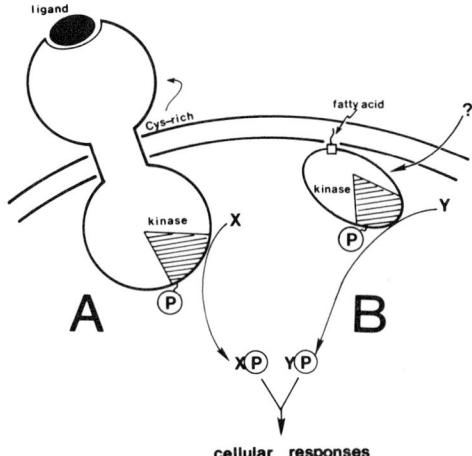

Figure 2. Protein-tyrosine kinases occur as transmembrane receptors (A) or membrane-associated proteins (B) that anchor in the lipid bilayer via a covalently bound fatty acyl moiety. The transmembrane receptor (A) consists of a ligand-binding domain and extracellular cysteine-rich domain that probably plays a role in conformational changes of the receptor. Information is transmitted through the transmembrane domain to activate the protein-tyrosine kinase activity, resulting in phosphorylation of protein X. Signals that activate the tyrosine kinase of (B) are not known.

which these factors stimulate cells to proliferate are not understood. However, it is known that growth factors act through binding specific membrane receptors. Extracellular stimuli arriving at the cell membrane must be accurately received and the message correctly transmitted inside the cell for appropriate responses to occur. These processes are referred to as signal transduction and are discussed below.

Transmembrane signal transduction

Several major biochemical pathways that transduce extracellular information and influence cell growth have been identified (figure 2–4): 1) membrane-associated protein kinases; 2) inositol phosphates, diacylglycerol, and protein kinase C; 3) guanine nucleotide-binding proteins and adenylate cyclase; and 4) calcium, calmodulin, and ion fluxes.

Membrane-associated protein kinases. Protein modification by phosphorylation plays an important role in signal transduction [6–8]. An example of a classical type of transmembrane receptor is the insulin receptor (figure 2). Upon interaction with insulin, tyrosine residues on the receptor protein are autophosphorylated [9]. Autophosphorylation of the receptor enhances its tyrosine kinase activity and permits it to phosphorylate target proteins, lead-

Table 1. Protein-tyrosine kinases

A. *src*-related
  fgr, fyn, lyn, lck, hck, src, yes
B. *abl*-related
  abl, arg, dash (Drosophila), *fes/fps*
C. Insulin-receptor-related
  INSR, IGF1R, DILR (Drosophila), *ros*, 7Less (Drosophila), *trk, met*
D. Epidermal growth factor receptor-related
  EGFR, *neu*, der (Drosophila)
E. Platelet-derived growth factor receptor-related
  PDGFR, CSF1R, *kit, ret*

---

ing to transfer of information across the membrane. Other similar receptors have been identified with protein kinase activity (table 1) [6].

Unlike the classical transmembrane receptors, a number of nontransmembrane proteins have been identified that have tyrosine-specific protein kinase activities (figure 2) [6]. Many of these proteins lack the extracellular domains and therefore probably transduce extracellular signals by interacting with classical receptors or with intermediary membrane proteins that relay the information across the cell membrane (table 1) [10]. Although the membrane-associated protein kinases are relatively well characterized, their physiologic and pathophysiologic protein substrates remain to be definitively identified.

Inositol phosphates, diacylglycerol, and protein kinase C. Activation of many membrane receptors result in the increase in intracellular Ca^{2+}. One of the mechanisms of increased intracellular Ca^{2+} is release of endoplasmic reticular Ca^{2+} stores. This process is mediated by the receptor activation of phospholipase C, which in turn hydrolyzes phosphatidyl inositol trisphosphate into inositol trisphosphate and diacylglycerol (figure 3) [11]. Inositol trisphosphate has been identified as the mediator for intracellular Ca^{2+} release. The effects of increased intracellular Ca^{2+} are numerous and include activation of protein kinase C (PKC) and calmodulin.

The other product of phospholipase hydrolysis, diacylglycerol, diffuse in the membrane and then binds to and activates PKC [12]. Increased intracellular calcium also appears to independently increase PKC activity. PKC has been shown to mediate the tumor-promoting effects of phorbol esters, which biologically resemble diacylglycerol. PKC is also known to activate other membrane receptors by phosphorylation, such as the EGF receptor. However, the substrates of PKC involved in cell growth or tumor promotion are not known definitively.

Guanine nucleotide-binding proteins and adenylyl cyclase. Adenylyl cyclase and phophodiesterase can transduce extracellular signals that influence cell growth by producing cAMP and degrading cAMP, respectively [13]. It has been proposed that cAMP levels reciprocally correlate with the state of cellular proliferation; however, this correlation is not universal. The mec-

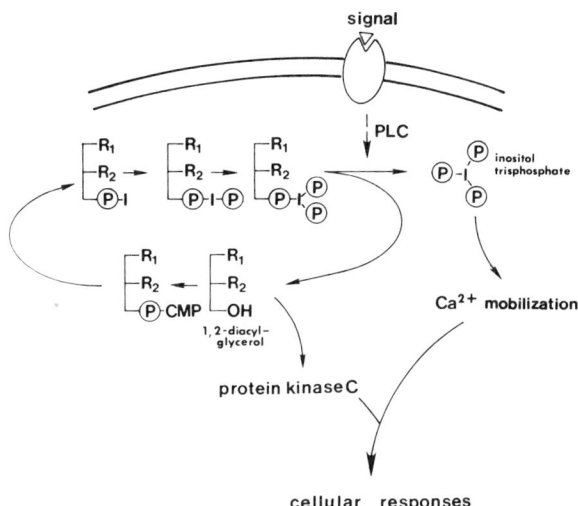

Figure 3. Inositol phosphate metabolism. Phosphatidyl inositol trisphosphate is hydrolyzed by signal-activated phospholipase C (PLC) to release inositol trisphosphate and 1,2-diacylglycerol, which stimulate calcium mobilization and protein kinase C, respectively. Diacylglycerol is recycled into phosphatidyl inositol (PI) monophosphate, to PI bisphosphate, and then to PI trisphosphate.

hanism of activation of adenylyl cyclase involves the transfer of information from membrane receptors by a group of GTP-binding proteins (figure 4) [14–16].

For example, it has been shown that binding of hormones to B-adrenergic receptors activates adenylyl cyclase through a communicator G protein. The G proteins, which are distinguished through differences in the α-subunit, are heterotrimers consisting of three subunits α, β and γ. The α-subunits contain GTPase activity and a guanine nucleotide-binding site that binds to GDP in the basal state [14–16]. Interaction of the hormone–receptor complex (H–R) with the G protein results in the dissociation of GDP. In the presence of high intracellular GTP, the G protein rapidly binds GTP. This reaction results in the dissociation of Gβ Gγ subunits from the Gα-GTP complex, which can interact with a target effector such as adenylyl cyclase. This activated GTP-bound G protein is short-lived due to the GTPase activity of G protein that converts GTP to GDP (figure 4). The G-proteins are a family of proteins that are involved in various receptor signal transductions (table 2). The *ras* oncoprotein (Ras) is related to this group of proteins; however, Ras does not appear to interact with the Gβ Gγ complex but rather with another protein that can enhance the intrinsic Ras GTPase activity [17].

The increase in intracellular cAMP is known to activate the cAMP-dependent protein kinase (PKA) [13]. It is established that glycogen synthesis and degradation is modulated by cAMP through the actions of PKA on the enzymes of glycogen metabolism. Presumably, the growth effects of cAMP

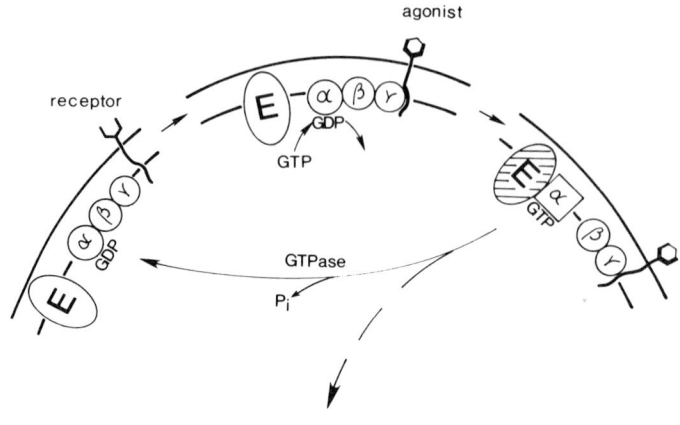

Figure 4. G proteins consist of three subunits α, β, and γ. The receptor–ligand complex interacts with the G-protein complex (through the α-subunit) to induce dissociation of GDP and the Gβ Gγ complex from Gα. The Gα–GTP complex activates the effector molecule (E), e.g. adenylyl cyclase. Intrinsic Gα GTPase hydrolyzes GTP and returns the Gα subunit to its basal state bound to GDP.

are also mediated by modification of proteins involved in cellular proliferation by PKA. The degradation of cAMP is also influenced by Ca^{2+}, since Ca^{2+} can activate phosphodiesterase.

Calcium, calmodulin, and ion fluxes. Stimulation of cell proliferation by mitogens is associated with increased intracellular Ca^{2+} and increased fluxes of Na^+, K^+, and H^+ that result in intracellular alkalinization [18]. The induction of cytoplasmic alkalinization is due to the activation of Na^+/H^+ exchange. The lack of this Na^+/H^+ antiport activity correlates with the inability of cells to be stimulated by mitogens. Hence, cytoplasmic alkalinization appears to be important for mitogenesis. In fact, introduction of a yeast proton-pump gene into fibroblasts can induce cytoplasmic alkalinization that is associated with tumorigenicity [19].

Table 2. G proteins

Subunits	MW (kDa)	Receptor	Role
Gsα	45, 52	β-adrenergic	Activates adenylyl cyclase
Giα	40	β-adrenergic GABA $α_2$-adrenergic muscarinic GABA	Inhibits adenylyl cyclase
Goα	40	$α_2$-adrenergic muscarinic rhodopsin	Pertussis-toxin sensitive
Gtα	40	β-adrenergic	Activates cGMP Phosphodiesterase
Gβ	37		
Gγ	9		Gβ Gγ complex deactivates Gα

The increase in intracellular Ca^{2+} transduces external stimuli in part by activation of calmodulin, which binds Ca^{2+} tightly [20]. Calmodulin, in turn, binds to and modulates protein kinase and other intracellular enzymatic activities. Additionally, Ca^{2+} influx appears to enhance PKC activity independent of diacylglycerol. The physiological significance of this alternative pathway for PKC activity remains to be established.

The existing evidence indicates that extracellular stimuli influence cell proliferation by interaction of growth factors with specific cell surface receptors. Another mode of cell stimulation is the direct interaction of steroid or thyroid hormones with intracellular receptors that can directly alter gene expression. Receptor–ligand interactions result in a number of modes of transmembrane signal transduction, including direct activation of receptor protein kinase activities or indirect activation of a variety of biochemical pathways discussed above. These pathways presumably lead to immediate cellular responses such as neuronal response to neurotransmitters or regulation of gene activity through modulation of transcriptional factors. Information on the latter is still fragmentary with much remaining to be investigated.

Transcription-regulating factors. Whichever intracellular signal transducing pathway is elicited by an external stimulus, one possible response is the activation or suppression of gene expression [21]. Modulation of gene expression can occur through intricate interactions between transcription-regulating proteins or factors. These factors may bind DNA directly or may bind to and modulate the DNA-binding activity of other proteins. While some transcription factors are constitutively present in certain cells, other factors require de novo protein synthesis after cellular stimulation.

The transcription of DNA to RNA is commonly controlled by multiple specific DNA sequences that interact with multiple protein factors. Promoter DNA sequences are required for RNA polymerase to bind to double-stranded DNA to initiate RNA synthesis. Enhancer sequences are *cis*-acting elements that increase the utilization of some eucaryotic promoters. The enhancers can function in any orientation and in any location relative to the promoter. Protein factors have been identified that bind specifically to promoter or enhancer sequences. A working hypothesis suggests that multiprotein complexes of transcription factors associate with promoter and enhancer sequences and catalyze the initiation of RNA synthesis from looped regions of DNA.

Studies with PDGF-stimulated cells demonstrate the increase expression of genes that encode proteins that bind DNA or proteins with significant homology with transcription factors. One such gene, *jun*B, encodes a protein that resembles an AP1 transcription factor [22]. The AP1 motif is found in the 5' sequence of many cellular genes and also in simian virus 40 (SV40) and polyoma enhancer sequences. Other genes activated by PDGF include the c-*fos* and c-*myc* proto-oncogenes. The c-*fos* protein was recently shown to associate with and enhance the binding of a transcription factor AP1 (c-Jun) protein to the AP1 site. Hence, it has been demonstrated that mitogenic stimulation can elicit the expression of certain transcription factors that result in a cascade of cellular responses.

The cancerous phenotype

The control of normal cell proliferation appears to involve regulated stimulation of cell surface and cytoplasmic receptors and activation or suppression of gene transcriptional activities. Derangement of any of these normal processes can theoretically result in uncontrolled cell growth. The cancerous phenotype most likely results from heritable changes that short-circuit normal pathways involved in normal cellular proliferation. In addition, cancer cells acquire the potential to metastasize, a phenotype which may be in part due to abnormal oncogene expression.

Several features of cultured cells associated with the cancerous or transformed phenotype are
1. Immortalization
2. Decreased serum dependency
3. Loss of contact growth inhibition
4. Anchorage-independent growth

The normal cell, like the intact organism, has a definite lifespan. In contrast to normal primary cells that have limited lifespan in culture, transformed cells can be passaged in culture indefinitely. This phenotype of immortalization appears to be associated with polyploidy that is acquired de novo or during culture. Cells in culture universally require serum for optimal growth, since serum contains many growth factors. Decreased serum requirement appears to be a common phenotype of transformed cells. Whether this phenomenon is related to autocrine stimulation of growth in transformed cells is not established as a universal mechanism.

Normal cells stop growing when cells contact each other at confluence. Apparently, cell–cell and cell–extracellular matrix interactions transduce signals that prevent cellular proliferation. In contrast, transformed cells tend to lose contact inhibition and are able to continue to grow and pile up upon one another. These piles of cells are recognized in culture as foci of transformed cells. A related phenotype is the ability of transformed cells to grow in suspension, whereas many normal cells require attachment to the substratum to grow. The ability to grow in suspension, or anchorage-independence, is yet another operational definition of the transformed phenotype.

Viral oncogenes and proto-oncogenes

Cellular transformation may occur spontaneously, result from mutagenic agents, or be caused by tumor viruses [23]. Many classes of DNA and RNA viruses can cause tumor. Among the RNA viruses are the retroviruses that carry viral oncogenes. These genes have homologous cellular counterparts or cellular proto-oncogenes. Other viruses can transform in the absence of a viral oncogene by insertionally activating cellular host genes. The DNA viruses appear to carry viral genes required for viral replication that are also oncogenic.

DNA tumor viruses

Among the DNA tumor viruses are the adenovirus, papovavirus, and herpes viruses [24]. Most notable is the simian virus 40 (SV40) that contains the large tumor (T) antigen. The T-antigen is a nuclear phosphoprotein of 708 amino acids that plays a role in SV40 DNA replication and gene transcription. However, the transforming activity of SV40 T-antigen does not appear to require nuclear location or DNA-binding activity [25]. Similarly, the adenovirus E1A protein-transforming activity does not appear to involve the ability of E1A to modulate adenoviral gene transcription, which is a normal function of E1A. Rather, E1A transforming activity appears to require domains of E1A that interact with cellular proteins [26,27]. In fact, it appears that both SV40 large T and E1A proteins interact specifically with the protein product of the retinoblastoma susceptibility (RB) locus [27,28]. This suggests that nuclear oncoproteins may induce transformation through protein–protein interactions instead of protein–nucleic-acid interactions.

There are various DNA viruses that are associated with human cancers. The hepatitis B virus is associated with hepatomas. Cervical cancers have been linked with papilloma virus infections. The molecular mechanisms by which these agents contribute to oncogenesis are unknown.

RNA tumor viruses

The study of RNA tumor viruses began with the discovery that avian leukemia can be transmitted horizontally by cell-free infectious agents [23]. The RNA tumor viruses are associated with a variety of neoplasms (table 3). The virion consists of an envelope derived from the plasma membrane of the host cells that encloses a nucleoprotein core. The viral genome and its propagation are depicted in figure 5.

The RNA tumor viruses can be classified as acutely and chronically transforming types. In general, the acutely transforming viruses carry with their incomplete genome transforming genes or viral oncogenes that have replaced part of the normal viral genome (table 3). The origin of viral oncogenes appears to be the capture or transduction of homologous host cellular genes or proto-oncogenes. It is noteworthy that viral oncogenes are significantly altered from their cellular counterpart. These changes can be viewed as acquired multiple mutations that cause the cellular counterpart to become oncogenic.

The protein product of viral oncogenes generally consists of fusions between

Table 3. RNA tumor viruses

A) Acutely transforming retroviruses

v-oncogene	Origin	Tumor
erb-A	Chicken	Erythroblastosis
erb-B	Chicken	Erythroblastosis
ets	Chicken	Erythroblastosis
fps	Chicken	Sarcoma
mil	Chicken	Myeloid leukemia
myb	Chicken	Myeloblastoma
myc	Chicken	Myelocytomatosis
ros	Chicken	Sarcoma
ski	Chicken	Sarcoma
src	Chicken	Sarcoma
yes	Chicken	Sarcoma
rel	Turkey	Reticuloendotheliosis
abl	Mouse	Leukemia
fos	Mouse	Osteosarcoma
mos	Mouse	Sarcoma
raf	Mouse	Sarcoma
Ha-*ras*	Rat	Sarcoma, erythroleukemia
Ki-*ras*	Rat	Sarcoma, erythroleukemia
fes	Cat	Sarcoma
fgr	Cat	Sarcoma
fms	Cat	Sarcoma
kit	Cat	Sarcoma
sis	Cat	Sarcoma

B) Retroviral insertionally activated oncogenes

Gene	Insertional agent	Tumor	Animal
c-*myc*	ALV, CSV, REV	B-cell lymphoma	Chicken
	MoMLV	T-cell lymphoma	Rat, mouse
	FeLV	T-cell lymphoma	Cat
c-*erb*B	ALV	Erythroblastosis	Chicken
Fis-1		Lymphoma	Mouse
c-Ha-*ras*	MAV	Nephroblastoma	Chicken
c-Ki-*ras*	F-MLV	Myeloid cell	Mouse
c-*mos*	IAP	Plasmacytoma	Mouse
c-*myb*	MLV	Lymphosarcoma	Mouse
Gin-1	G-MLV	T-cell lymphoma	Mouse
IL-2	GaLV	T-cell lymphoma	Monkey
IL-3	IAP	Myelomonocytic leukemia	Mouse
int-1	MMTV	Mammary cancer	Mouse
int-2	MMTV	Mammary cancer	Mouse
int-41	MMTV	Mammary cancer	Mouse
Mlvi-1	M-MLV	T-cell lymphoma	Rat
Mlvi-2	M-MLV	T-cell lymphoma	Rat

Table 3. (Continued)

Gene	Insertional agent	Tumor	Animal
Mlvi-3	M-MLV	T-cell lymphoma	Rat
pim-1	M-MLV	T-cell lymphoma	Mouse
pvt-1	M-MLV	Plasmacytoma	Mouse/rat
tck	M-MLV	Thymoma	Mouse

the viral *gag* protein and the oncogene protein. In a variety of retroviruses the viral oncogene appears to be sufficient for transformation.

By contrast, the chronically transforming viruses do not contain oncogenes (table 3). The mechanism of transformation by the chronically transforming viruses involves insertional activation of cellular "cancer genes" or proto-oncogenes. That is, integration of the viral genome into host DNA can activate host genes flanking the inserted viral genome either by viral promoter or enhancer activities.

The only human retroviruses that cause in vivo transformation are the HTLV-I and HTLV-II viruses. These viruses have been isolated from T-cell malignancies. The transforming activity of HTLV-I appears to be related to

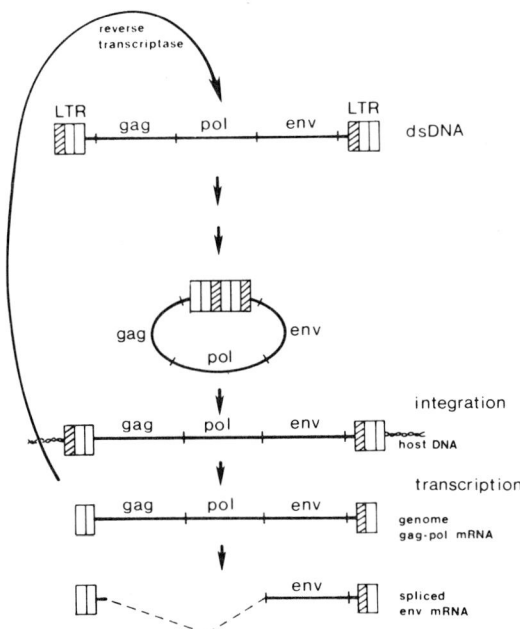

Figure 5. Life cycle of retroviruses. The genomic retroviral RNA is duplicated by reverse transcriptase to double-stranded DNA (dsDNA), which circularizes and integrates into the host cellular DNA. Transcription from the integrated provirus results in the genomic RNA or *gag-pol* mRNA and the spliced *env* mRNA.

the *trans*-activating activity of the virally encoded *tat* protein [29]. The cellular target(s) for the *tat* protein is(are) presently unknown.

Human oncogenes

Studies of viral oncogenes led to the discovery of the cellular counterparts or proto-oncogenes. Although it is quite evident that retroviruses carrying oncogenes can cause tumor formation, it remains to be proven that the cellular counterparts are also contributory to oncogenesis. To this end, in vitro transformation of NIH 3T3 cells (a mouse fibroblast cell line) by transfection with DNA isolated from various human tumor cells has identified a number of human transforming genes [30]. This technique is most sensitive for the detection of activated *ras* oncogenes; however, other transforming genes have also been identified by this technique (table 4) [31]. It is noteworthy that point mutations can occur with transfection of tumor DNA into NIH 3T3 cells. More recently activated *ras* oncogenes can be detected in primary tumor tissues by using the polymerase chain reaction to amplify the DNA of interest and hybridizing with specific oligonucleotides.

Oncogenes that are not detected by the transfection method, such as the *myc* family, have been implicated in oncogenesis of human tumors by their aberrant expression (table 5). Aberrant expression may result from gene amplication, rearrangement, or mutations that affect gene expression.

Another group of putative transforming genes localizes to chromosomal translocation breakpoints that are frequently associated with distinct types of neoplasms. Exemplary of this group is the human follicular lymphoma *bcl-2* gene, which fuses with an immunoglobulin gene [32]. Other putative proto-oncogenes associated with breakpoints are *bcl-1*, found in chronic lymphocytic lymphoma [33], and *tcl-1* and *tcl-2*, which are isolated from T-cell lymphoma/leukemia [34,35]. The *bcl-1* and *bcl-2* genes on chromosomes 11 and 18,

Table 4. Activated oncogenes in human cancers detected by transfection

Gene	Tumor
dbl	Diffuse B-cell lymphoma
hst	Stomach
lca	Hepatoma
mas	Epidermoid carcinoma
mcf2, *mcf3*	Breast
oncD (*trk*)	Colon
raf	Stomach
H-*ras*	Bladder, lung, breast
K-*ras*	Bladder, lung, colon, pancreas, stomach, gall bladder, ovary, rhabdomyosarcoma, acute lymphocytic leukemia
N-*ras*	Bladder, lung, colon, melanoma, neuroblastoma, fibrosarcoma, rhabdomyosarcoma, promyelocytic leukemia, chronic myelogenous leukemia, T-cell acute myelogenous leukemia
ret	T-cell lymphoma

respectively, are translocated to the immunoglobulin heavy-chain locus of chromosome 14 [32,33]. The *tcl*-1 and *tcl*-2 loci on chromosomes 7 and 11, respectively, are translocated to the T-cell receptor β- and α-chain loci on chromosome 14. Future investigations into the other pathognomonic chromosomal translocations in other tumors will yield additional loci of putative oncogenes.

Classes and functions of oncogenes

The classification of oncogenes is based on properties of the oncogene product such as a particular biochemical property or activity or the subcellular location of the oncoprotein. In keeping with the general scheme of signal transduction from the cell membrane to the nucleus, the classes of oncogenes will be discussed starting on the outside of the cell with growth-factor-like oncoproteins and ending with the nuclear oncoproteins (table 5).

Growth-factorlike oncogenes

It is conceivable that the abnormal expression of genes encoding growth-factorlike substances may result in either elevated amounts of growth factors or altered growth-factorlike proteins leading to aberrant cell growth. In fact, the p28 v-*sis* protein was the first oncoprotein discovered to display striking homology to the platelet-derived growth factor B chain [36]. This observation suggests that cells transformed by v-*sis* may be stimulated to grow via an autocrine mechanism whereby the transformed cells produce a growth factor that in turn stimulates the cells to proliferate further. This positive feed-back loop has been substantiated by the finding that cells transformed by v-*sis* are

Table 5. Classes of oncogenes

I)	*Growth-factor-related oncogenes*						
	sis	hst (Kaposi's *fgf*-like oncogene)					
	int-1	int-2					
II)	*Growth-factor-receptorlike oncogenes*						
	erbB1	erbB2 (neu)	met				
	ros	trk	fms	kit			
III)	*Protein-tyrosine kinase oncogenes*						
	abl	kit	src	erb1	met	yes	fgr
	neu	syn	fms	trk	lck	ros	lyn
	fps/fes						
IV)	*Protein-serine/threonine kinase oncogenes*						
	mos	pks	raf/mil	A-raf			
V)	*G-proteins-like oncogenes*						
	H-*ras*	N-*ras*	K-*ras*				
VI)	*Nuclear oncogenes*						
	fos	erb-A	jun	gli	ski	rel	
	c-*myc*	L-*myc*	N-*myc*	B-*myc*			

not stimulated by the secreted product, but instead the v-*sis* product probably stimulates the cells internally [37].

Another oncogene *int*-1, which is not transduced by transforming viruses but is insertionally activated by the mouse mammary tumor virus (MMTV), appears to produce a growth-factor-like product. The *int*-1 oncoprotein displays remarkable homology to the predicted protein sequence of the Drosophila *wingless* gene that is involved in the normal development of Drosophila appendages [38]. Although rigorous proof remains scarce, initial observation that *int*-1 is a secreted glycoprotein suggests that it is a soluble growth factor.

A number of human transforming genes display striking homology to fibroblast growth factor (FGF) [39]. Among these are the transforming gene isolated from Kaposi's sarcoma [40] and the *hst* oncogene isolated from human stomach cancer [41]. Yet another oncogene insertionally activated by MMTV is *int*-2, which also displays significant homology with FGF. These obvious homologies strongly suggest that these oncogenes also produce growth-factorlike materials.

Growth-factor-receptorlike oncogenes

Intracellular events can be triggered by the interaction of growth factors with specific receptors, resulting in conformational changes of the receptors. With this notion, it is conceivable that mutations in the growth-factor receptor, leading to increased affinity for growth factors or resulting in receptors with conformations resembling the activated ligand-bound receptor, can culminate in uncontrolled cell growth.

The first oncogene product recognized to resemble a growth-factor receptor is the v-*erb*B protein [42]. This protein corresponds to a truncated form of the EGF receptor with deletion of the extracellular amino-terminal end. The v-*erb*B protein contains the transmembrane and the cytoplasmic tyrosine kinase domain of the EGF receptor. Hence, it is a receptor that lacks the ligand-binding domain but retains the transducing domains, suggesting an unregulated receptor that may be constitutively in the activated state. Similar to *erb*B is the c-*neu* (*erb*B2) oncogene protein, which is the transforming gene isolated from ethylnitrosourea-induced rat neuroglioblastoma by DNA transfection experiments. The ligand for *neu* is unknown; however, amplication of *neu* has been reported in a subclass of human breast cancer [43].

Hematopoiesis involves the generation of blood cells from precursors that are stimulated to grow by specific growth factors [44]. Progenitor cells committed to the granulocyte–macrophage lineage are stimulated to grow by colony stimulating factor-1 (CSF-1). Specific receptors for CSF-1 are found on mononuclear phagocyte, macrophage, and myelomonocytic cell lines. The feline sarcoma virus (FeSV) transduces the oncogene v-*fms* whose product is a glycoprotein gp 140 v-*fms* [45]. The v-*fms* protein has characteristics of a membrane receptor with tyrosine kinase activity and resembles the CSF-1 receptor. The v-*fms* product has a C-terminal alteration that removes a site of tyrosine phosphorylation important for regulating the protein kinase activity. This alteration results in a constitutively active receptor that normally requires receptor–ligand interaction for activation. Although CSF-1 is specific for the monocytic cells, transgenic mice expressing v-*fms* display multilineage hematopoietic abnormalities.

Other potential growth-factor-receptorlike oncogenes are the *ros* and *trk* genes [46,47]. An unusual characteristic of the *ros* gene is that activation by gene rearrangement can occur during gene transfer, which is used as an assay for human oncogenes. The rearrangement results in the loss of the ligand-binding domain in a manner similar to activated genes of *erb*B and v-*fms*. ROS1 rearrangement and increased expression have been detected in a human glioblastoma cell line. Remarkably, when the ROS oncogene is replaced by the human insulin-receptor gene in the avian sarcoma virus UR2, the resulting virus is capable of transforming chicken embryo fibroblast [48]. The genome codes for a membrane-associated *gag*–human-insulin-receptor fusion protein. These findings indicate that specific mutations of normal growth-factor receptors can result in transforming genes. The *trk* oncogene was identified in a human colon carcinoma biopsy. This oncogene is activated by a rearrangement that fuses part of the nonmuscle tropomyosin gene with the sequences from a tyrosine kinase locus *trk*. The tyrosine kinase activity appears to be required for transformation, since various rearrangements of *trk*, which transforms fibroblasts, retain the tyrosine kinase domain [49]. The tropomyosin component of the fusion protein is not required for transformation. These observations substantiate the hypothesis that alterations of membrane receptors leading to a virtual activated receptor may be sufficient for transformation.

Protein–tyrosine-kinase oncogenes

Another class of oncogenes that is related to growth-factor receptors are the peripheral membrane-associated oncoproteins with tyrosine kinase activity. The prototype *src* oncogene was among the first to be discovered in this class of oncogenes. Presumably, these proteins receive signals from transmembrane receptors or membrane signal-transducing intermediary proteins, resulting in activation of the tyrosine kinase activity. Specific phosphorylation of substrates by this class of proteins is believed to lead to appropriate cellular responses such as cell proliferation.

The v-*src* oncogene produces a fatty-acid-bound or myristylated membrane-associated protein that appears to phosphorylate specific cellular proteins. Myristylation appears to be important for transforming activity, since site-directed mutagenesis of *src* leading to the lack of myristylation results in the loss of transforming activity. The events following protein phosphorylation that lead to the transformed phenotype are not yet known. In fact, one of the major *src* phosphorylated proteins, p36, does not appear to be necessary for transformation [50].

The c-*abl* oncogene, which encodes a membrane-associated tyrosine kinase, is translocated in over 90% of chronic myelogenous leukemias (CMLs) and results in production of a fusion protein consisting of *bcr* and *abl* [51]. Although the c-*abl* protein has low intrinsic tyrosine kinase activity, both the *bcr-abl* and the v-*abl* proteins, which have an N-terminal segment encoded by the viral genome fused to *abl*, have high levels of tyrosine kinase activity. Although the *bcr-abl* product is assumed to contribute to the pathogenesis of CML, this hypothesis remains to be substantiated. In fact, the *bcr-abl* product does not transform fibroblasts [52]. Perhaps fibroblasts are not suitable hosts for the expression of the transformed phenotype.

Other membrane-associated tyrosine kinases have been implicated in the genesis of a variety of tumors (table 1). In general, these oncogenes are activated by mutations that lead to enhanced tyrosine kinase activity. Since the pathogenic substrate(s) for these tyrosine kinases are not yet known, the significance of tyrosine-specific phosphorylation remains to be delineated.

Protein-serine/threonine kinase oncogenes

Phosphorylation of proteins catalyzed by protein–serine/threonine kinases constitutes one of the major processes that control cellular functions [53]. Some of these protein kinases play a role in the regulation of cell proliferation; among these are the cAMP-dependent protein kinases, the calcium/calmodulin-dependent protein kinases, and protein kinase C. Not suprisingly, several onocoproteins have serine/threonine kinase activities.

The *raf* family of proto-oncogenes encodes cytoplasmic serine/threonine-specific protein kinases that have partial homology to the *src* family of tyrosine kinases [54]. Oncogenicity of the *raf* genes may involve altered gene products [55]. It is most likely, but presently unclear, that the protein kinase activity is involved in transformation.

The *mos* proteins have been shown to have serine/threonine autophosphorylation activity and to localize in the cytoplasm. In addition, the p40 Mos has ATPase, ATP-binding, and DNA-binding activities [56]. Whether any of these biochemical properties are relevant for transforming activity is unknown.

The major challenge in understanding this group of onco-proteins appears to be establishing the functional importance of phosphorylation and identification of the pathophysiologic substrates.

G-protein-related oncogenes

The *ras* family of oncoproteins represents an intriguing group of oncoproteins all of which appear sufficient by themselves when mutated to transform certain cells [57]. Moreover, mutations of these genes appear to be a major factor in the genesis of many different human cancers [58]. Biochemically, these proteins bind guanine nucleotides and resembles the G-proteins group.

The four types of *ras* genes that encode proteins of 21 kDa are H-, K-, N-, and R-*ras*. Conversion of H-, K-, and N-*ras* genes to transforming genes appears to involve mutations of specific amino acids at positions 12, 13, and 61. Recently, crystal structure of recombinant c-H-*ras* protein demonstrates that these amino acids are in close proximity to the guanine nucleotide-binding site [59]. Theoretically, the mutations at these sites can contribute to the enhanced binding of GTP and/or decrease GTPase activity. Experimentally, decreased GTPase activity appears to be the lesion responsible for the abnormal behavior of these mutant molecules. These biochemical changes result in a constitutive activated state of the *ras* proteins that appears to contribute to oncogenesis. The cellular targets for activated *ras* proteins are unknown. The *ras* protein may interact directly with a cytoplasmic protein, GTPase-activating protein (GAP), that enhances the GTPase activity of normal but not mutated *ras* [17]. Furthermore, reports suggest that *ras* may be involved in the phosphoinositide metabolism.

In contrast to the human *ras* genes, the yeast homologs *NRAS1* and *NRAS2* stimulate adenylate cyclase activity, a function not associated with the mammalian *ras* proteins [60]. Another *ras*-related yeast protein *YPT1* has been identified and appears to be involved in the organization of microtubules [61]. Clues from yeast homologs of mammalian *ras* may yield avenues to attack the biochemical mechanisms of oncogenesis by the *ras* proteins.

The ability of the *ras* proteins to cooperate with nuclear oncogenes in transforming primary embryo cells is an intriguing phenomenon. The mechanism by which this occurs is unknown.

Nuclear oncogenes

The nuclear oncoproteins are most likely involved in the final steps of signal transduction that can lead to cell growth [62]. Initially, the nuclear oncogenes were classified together because their products localize to the nucleus. However, recent work from many laboratories have provided evidence for the involvement of some of the nuclear oncoproteins in transcriptional regulation. More controversial is the direct role of some of the nuclear oncoproteins in DNA replication. Among the better studied nuclear oncoproteins are c-*myc*, N-*myc*, c-*myb*, c-*fos*, c-*erb*-A, c-*rel*, and c-*jun*.

Nuclear location, a property shared by all nuclear oncoproteins, is determined by specific peptide sequence(s) that is (are) found in the oncoprotein (or possibly proteins associated with the oncoprotein). A definitive identification of such sequence in a nuclear oncoprotein was carried out with the human c-*myc* protein [63]. This sequence resembles nuclear targeting sequences of viral proteins. It consists of a short peptide that starts at the N-terminal end with a helix-breaking amino acid, followed by several positively charged amino acids. Proper nuclear location of c-*myc* is not required for its co-transforming activity with EJ-*ras*. Similarly, nuclear location of SV40 T-Ag or c-*rel* is not required for transforming activity [64].

Another property shared by some of the nuclear oncoproteins is the ability to bind DNA in vitro. Whether this property is relevant for transforming activity remains unclear for most oncoproteins except possibly for the c-*jun*/ c-*fos* protein complex [65–67]. It has become clear that the c-*jun*/c-*fos* complex binds specifically to AP-1 DNA sites. How this may be related to transformation remains to be elucidated. Interestingly, a number of nuclear oncoproteins, namely c-*fos*, c-*jun*, c-*myc*, N-*myc*, and L-*myc*, share an intriguing heptad repeat of leucines in regions of the proteins predicted to be alpha-helical. It has been proposed that such a motif can mediate protein–protein interaction important for the recognition of specific DNA binding sites [68]. This hypothesis remains to be substantiated, but it does raise the possibility that transformation may be mediated in part by protein–protein interactions involving nuclear oncoproteins. Recently, the viral transforming proteins SV40 T and E1A were shown to bind specifically to the protein product of the retinoblastoma gene through regions of SV40 T or E1A that are important for transformation [27,28]. Whether the other nuclear oncoproteins interact specifically with other cellular proteins is a subject of current and future investigations.

Although the exact biochemical functions of nuclear oncoproteins other than *jun*, *fos*, and *erb*-A remain unclear, it appears that in most cases the presence of an elevated level of the nuclear oncoprotein is contributory to the transformed phenotype. This may occur through many different mechanisms including gene amplification, enhanced transcriptional rate, and prolonged mRNA half-lives. Even though many different genetic mechanisms lead to an elevated level of protein, the biochemical consequences of this elevation remain a mystery since the immediate and relevant targets for many nuclear oncoproteins are not known.

The c-*erb*-A gene is a unique member of the nuclear oncogenes, since it has been identified as the thyroid hormone receptor or a closely related gene [69,70]. The c-*erb*-A protein binds to thyroxine and tri-iodothyronine, which appears to be required for the growth of certain cells in culture. The retroviral homolog v-*erb*-A can inhibit the expression of band 3, a major anion transporter of chicken erythrocytes [71]. Whether band 3 expression is altered by the direct or indirect interaction of v-*erb*-A protein on the band 3 gene is unclear. It is likely that the pathophysiologic effect of *erb*-A is related to its ability to specifically bind DNA through the zinc-finger motif. The c-*erb*-A gene is nontransforming by contrast to v-*erb*-A, which cooperates with v-*erb*-B to transform chicken cells [72]. The v-*erb*-A protein consists of the viral *gag* protein fused with the DNA and ligand binding domains of *erb*-A that contain several point and deletion mutations. v-*erb*-A does not bind thyroid hormones, suggesting that it is a constitutively 'on' hormone receptor.

Mechanisms of proto-oncogene activation

The mechanism of proto-oncogene activation varies with the type or class of proto-oncogene described above. It is clear that mutations in the genome can result in a variety of gene-regulatory and/or protein-structure abnormalities. Mutations may vary from single point alterations, as found in *ras*, to chromosomal translocation, as exemplified by *bcr-abl* fusion that occur in chronic myelogenous leukemia.

Clearly, the most dramatic case of proto-oncogene activation by point mutation is exemplified by the altered gene product of the *ras* oncogenes. The result is a profound disturbance of the biochemical properties of the *ras* proteins. By contrast, many other oncoproteins appear to require more extensive alteration of protein structure for activation of transforming activity. This feature is exemplified by many viral oncoproteins that are fusions of viral *gag* protein and the transduced oncogene sequences such as *myc*, *myb*, and *abl*. For *abl*, the human oncogenic equivalent may be the fusion of *bcr* and *abl*. It has been proposed that the oncogenic retroviral genes may be viewed as multiply mutated transduced 'proto-oncogenes' [73].

On the other hand, the group of oncogenes that contributes to oncogenesis through elevated levels of normal protein product requires gene amplification, activation of transcriptional rate, or enhancement of mRNA stability through specific mutations. For *myc* and *fos*, mutations that alter transcriptional rate, including chromosomal translocation, changes in transcriptional attenuation in *myc* exon I, or mutations that change mRNA stablility leading to increased protein level, play a central role in oncogenic activation.

To summarize, two major modes of activation of proto-oncogenes appear to exist: mutations that lead to abnormalities in protein structure and mutations that lead to enhanced levels of normal protein product. It is noteworthy that the class of anti-oncogenes (not discussed above) is also involved in oncogenesis. In contrast to the oncogenes, the loss or inactivation of anti-oncogenes or their products may be contributory to transformation. The protein products of these genes theoretically play a role in the suppression of abnormal cell growth.

Acknowledgments

Research is supported in part by PHS Biomedical Research Support, American Cancer Institutional Research, and Henry M. and Lillian Stratton Foundation Grants.

References

1. Varmus HE: Cellular and viral oncogenes. In: Stamatoyannopoulos G, Nienhuis AW, Leder P, Majerus PW (eds): The Molecular Basis of Blood Diseases. Philadelphia, WB Saunders, 1987, pp 271–346.
2. Bishop JM: The molecular genetics of cancer. Science 235:305–311, 1987.
3. Baserga R: The Biology of Cell Reproduction. Cambridge, Havard University Press, 1985.
4. Sporn MB, Roberts AB: Peptide growth factors are multifunctional. Nature 332:217–219, 1988.

5. Evans RM: The steroid and thyroid hormone receptor superfamily. Science 240:889–895, 1988.
6. Hanks SK, Quinn AM, Hunter T: The protein kinase family: conserved features and deduced phylogeny of the catalytic domains. Science 241:42–52, 1988.
7. Hunter T, Cooper JA: Protein tyrosine kinases. Annu Rev Biochem 54:897–930, 1985.
8. Sherr CJ: Growth factor receptor and cell transformation. Mol Biol Med 4:1–10, 1987.
9. Czech MP, Klarlund JK, Yagaloff KA, Bradford AP, Lewis RE: Insulin receptor signalling. J Biol Chem 263:11017–11020, 1988.
10. Yarden Y, Ullrich A: Molecular analysis of signal transduction by growth factors. Biochemistry 27:3113–3119, 1988.
11. Majerus PW, Connolly TM, Bansal VS, Inhorn RC, Ross TS, Lips DL: Inositol phophates: synthesis and degradation. J Biol Chem 263:3051–3054.
12. Kikkawa U, Nishizuka Y: Role of protein kinase C in transmembrane signalling. Annu Rev Cell Biol 2:149–178, 1986.
13. Roesler WJ, Vanderbark GR, Hanson RW: Cyclic AMP and the induction of eukaryotic gene expression. J Biol Chem 263:9063–9066, 1988.
14. Neer EJ, Clapham DE: Roles of G protein subunits in transmembrane signalling. Nature 333:129–134, 1988.
15. Gilman AG: G proteins: transducers of receptor-generated signals. Annu Rev Biochem 56:615–649, 1987.
16. Casey PJ, Gilman AG: G protein involvement in receptor–effector coupling. J Biol Chem 263:2577–2580, 1988.
17. Cales C, Hancock JF, Marshall CJ, Hall: The cytoplasmic protein GAP is implicated as the target for regulation by the *ras* gene product. Nature 332:548:551, 1988.
18. Rozengurt E: Early signals in the mitogenic response. Science 234:161–166, 1986.
19. Perona R, Serrano R: Increased pH and tumorigenicity of fibroblasts expressing a yeast proton pump. Nature 334:438–440, 1988.
20. Klee CB, Gouch TH, Richman PG: Calmodulin. Annu Rev Biochem 49:489–515, 1980.
21. McKnight S, Tjian R: Transcriptional selectivity of viral genes in mammalian cells. Cell 46:795–805, 1986.
22. Ryder K, Lau LF, Nathans D: A gene activated by growth factors is related to the oncogene v-*jun*. Proc Natl Acad Sci USA 85:1487–1491, 1988.
23. Varmus HE: Retroviruses. Science 240:1427–1435, 1988.
24. Levine AJ: Oncogenes of DNA tumor viruses. Cancer Res 48:493–496, 1988.
25. Colledge WH, Richardson WD, Edge MD, Smith AE: Extensive mutagenesis of the nuclear location signal of simian virus 40 large T antigen. Mol Cell Biol 8:2177–2183, 1986.
26. Velcich A, Ziff E: Adenovirus Ela *ras* cooperation activity is separate from its positive and negative transcription regulating functions. Mol Cell Biol 8:2177–2183, 1988.
27. Whyte P, Buchkovich KJ, Horowitz JM, Friend SH, Raybuch M, Weinberg RA, Harlow E: Association between an oncogene and an anti-oncogene: the adenovirus E1A products bind to the retinoblastoma gene product. Nature 334:124–129, 1988.
28. DeCaprio JA, Ludlow JW, Figge J, Shew JY, Huang CM, Lee WH, Marsilio E, Paucha E, Livingston D: SV40 large tumor antigen forms a specific complex with the product of the retinoblastoma susceptibility gene. Cell 54:275–283, 1988.
29. Yoshida M, Seiki M: Recent advances in the molecular biology of HTLV-1: transactivation of viral and cellular genes. Annu Rev Immunol 5:541–559, 1987.
30. Shih C, Shilo B, Goldfarb MP, Dannenberg A, Weinberg RA: Passage of phenotypes of chemically transformed cells via transfection of DNA and chromatin. Proc Natl Acad Sci USA 76:5714–5718, 1979.
31. Nishimura S, Sekiya T: Human cancer and cellular oncogenes. Biochem J 243:313–327, 1987.
32. Tsujimoto Y, Cossman J, Jaffe E, Croce CM: Involvement of the *bcl*-2 gene in human follicular lymphoma. Science 228:1440–1443, 1985.
33. Tsujimoto Y, Jaffe E, Cossman J, Gorham J, Nowell PC, Croce CM: Clustering of break-

points on chromosome 11 in human B-cell neoplasms with the t[11;14] chromosome translocation. Nature 315:340–343, 1985.
34. Morton CC, Duby AD, Eddy RL Show TB, Seidman JG: Genes for beta gene of human T-cell antigen receptor map to regions of chromosomal rearrangement in T cells. Science 228:582–585, 1985.
35. Lewis WH, Michalopoulos EE, Williams DL, Minden MD, Mak TW: Breakpoints in the human T-cell antigen receptor alpha-chain locus in two T-cell leukaemia patients with chromosomal translocations. Nature 317:544–546, 1985.
36. Doolittle RF, Hunkapiller MW, Hood LE, Devare SG, Robbins KC, Aaronson SA, Antonaides HN: Simian sarcoma virus *onc* gene, v-*sis*, is derived from the gene (or genes) encoding a platelet-derived growth factor. Science 221:275–277, 1983.
37. Keating MT, Williams LT: Autocrine stimulation of intracellular PDGF receptors in v-*sis* transformed cells. Science 239:914–916, 1988.
38. Rijsewijk F, Schuermann M, Wagenaar E, Parren P, Weigel D, Nusse R: The Drosophila homolog of the mouse mammary oncogene *int*-1 is identical to the segment polarity gene wingless. Cell 50:649–657, 1987.
39. Jaye M, Lyall RM, Mudd R, Schlessinger J, Sarver N: Expression of acidic fibroblast growth factor cDNA confers growth advantage and tumorigenesis to Swiss 3T3 cells. EMBO J 7:963–969, 1988.
40. Delli Bovi P, Curatola AM, Kern FG, Breco A, Ittman M, Basilico C: An oncogene isolated by transfection of Kaposi's sarcoma DNA encodes a growth factor. Cell 50:729–737, 1987.
41. Taira M, Yoshida T, Miyagawa K, Sakamoto H, Terada M, Sugimara T; cDNA sequence of human transforming gene *hst* and identification of the coding sequence required for transforming activity. Proc Natl Acad Sci USA 84:2980–2984, 1987.
42. Downward J, Yarden Y, Mayes E, Scrace G, Totty N, Stockwell P, Ullrich A, Schlessinger J, Waterfield MD: Close similarity of epidermal growth factor receptor and v-*erb*-B oncogene protein sequences. Nature 307:521–527, 1984.
43. Slamon DJ, Clark GM, Wong SG, Levin WJ, Ullrich A, McGuire WL: Human breast cancer: correlation of relapse and survival with amplification of the HER-2/*ner* oncogene. Science 235:177–182, 1987.
44. Sieff CA: Hematopoietic growth factors. J Clin Invest 79:1549–1557, 1987.
45. Sherr CJ, Rettenmier CW, Sacca R, Roussel MF, Look AT, Stanley ER: The c-*fms* proto-oncogene product is related to the receptor for the mononuclear phagocyte growth factor CSF-1. Cell 41:665–676, 1985.
46. Birchmeier C, Sharma S, Wigler M: Expression and rearrangement of the ROS1 gene in human glioblastoma cells. Proc Natl Acad Sci USA 84:9270–9274, 1987.
47. Oskam R, Coulier F, Ernst M, Martin-Zanca D, Barbacid M: Frequent generation of oncogenes by *in vitro* recombination of *Trk* protooncogene sequences. Proc Natl Acad Sci USA 85:2964–2968, 1988.
48. Wang LH, Lin B, Jong SMJ, Dixon D, Ellis L, Roth RA, Rutter WJ: Activation of transforming potential of the human insulin receptor gene. Proc Natl Acad Sci USA 84:5725–5729, 1987.
49. Kozma SC, Redmond SMS, Xiao-Chang F, Saurer SM, Groner B, Hynes NE: Activation of the receptor kinase domain of the *trk* oncogene by recombination with two cellular sequences. EMBO J 7:147–154, 1988.
50. Kamps MP, Buss JE, Sefton BM: Rous sarcoma virus transforming protein lacking myristic acid phosphorylates known peptide substrates without inducing transformation. Cell 45: 105–112, 1986.
51. Dreazen O, Canaani E, Gale RP: Molecular biology of chronic myelogenous leukemia. Semin Hematol 25:35–49, 1988.
52. Daley GQ, McLaughlin J, Witte ON, Baltimore D: The CML-specific P210 *bcr/abl* protein, unlike v-*abl*, does not transform NIH/3T3 fibroblasts. Science 237:532–535, 1987.
53. Edelman AM, Blumenthal DK, Krebs EG: Protein serine/threonine kinases. Annu Rev Biochem 56:567–613, 1987.

54. Kasid U, Pfeifer A, Weichselbaum RR, Dritschilo A, Mark GE: The *raf* oncogene is associated with a radiation-resistant human laryngeal cancer. Science 237:1039–1041, 1987.
55. Stanton VP, Cooper GM: Activation of human *raf* transforming genes by deletion of normal amino-terminal coding sequences. Mol Cell Biol 7:1171–1179, 1987.
56. Seith A, Priel E, Vande Woude GF: Nucleotide triphosphate-dependent DNA-binding properties of *mos* protein. Proc Natl Acad Sci USA 84:3560–3564, 1987.
57. Barbacid M: *ras* genes. Annu Rev Biochem 56:779–827, 1987.
58. Bos JL, Fearon ER, Hamilton SR, Verlaan-deVries M, van Boom JH, van der Eb AT, Volgelstein B: Prevalence of *ras* gene mutations in human colorectal cancers. Nature 327:293–297, 1987.
59. deVos A, Tong L, Milburn MV, Matias PM, Jancarik J, Noguchi S, Nishimura S, Miura K, Ohtsuka E, Kim SH: Three dimensional structure of an oncogene protein: catalytic domain of human c-H-*ras* p21. Science 239:888–893, 1988.
60. Toda T, Uno I, Ishikawa T, Powers S, Kataoka T, Broek D, Cameron S, Broach J, Matsumoto K, Wigler M: In yeast, *RAS* proteins are controlling elements of adenylate cyclase. Cell 40:27–36, 1985.
61. Schmitt HD, Wagner P, Pfaff E, Gallwitz D: The *ras*-related *YPT*1 gene product in yeast: a GTP-binding protein that might be involved in microtubule organization. Cell 47:401–412, 1986.
62. Alt FW, Harlow E, Ziff EB: Nuclear Oncogenes. Current Communications in Molecular Biology. Cold Spring Harbor, NY, Cold Spring Harbor Laboratory, 1987.
63. Dang CV, Lee WMF: Identification of the human c-*myc* protein nuclear translocation signal. Mol Cell Biol 8:4048–4054, 1988.
64. Gilmore TD, Temin HM: v-*rel* oncoproteins in the nucleus and cytoplasm transform chicken spleen cells. J Virol 62:703–714, 1988.
65. Franza BR JR, Rauscher III FJ, Josephs SF, Curran T: The Fos complex and Fos-related antigens recognize sequence elements that contain AP1 binding sites. Science 239:1150–1153, 1988.
66. Bohmann D, Bos TJ, Admon A, Nishimura T, Vogt PK, Tjian R: Human proto-oncogene c-*jun* encodes a DNA binding protein with structural and functional properties of transcription factor AP-1. Science 238:1386–1392, 1988.
67. Angel P, Allegretto EA, Okino ST, Hattori K, Boyle WT, Hunter T, Karin M: Oncogene *jun* encodes a sequence-specific trans-activator similar to AP-1. Nature 332:166–170, 1988.
68. Landshulz WH, Johnson PF, McKnight SL: The leucine zipper: a hypothetical structure common to a new class of DNA binding proteins. Science 240:1759–1764, 1988.
69. Weinberger C, Thompson EC, Ong ES, Lebo R, Gruol DJ, Evans RM: The c-*erb*-A gene encodes a thyroid hormone receptor. Nature 324:641–646, 1986.
70. Munoz A, Zenke M, Gehring U, Sap J, Beug H, Vennstrom B: Characterization of the hormone-binding domain of the chicken c-*erb*-A/thyroid hormone receptor protein. EMBO J 7:155–159, 1988.
71. Zenke M, Kahn P, Disela C, Vennstrom B, Lentz A, Keegan K, Hayman MJ, Choi HR, Yew N, Engel JD, Beug H: v-*erb*-A specifically suppresses transcription of the avian anion transporter (band 3) gene. Cell 53:107–119, 1988.
72. Kahn P, Fryberg L, Brady C, Stanley IJ, Beug H: v-*erb*-A cooperates with sarcoma oncogenes in leukemia cell transformation. Cell 45:349–356, 1986.
73. Temin HM: Evolution of cancer genes as a mutation-driven process. Cancer Res 48: 1697–1701, 1988.

2. Molecular biology: Concepts and techniques

Edison Liu and James W. Larrick

This chapter briefly reviews the principles of molecular biology, and the techniques that frequently are mentioned in this volume. The nuances of molecular biology are not explored, and the discussions of certain biological processes are necessarily dogmatic. The reader is referred to more lengthy texts for detailed discussions [1–3].

Concepts of molecular biology

Introduction

All genetic information is encoded in deoxyribonucleic acid or DNA, which is comprised of four bases—adenine, thymine, cytosine, and guanine (designated A, T, C, G)—linked together by a sugar backbone (deoxyribose) into a long linear molecule. These four bases can be viewed as the alphabet in which the genetic code is written. Just as the alphabet is meaningless until grouped together as words, these bases attain a higher meaning when placed in groups of three called *codons*. Each codon determines a specific amino acid, and a string of codons on a DNA molecule then determines the sequence of amino acids in a protein. The flow of genetic information within a cell is from DNA to RNA (ribonucleic acid) to protein and provides a process by which information can be transmitted from the nucleus, where the DNA resides, to the cytoplasm, where all the machinery to assemble proteins is situated. RNA differs from DNA in that it substitutes uracil for thymidine and in that its sugar backbone has an extra -OH group. The transfer of information from DNA to RNA is called *transcription* and the transfer of information from RNA to protein is designated *translation*.

When the bases are grouped together into strings of codons that ultimately may become translated into proteins, they encode structural information. There must, however, be DNA sequences that control this transfer of information. These sequences do not determine the ingredients that make up the proteins, but rather dictate to the cell when these ingredients should be assembled and how much should be produced. There are sequences that

Benz, C. and Liu, E., (eds.), Oncogenes. © 1989 Kluwer Academic Publishers.
ISBN 0-7923-0237-0. All rights reserved.

determine where transcription of RNA begins; these are called *promoters*. Sequences that enhance the transcription of a gene and determine the tissues in which a gene can be expressed are called *enhancers*. The sequence AATAAA frequently signals the RNA polymerase (the enzyme that reads DNA into RNA) to *terminate* the transcription process is called *polyadenylation* and is thought to permit the RNA molecule to transfer from the nucleus to the cytoplasm.

RNA splicing

With some exceptions, it is thought that the initial RNA transcript from a DNA segment is a direct copy of the DNA sequence. However, in most human genes this nuclear RNA undergoes the removal of very specific segments by a process called RNA splicing. This spliced RNA, called messenger RNA or mRNA, then appears in the cytoplasm and is subsequently translated into protein. The signals for splicing to occur are encoded in common or *consensus* DNA sequences that determine the splice donor and the splice acceptor. This means that a linear DNA molecule carrying information to be translated also has sequences that will be removed or spliced out in the RNA stage of the information transfer. Those DNA sequences encoding the final polypeptide are called *coding sequences*. Sequences that are not ultimately translated into a protein are called *noncoding sequences*. It should be noted that mature, cytoplasmic mRNAs frequently carry coding sequences flanked by noncoding sequences that are thought to help control the process of translation. Coding and noncoding regions of mature mRNA are represented in DNA segments called *exons*. Those DNA sequences that will be spliced out are called *introns*. Thus a *gene* now can be defined as a segment of DNA that contains control elements (promoter, enhancer, terminator), introns and exons, which would include the coding regions of the gene.

Orientation of a gene

The beginning of a gene resides in the 5' portion of the gene, and the end is in the 3' portion. This designation is based on the positions of the carbons within the sugar backbone where the linking phosphodiester bonds are made. Thus the promoter of a gene is always in the 5' end and the polyadenylation site is always in the 3' end.

A DNA molecule is always paired with another, complementary DNA molecule, and the two strands coexist in a spiral called the double helix. The pairing is due to hydrogen bonds between complementary bases: A is paired with T and G is paired with C. Thus a segment with the sequence 5'-AATGGC-3' will have a complementary strand with a sequence 3'-TTACCG-5'. For any individual gene, only one strand is transcribed and translated. By convention, the plus (+) DNA strand reflects the sequence of the transcribed RNA.

The RNA template is 'read' by the ribosome from a 5' to 3' direction to produce a protein. The beginning of the protein, corresponding to the 5' portion of the mRNA, is the amino terminus, and the end of the protein is the carboxy terminus.

Techniques in molecular biology

DNA studies: restriction endonucleases

Restriction endonucleases are enzymes, isolated from a variety of bacteria that recognize specific DNA sequences and cut the target DNA, usually within the recognition sites. For example, the enzyme Eco RI recognizes the sequence

$$\text{nucleotide:} \quad 1\ 2\ 3\ 4\ 5\ 6$$
$$5'\text{-GAATTC-}3'$$
$$3'\text{-CTTAAG-}5'$$

and cleaves the upper strand between nucleotides 1 and 2 (G and A), and the lower strand between nucleotides 5 and 6 (A and G). Therefore, in the presence of Eco RI, wherever the GAATTC sequence appears, a break will occur in the double-stranded DNA molecule.

This ability to cut DNA at sequence-specific sites was pivotal in allowing DNA cloning (see below) to take place. Furthermore, restriction enzymes can be used to determine the identity of plasmids and other DNA fragments by comparing the size of the DNA fragments after endonuclease cleavage.

Southern hybridization [4] (figure 1)

In this procedure, DNA is cleaved with a specific restriction enzyme and the resultant fragments are electrophoretically separated according to size (and therefore length as well) in agarose gels. This DNA is then denatured and transferred to nitrocellulose or nylon paper. On the paper, the DNA can be hybridized to specific probes, which are cloned DNA fragments labeled with radioactive ^{32}P. The hybridization process takes into account the propensity of single-stranded DNA fragments to form hydrogen bonds with other DNA strands of complementary sequence. Thus, under the correct conditions, a proble will hybridize only with DNA with near identical sequence. In this manner, the presence and the size of a gene can be discerned from a sample of total cellular DNA.

Restriction fragment length polymorphism (RFLP) analysis

The human genome is highly redundant, containing many repetitive DNA sequences that have unknown functions. In these sequences, nucleotide

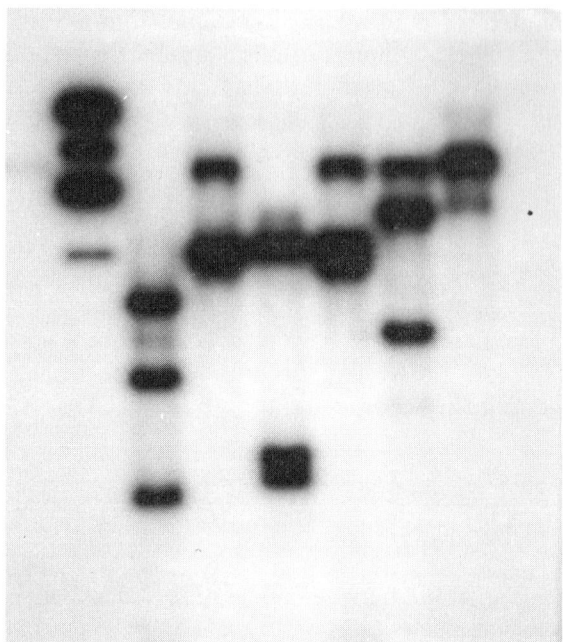

Figure 1. Autoradiograph of a Southern blot. DNA fragments generated by restriction endonuclease cleave of DNA are electrophoresed in an agarose gel. DNA molecules are negatively charged owing to their phosphate groups. When an electric field is applied across the gel, the DNA fragments migrate at a rate inversely proportional to their size: the smallest fragments migrate most quickly. DNA 'marker' fragments of known size are frequently run in parallel with the unknown fragments. Separated DNA fragments are transferred to a nitrocellulose or nylon membrane that is hybridized with radioactive probes. Southern blotting refers to transfer of DNA. Northern blotting refers to transfer of RNA. Transfer of proteins to filters is called a Western transfer or blot. (Courtesy of Dr. Jungsuh Kim, Genelabs Inc.)

changes may occur without affecting the viability of the individual and therefore can be inherited from generation to generation in a random fashion. If such a sequence makes up the recognition site for a restriction enzyme, then Southern analysis will show banding patterns for a segment of DNA that will differ from person to person, and frequently from one allele to the other within an individual. This ability to distinguish one allele from the other has been employed to 'tag' an affected gene or chromosome so that patterns of inheritance of a diseased gene can be studied.

DNA sequencing (figure 2a and 2b)

One of the major advances in molecular biology is the development of techniques to determine the exact nucleotide sequence of cloned genes. Though there are several methods to accomplish this, only one, the chain termination method (also known as the Sanger method or the dideoxynuc-

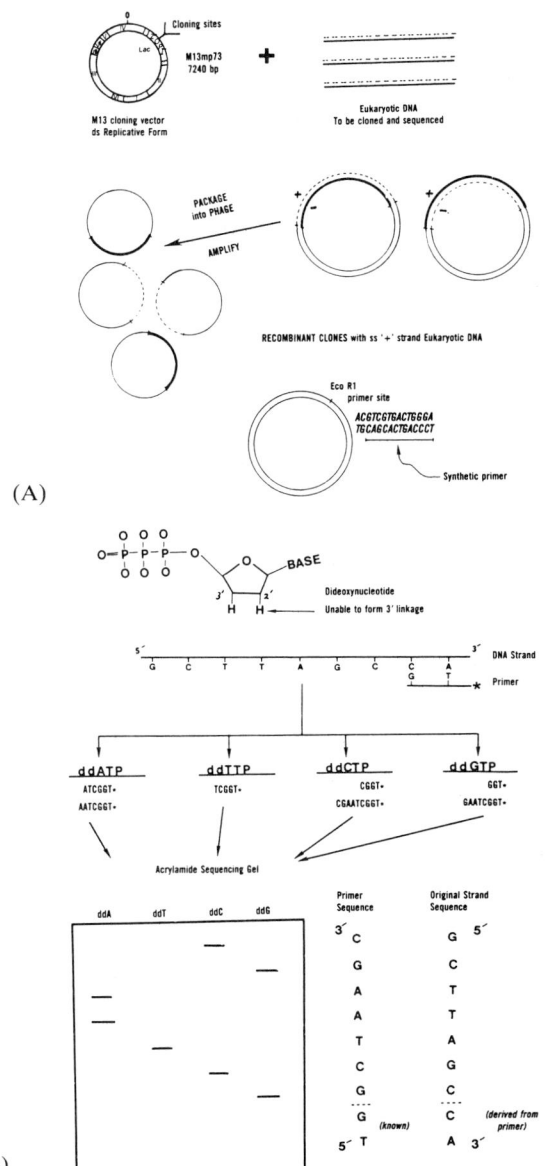

Figure 2. M13 bacteriophage cloning and dideoxy sequencing. A) M13, an E. coli bacteriophage, has been modified to facilitate cloning and sequencing. One such modified M13 vector, M13 mp73, takes advantage of an engineered segment of the E. coli lac operon inserted into the phage. This segment contains cloning sites for various restriction enzymes. DNA is cut with one these enzymes and mixed with the double-stranded replicative for (RF) of the phage. After amplification, single-stranded DNA is packaged into the phage particle; only the '+' strand is packaged. The amplified single strand is then sequenced using the Sanger dideoxy method. B) Dideoxy sequencing (Sanger method) takes advantage of nucleotides missing both 2' and 3' OH groups. A primer hybridizes to the 3' end of the DNA to be sequenced. Four reaction mixtures are set up, each containing the same DNA strand and primer, the four normal deoxynucleotides, a polymerase, and one each of the four dideoxynucleotides. The polymerase adds nucleotides to the primer until a dideoxynucleotide is incorporated, after which the chain cannot further elongate. Following the reaction, each mixture is run on a separate lane of a polyacrylamide sequencing gel. The sequence is read directly from the gel. (Courtesy of Dr. Kathy Burck, University of Washington, Seattle WA.)

leotide incorporation method), will be described. In this technique, the DNA to be sequenced is almost always a cloned gene in a bacterial vector. A single-stranded version of this clone is generated, and a sequencing primer consisting of a short synthetic oligonucleotide complementary to a known sequence in the target DNA is allowed to anneal to the appropriate sequences. Most commonly, the sequencing primer is complementary to vector sequences that adjoin the junction between the vector and the cloned insert to be sequenced. Four reaction mixes are established, each containing all four deoxynucleotides but only one individual dideoxynucleotide. Dideoxynucleotides can be incorporated into an elongating DNA strand by DNA polymerase, but unlike their normal deoxynucleotide counterparts, once incorporated, DNA synthesis stops. This is because dideoxynucleotides lack the 3' linkage site necessary for further elongation of the nascent DNA strand. Thus when a DNA polymerase is added to each reaction mixture, nucleotides are added to the sequencing primer using the cloned DNA as template until a dideoxynucleotide is incorporated. Since the chain termination is a semirandom procedure dependent on the concentration of the dideoxynucleotides, a series of DNA strands will be generated whose lengths are determined by where a particular dideoxynucleotide has been incorporated. Therefore, in the reaction mixture containing dideoxyadenylate, fragments will be synthesized whose lengths are determined by wherever a T occurs in the sequence of the complementary strand. When such fragments are radiolabeled and electrophoresed in a denaturing polyacrylamide gel capable of resolving one-base differences in fragments lengths, the relative position of each 'A' in the sequence can be identified. These sequencing reactions for all the dideoxynucleotides (dideoxy A, T, C, G) can be electrophoresed side by side, and the complete nucleotide sequence of the clone of interest can be determined.

DNA cloning (figures 3 and 4)

The power of DNA cloning lies in its ability to identify DNA fragments from a pool of fragments and to expand the segments of interest so that structural and functional analyses can be performed.

A general outline of DNA cloning techniques includes the following procedures:
1. DNA is cut with a restriction endonuclease and the resultant DNA fragments are ligated with DNA segments (vectors) that replicate in prokaryotic organisms as plasmids or bacteriophages.
2. These recombinant DNA fragments are then introduced into the appropriate organism and allowed to replicate, thereby expanding the number of copies of the DNA fragments. Different vectors carry different sizes of DNA fragments: plasmid vectors from 0.5 to 10 kbs, phage vectors from 5 to 20 kbs, and cosmid vectors from 30 to 50 kbs. Each bacterium or phage represents a 'cloned' copy of a fragment of DNA; a pool of such

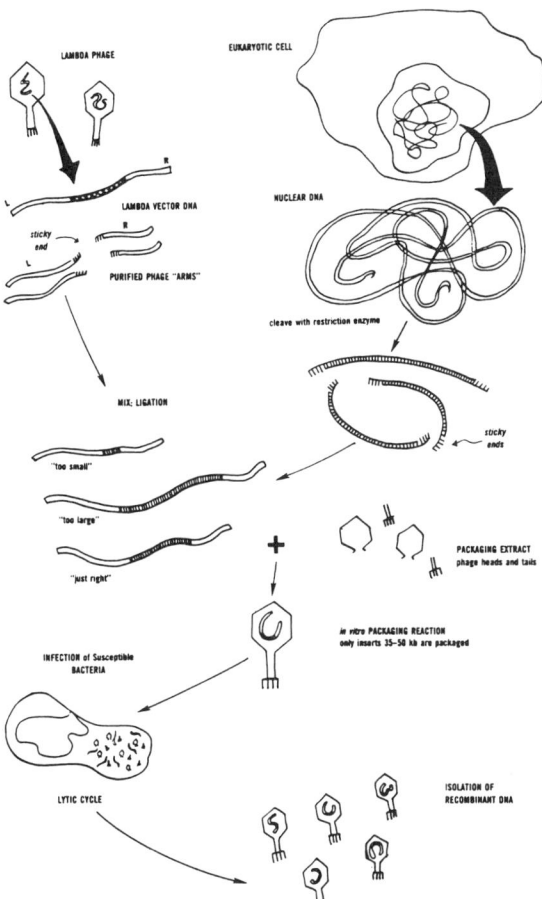

Figure 3. Bacteriophage lambda cloning. Phage 'arms' containing lytic function genes are mixed with restriction-endonclease-cleaved foreign DNA fragments. Inserts are ligated to the arms, and the recombinant DNA is mixed with a 'packaging extract' containing phage structural proteins. After packaging, fresh bacterial host cells are infected with the recombinant phage; the latter undergo a lytic life cycle and are plated to give single 'plaques' (clear spaces) in a 'lawn' of bacteria representing lysed bacteria and released progeny phage particles. DNA from the plaques is transferred to filters that are hybridized with radioactive probes or antibodies to select particular clones. (Courtesy Dr. Kathy Burck, University of Washington, Seattle, WA.)

clones containing copies of DNA segments from a virus, bacterium, or cell is called a *'library'*.
3. When a specific gene or DNA fragment is desired, the library is *screened* by hybridizing with a radiolabeled probe containing sequences complementary to the gene of interest. Those clones that are positive on the screen can be picked and expanded for further studies (e.g., restriction mapping, sequencing, etc.).

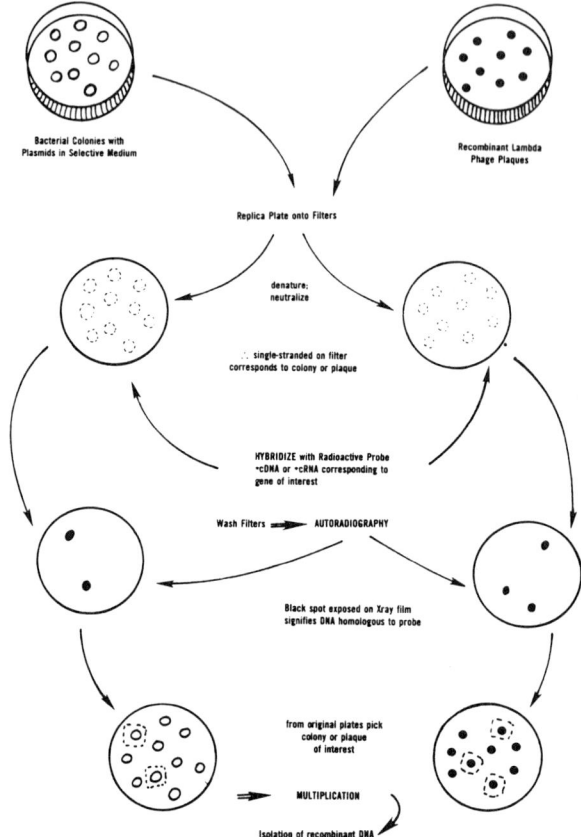

Figure 4. Selection with radioactive probes. DNA from recombinant clones is transferred to filters, denatured to single strands, then neutralized and hybridized in solution with radioactive single-stranded probe DNA or RNA. The probe hybridizes specifically with complementary single strands on the filter. Filters are washed to remove nonspecifically bound radioactivity and placed in proximity to X-ray film. Radioactivity from probe nucleic acid exposes the film in a pattern corresponding to the desired clones, which thus are identified and selected for further propagation. It is also possible to use antibodies to identify positive clones. (Courtesy of Dr. Kathy Burck, University of Washington, Seattle, WA.)

Polymerase chain reaction

Detection methods using Southern hybridization techniques require between 5–15 micrograms of genomic DNA. This technique can detect the presence of a new DNA fragment (e.g., a gene rearrangement) when the molar ratio of the fragment to a single copy gene is greater than 1:100. To have exact sequence data, however, requires making a genomic library, cloning out the fragment of interest, and sequencing that fragment—a procedure that is time-consuming and that demands a large amount of genomic DNA. The

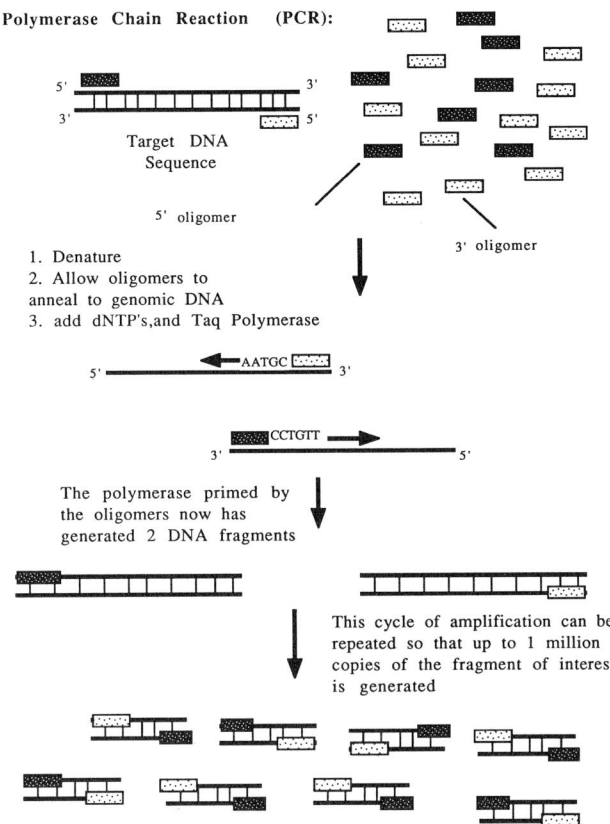

Figure 5. Polymerase chain reaction: oligonucleotide-directed enzymatic amplification of selected segments of DNA. A) Representation of two antiparallel strands of DNA. B) The DNA is heated to separate the strands, and two primers, 20 bases, in length, bind to the ends of the region to be amplified. Using these primers, a DNA polymerase makes a copy of each strand. C) The process of denaturation, annealing, and primer-extension continues, with doubling of the amount of target DNA in every cycle. Ten cycles of amplification gives a 1000-fold amplification; 20 cycles a theoretical million-fold amplification.

polymerase chain reaction (PCR) dramatically improves the sensitivity and specificity of DNA analysis [5]. With PCR, less than 50 nanograms of genomic DNA are necessary for analysis, and fragment:single copy gene ratios of 1:100,000 are sufficient for detection [6]. In the PCR method, short synthetic oligonucleotides (chains of nucleotides linked together in specific sequences) are constructed that are complementary to sequences on opposite strands bracketing a DNA segment of interest (figure 5). These oligonucleotides are mixed with target genomic DNA and the solution is heated to denature the double-helical DNA. Upon lowering the temperature, the oligonucleotides hybridize to the target sequences, and in the presence of the four nucleotides and a DNA polymerase, new DNA will be synthesized using the oligonucleotides as primers and the genomic DNA as template. Thus from one copy of a DNA segment present in the genomic DNA, two are formed. The number of copies increase by two-fold each time the process is repeated, and after 30 cycles of denaturation, annealing, and polymerization, one segment is copied over a million times. This increase in the signal-to-noise ratio then allows for sequence analysis either by oligonucleotide hybridization or by direct sequencing. Furthermore, direct cloning of the PCR-amplified fragments require only minimal screening efforts. Thus PCR represents a major advance in the genetic analysis of human tumors, since it permits the detection of gene mutations in many samples using only miniscule amounts of genomic DNA.

RNA studies

In principle, RNA techniques are similar to those employing DNA, taking into account the differences between RNA and DNA; i.e., RNA is single-stranded, exhibits secondary structure (and therefore needs denaturing conditions in gel electrophretic studies), and is sensitive to different enzymes. The RNA counterpart to Southern blot hybridization is the *Northern blot* analysis, where RNA is separated electrophoretically by size, transferred onto nylon or nitrocellulose paper, and probed with labeled nucleic acid probes. The RNA counterpart to genomic cloning is cDNA cloning. Here, the special properties of the enzyme reverse transcriptase are employed to synthesize a DNA copy (cDNA) of the RNA isolated from the tissues or cells of interest. The resultant cDNA fragments can be cloned into phage or plasmid vectors and can then be screened in a fashion identical to that of genomic libraries. An added advantage of cDNA libraries is that, given the appropriate transcriptional start and stop signals, protein can be synthesized in the vector containing a full-length cDNA. Such *expression* libraries can be screened using antibodies to a particular protein of interest rather than using DNA probes. Alternatively, the expressed product can be detected directly in a bioassay.

Protein studies

The presence of a particular protein species in a cell extract can be detected by several methods. All such techniques require the separation of the different proteins by size, charge, isoelectric point, or hydrophobicity characteristics. The most frequently used analytical techniques separate proteins by size in polyacrylamide gels. Since proteins fold into a tertiary structure that will affect the mobility in polyacrylamide gels, most common methods use detergents such as sodium dodecyl sulfate (SDS) to denature the protein so as to normalize the migration patterns. When an electrical field is applied across the gel, the proteins will migrate at a speed inversely proportional to their molecular weights.

Once the proteins are separated, the presence of a particular species can be determined by *Western blot hybridization*. In this technique, the proteins in the electrophoresed gel are transferred onto nylon or nitrocellulose paper in a fashion similar to that for Northern and Southern blots. Antibodies directed against the protein of interest are then hybridized onto the filter, and these attached antibodies are visualized by anti-immunoglobulin antibodes labeled radioactively or enzymatically.

An alternative to Western blot hybridization is *immunoprecipitation*, where all the proteins in a cell are labeled by incorporation of a radioactively labeled amino acid (e.g., ^{35}S-methionine). The cell lysate is then incubated with a specific antibody and the antibody/antigen (protein) precipitated with Staphylococcal protein A. This precipitate is washed to eliminate nonspecific hybridization, and the radiolabeled protein electrophoresed on polyacrylamide gels.

By combining a variety of protein isolation techniques (such as gel permeation chromatography, ion exchange chromatography, hydrophobic chromatography, and affinity chromatography), sufficient quantities of specific proteins can be isolated and their primary amino acid sequence determined using available automated procedures. This amino acid sequence can be translated back to the original nucleotide sequence, which in turn can be used to construct oligonucleotide probes. These probes can then be employed to screen cDNA libraries and ultimately to isolate the gene from which the protein originated.

Cell culture

Cells grown in culture can be *primary cells* or *cell lines*. In the first case, the cells are derived immediately from fresh animal tissue and have not undergone many passages. Primary cells cannot grow indefinitely in culture and in fact will senesce after a finite number of passages and die. A small number of these primary cells may acquire genetic or epigenetic changes that allow them to grow indefinitely in culture or become immortalized. These are then called cell lines.

The criteria for transformation in cell culture include:
1. Loss of contact inhibition, i.e., cells do not cease to divide once they contact adjacent cells in culture;
2. The ability to grow without anchoring onto a solid matrix (anchorage-independent growth), and thus the ability to divide suspended in semisolid agar; and
3. The capability of forming tumors in syngeneic or athymic nude mice.

Fully transformed cell lines fulfill all three criteria, but more weakly tranformed cells can exhibit only one or two of these characteristics. Cell lines can be either untransformed, as in the case of the murine NIH3T3 fibroblast cell line, or transformed.

DNA transfection

A major technical tool in the study of oncogenes is the ability to transfer cloned DNA into the genetic make-up of recipient cells. This process of gene transfer can be accomplished by a variety methods, but the most common is $CaPO_4$-mediated DNA transfection [7]. In this method, purified DNA is complexed with a $CaPO_4$ precipitate formed in solution and applied to cells in culture. The exact mechanism of this gene transfer is unknown, but the transfected DNA is taken up by recipient cells, integrated into the genetic material of the target cells, and expressed to a varying degree. This technique was used to identity several of the dominantly acting oncogenes e.g., *ras*. In recent years, cloned oncogenes have been altered and reinserted back into living cells to determine any associated phenotypic changes. In this fashion, the mechanisms for conversion of a proto-oncogene to a transforming oncogene can be ascertained.

References

1. Davis LG, Dibner MD, Batley JF: Basic Methods in Molecular Biology. New York, Elsevier, 1986.
2. Watson JD, Tooze J, Kurtz DT: Recombinant DNA: A Short Course. New York, Scientific American Books, W.H. Freeman 1983.
3. Berger SL, Kimmel AR (eds): Guide to Molecular Cloning Techniques: Methods in Enzymology, volume 152. New York, Academic Press, 1987.
4. Southern EM: Detection of specific sequences among DNA fragments separated by gel electrophoresis. J Mol Biol 98:590–513, 1975.
5. Saiki RK, Gelfand DH, Stoffel S, et al.: Primer-directed enzymatic amplification of DNA with a thermostable DNA polymerase. Science 239:487–491, 1988.
6. Mullis KB, Faloona F: Specific synthesis of DNA in vitro via a polymerase catalyzed chain reaction. Methods Enzymology 155:335–350, 1987.
7. Wigler M, Pellicer A, Silverstein S, et al.: Biochemical transfer of single-copy eukaryotic genes using total cellular DNA as donor. Cell 14:725–734, 1978.

3 The *myc* family of nuclear proto-oncogenes

William M.F. Lee

The *myc* family of genes is made up of several members that share common characteristics both at the DNA level and at the level of their protein product. c-*myc*, the senior member of this group of genes, is among the best studied of all cellular genes; N-*myc*, the next gene to be discovered, established the existence of genes closely resembling c-*myc* in the mammalian genome; L-*myc*, the third gene of the group to be described, confirmed some of the *myc* famiiial characteristics but also demonstrated some intriguing differences; and finally, B-*myc* has been described only recently and its characterization is incomplete. Reference has been made to the existence of yet other members of this family of genes, but no detailed descriptions have appeared thus far. In commonly used classifications of proto-oncogenes, the *myc* genes with demonstrated oncogenic potential (c-, N-, and L-*myc*) are grouped with the nuclear proto-oncogenes by virtue of the nuclear location of their protein products. Although two members, c-*myc* and N-*myc*, have been studied for many years, they remain among the most enigmatic of cellular genes, with functions and mechanisms of action that have yet to be elucidated. The effects of their proteins on cells have been described only in generic terms, and this poor understanding is at least partly due to our ignorance of the functional biochemical organization of the nucleus. Since oncogenic forms of members of the *myc* family of proto-oncogenes participate in the development of neoplasia, a state characterized by disordered regulation of cell proliferation and differentiation, speculation about their general cellular activity has centered around their involvement in either the replication or expression of genes. These two primary functions of the cell nucleus must be coordinately regulated for normal cell growth and differentiation to occur, and it is not unreasonable to assume that *myc* proto-oncoproteins (Myc) participate in these two events. However, since the mechanisms of cellular gene replication and expression are understood only poorly, these speculations do not clarify the specifics of Myc activity.

c-*myc*

One of the most intensively studied of proto-oncogenes, c-*myc* was first isolated and characterized as the chicken cellular homolog [1,2] of the viral

Benz, C. and Liu, E., (eds.), Oncogenes. © *1989 Kluwer Academic Publishers.*
ISBN 0-7923-0237-0. All rights reserved.

oncogene (v-*myc*) present in MC29 [3–6] and several other independently isolated and highly oncogenic avian retroviruses (MH2 [7,8], OK10 [9], and CM2 [10]). The presence of v-*myc* endows these viruses with the ability to induce a variety of neoplasms, including leukemias, carcinomas, and sarcomas, in the appropriate hosts (reviewed in [11]). c-*myc* has been found in the genome of many vertebrate species [12], including humans [13–15], mice [16], rats [17,18], cats [19,20], dogs [21], frogs [22–24], and trout [25], but so far it has not been identified in invertebrate genomes. It is a widely expressed gene, and c-*myc* mRNA can be detected in almost all cell types examined, both in adult animals and at different stages of embryonic development.

Gene

In those species in which it has been extensively characterized, c-*myc* is organized into three exons [16,18,20,26–29] (see figure 1 for a summary of the ensuing discussion.) Until recently, the protein-coding domain was thought to reside exclusively within the second and third exons, and the first exon was believed to form most of the untranslated leader sequence of the mature c-*myc* mRNA [16,26]. This assumption was based on published c-*myc* sequences showing that the only AUG preceding a long open reading frame (ORF) lies at the 5' end of exon 2, with all reading frames in exon 1 closed by termination codons. Furthermore, the active c-*myc* allele in some tumors has lost exon 1 by rearrangement, which therefore seems superfluous for formation of the encoded protein. However, a recent study showed that coding sequences exist within exon 1 and that translation of these sequences (which are in the traditional c-*myc* reading frame) initiates at a CUG codon rather than at the usual AUG, leading to the production of two c-*myc* proteins differing only at their N-termini [30].

Two major promoters at the 5' end of the gene (P1 and P2) are responsible for initiation of transcription of the vast majority of c-*myc* mRNAs [31,32]. The apparently unrearranged c-*myc* genes of Friend murine erythroleukemia and other transformed cells can also initiate transcription from a promoter in intron 1 (designated P3) [33]. A fourth promoter (P0), over 500 base-pairs upstream of P1, has been found to be operative in a variety of human cells [32,34]. Unlike P1 and P2, P0 initiates transcription at multiple sites and appears to produce small amounts of one or more larger-sized c-*myc* mRNAs [32]. Analysis of the longest of these mRNAs reveals that it has a 5' ORF with the potential to encode a 114-amino-acid protein, a middle ORF that could encode a 188-amino-acid protein, and a 3' ORF that encodes the well-accepted 439-amino-acid c-*myc* protein [32]. The 188-codon ORF, which lies almost entirely within exon 1, actually was detected previously [35,36], but since its AUG lay just upstream of the 5' end of exon 1, the utility of this ORF awaited description of mRNAs that encompassed its initiation codon (e.g., those initiated at P0) [32]. The enthusiasm generated by the coding potential of these novel c-*myc* ORFs is tempered by the fact that 1) some human c-*myc*

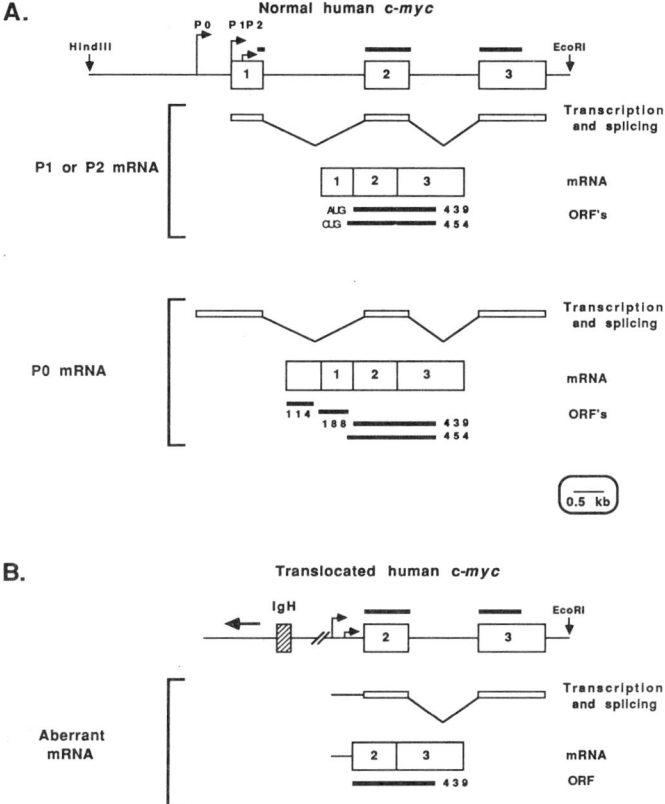

Figure 1. The human c-*myc* gene, mRNA, and open reading frames. (A) The normal human c-/*myc* gene (between the HindIII and EcoRI restriction sites) is shown at the top with the three exons indicated by boxes and numbered. The P0, P1 and P2 promoters are indicated by arrows, and the extent of the major open reading frame (ORF) is indicated by the dark line above the exons. Below are shown the primary transcript with splicing pattern, the mature mRNA, and the ORFs for transcripts from the P1/P2 promoters (2.3 kb) and for the long transcript from P0 (3.0 kb) [32]. The number of codons in each ORF is indicated, as well as the alternative initiation codons (AUG and CUG) used to produce the 439- and 454- amino-acid proteins from the major ORF [30]. (B) An example of a human c-*myc* allele that has been translocated to the IgH locus (exon hatched), which is in the opposite transcriptional orientation. c-*myc* exon 1 has become separated during translocation, and transcription initiates from cryptic promoters in intron 1. The aberrant *myc* mRNA produced has lost potential ORFs and the ability to synthesize the longer, CUG-initiated protein. See the text for a more detailed discussion.

clones and mouse c-*myc* do not have the 188-codon ORF [36], 2) mouse c-*myc* does not have the 114-codon ORF [32], and 3) there has been no convincing demonstration of the existence of either protein in cells.

The production of transcripts by the c-*myc* gene can be controlled at two levels, transcript initiation and transcript elongation. Transcription of c-*myc* is influenced by both positive and negative *cis*-acting sequences lying within a 3-kb stretch upstream of the promoters and within exon 1 [37–40]. The activity of P0 does not appear to be subject to the same forces that govern P1 and P2 activity [32]. It is clear, however, that regulation of the activity of these promoters and enhancers constitutes a mechanism by which c-*myc* expression can be modulated by external stimuli and during cell differentiation [41–44]. Somewhat unexpectedly, exon 1 not only provides sites for RNA polymerase-II-initiated transcription, but also for polymerase-III-initiated transcription [45]. However, since treatment with polymerase II inhibitors blocks c-*myc* mRNA expression [34], the contribution of polymerase III transcription is questionable. In addition to transcription of the coding strand of the c-*myc* gene, there is also transcription of the opposite, non-coding strand [34,46–48]. The regulation of this anti-sense transcription appears to be dissociated from the regulation of sense transcription, and its significance is unclear [48].

After c-*myc* transcription is initiated, its continuation to form full-length primary transcript can be regulated. HL60 cells, induced to differentiate in vitro by treatment with a variety of agents, markedly decrease their level of c-*myc* mRNA within 24 hours [49] due to diminished transcription of the gene [50]. When detailed nuclear run-on assays are performed on these cells to carefully assess c-*myc* transcription, one finds that transcription of exon 1 sequences remains constant, but transcription of downstream sequences is markedly decreased [34,46]. This implies that induction of HL60 differentiation diminishes neither initiation of c-*myc* transcription nor elongation of the transcript through most of exon 1. However, near the boundary of c-*myc* exon 1 and intron 1, elongation of the transcript stops or slows dramatically, resulting in the production of far lower levels of full-length message. The abortive, short c-*myc* transcripts are not detected in RNA isolated from induced HL60 cells, and are presumed to be degraded rapidly within the nucleus [34]. Regulation of c-*myc* expression by this process of "transcription attenuation", "premature termination", "elongation blockade", or "intragenic pausing" (as the phenomenon has been variously called) is not limited to HL60 cells and has been described in murine fibroblasts [47], differentiating Friend murine erythroleukemia (MEL) cells [44], B-lymphoid cells [51], and small-cell lung carcinoma (SCLC) cells [52]. The mechanism underlying premature c-*myc* transcription termination is unknown, but recent studies of transcription of microinjected human c-*myc* genes in *Xenopus* oocytes demonstrate that specific sequences in the vicinity of the exon 1–intron 1 junction are necessary [53], and the intron 1 sequences appear to halt the progression of purified mammalian RNA polymerases during in vitro transcription [54]. Premature transcription termination may be only one of several ways by which certain cells regulate c-*myc* expression. For example, in differentiating Hl60 cells, it is responsible only for the initial rapid decline in c-*myc* mRNA levels, and other mechanisms appear to be responsible for the sustained suppression of c-*myc* expression seen at later time points [55].

mRNA

The majority of c-*myc* mRNA arises from transcription initiated at P1 and P2, is approximately 2.3 kb in length, and has a short half-life of 10–30 minutes in many cell types [56,57]. Species that originate from P0 may constitute a few percent of total *myc* mRNA, are 2.5 and 3.1 kb in size, and appear to be significantly more stable [32]. Speculation about the *cis*-acting sequences responsible for c-*myc* mRNA instability has focused on sequences within exon 1 and 3. Aberrant c-*myc* mRNAs that have lost exon 1 are found in tumors that have decapitated one of their c-*myc* alleles by gene rearrangement. These mRNAs are frequently more stable than the normal c-*myc* transcript [58–60], a finding that has led some to conclude that sequences within exon 1 destabilize the message. However, a more thorough study showed that sequences within the 3′ untranslated region (UTR) of exon 3, which contains potentially destabilizing AU-rich stretches and the AUUUA motif [61], appear to be most responsible for c-*myc* mRNA lability [57]. The presence of exon 1 sequences appears to have only a minor destabilizing effect upon the mRNA [57]; but curiously, when it is not at the very 5′ end of the c-*myc* mRNA (as in P0 transcripts) or when it has been replaced at the 5′ end of the mRNA with intron 1 sequences (as frequently happens after tumor-associated c-*myc* gene rearrangements), the mRNA is much more stable [32,57], and the destabilizing effect of c-*myc* 3′ UTR sequences appears to be counteracted [57]. These data suggest that the enhanced stability of certain tumor-associated abnormal c-*myc* mRNAs [58–60] may not simply be due to the loss of exon 1 sequences, and the acquisition of intron 1 sequences may be even more important. A population of c-*myc* mRNA is not polyadenylated, and the poly(A)-fraction has been shown to have a much longer half-life than the poly(A)+ fraction [62]; the significance of these two species of transcripts is unclear at this time.

The rate of posttranscriptional turnover of c-*myc* mRNA may change in response to growth factors [63] or when cells are induced to differentiate [64–67], and provides another mechanism for regulating c-*myc* expression in cells. For example, both Daudi Burkitt's lymphoma cells whose growth is arrested by treatment with interferon [64,65] and F9 murine teratocarcinoma cells induced to differentiate by retinoic acid and dibutyryl cAMP [66,67] decrease their level of c-*myc* mRNA by posttranscriptional mechanisms.

The presence of a long untranslated leader sequence derived from exon 1 in normal c-*myc* mRNA has fueled speculations that it might play a role in controlling c-*myc* expression at the level of translation. Based on sequence analysis, intramolecular secondary structure formation within exon 1 [31] or between exon 1 and exon 2 [68] sequences has been postulated to affect the translational efficiency of c-*myc* mRNA. Although one in vitro translation study supports a negative effect of exon 1 upon c-*myc* translation [69], other studies find little effect [70,71].

Protein

c-Myc initiated by the methionine AUG at the 5' end of exon 2 is predicted to be over 410 amino acids in length and to have a molecular weight of 47–49 kDa, depending on the species. The cellular protein migrates on SDS-polyacrylamide gels as a doublet with apparent molecular weights of 62–66 kDa [72–74], and this disparity between its migration in gel and its molecular mass has been attributed to c-Myc's high content of proline and basic residues. The origin of the c-Myc doublet was recently shown not to be due to differences in posttranslational modification but to be due to the presence of an additional 15 N-terminal amino acids in the larger specie arising from the use of an in-frame non-AUG initiation codon within exon 1 [30].

c-Myc is a labile nuclear protein with a half-life of 15–30 minutes and is phosphorylated on serine and threonine, but not tyrosine, residues [72–75]. Although c-Myc can bind sequence-nonspecific DNA in vitro [76,77], neither its ability to bind DNA in vivo nor the functional significance of this in vitro property is clear. Within the nucleus, immunofluorescent staining has shown that c-Myc is distributed in a punctate pattern that coincides with the pattern seen when the nucleus is stained for small nuclear ribonucleoprotein particles (snRNPs) [78]. However, a biochemical association between c-Myc and snRNPs has not been demonstrated [78]. Elution of nuclear proteins with solutions of increasing salt concentrations shows that c-Myc belongs to a discrete subset of extractable nuclear proteins [79,80]. The interaction(s) of c-Myc with other nuclear components in situ is unknown. However, recent in vitro studies on purified, bacterially synthesized c-Myc [77] indicate that it exists as a tetramer in its native state [81]. Although these studies do not demonstrate the oligomeric state of c-Myc in cells, nor whether homo- or hetero-oligomers are formed, the ability of an inactive c-Myc mutant that can oligomerize in vitro to inhibit the transforming activity of wild-type c-Myc (i.e., a *dominant* negative phenotype) and the failure of inactive mutants that fail to oligomerize in vitro to inhibit (i.e., a *recessive* negative phenotype) suggest that oligomerization occurs in vivo and is necessary for activity [81]. An earlier study of v-Myc isolated from infected cells indicated that the retroviral homologue probably exists as an oligomer in vivo [82].

c-myc mutagenesis studies have been carried out in an attempt to define functionally important regions within c-Myc. Using transformation assays to assess protein activity, certain regions of c-Myc have been shown to be essential and others unimportant for activity [83,84]. Somewhat surprisingly, regions of c-Myc that are highly conserved through evolution are not necessarily essential for activity [83,84]. In addition, regions essential for activity in one transformation assay may not be necessary for activity in another assay of activity [84]. These mutants have been used to define regions of the protein responsible for certain for its properties. Thus, the peptides responsible for c-Myc nuclear localization [85], oligomerization [81], and sequence-nonspecific DNA binding (C.V. Dang and W.M.F. Lee, unpublished observations) have been determined. The transforming potential of c-Myc mutants that have deleted the regions responsible for each of these properties indicates that the ability to oligomerize is essential for activity [81] but that the ability to bind DNA is not (C.V. Dang and W.M.F. Lee, unpublished observations).

The presence of additional ORFs 5' to the main c-*myc* ORF (determined by exons 2 and 3) in some human c-*myc* mRNAs has led to speculation that additional proteins of 114 and 188 amino acids may be encoded by the c-*myc* locus [32,35,36]. The translatability of these ORFs has been demonstrated in vitro [32,36], but the presence of these proteins in cells remains unproven. The predicted amino acid sequence of the proteins shows no homology with other proteins of known sequence [32,35]. Thus, although it is tempting to speculate about the polycistronic nature of c-*myc* mRNA and the possible roles played by these additional ORFs and proteins, their significance currently remains hypothetical.

Involvement in neoplasia

No other oncogene has a more clearly established role in oncogenesis than c-*myc*. It is implicated in the pathogenesis of many tumors in diverse species, although there is a special association between c-*myc* activation and lymphoid tumors, particularly those that arise from B-cells. The association of c-*myc* activation with specific malignancies will be covered in a separate chapter, and the following discussion will focus on general principles of c-*myc* activation, highlighting those tumors that illustrate these principles. c-*myc* activation in tumors appears to occur by one of three general mechanisms: proviral insertion, chromosomal translocation, and gene amplification. Each of these mechanisms serves to alter or augment c-*myc* expression, which is normally under stringent regulatory control.

In the great majority of chicken bursal (B-cell) tumors induced by infection with avian leukosis virus (ALV, a replication-competent retrovirus that does not carry an oncogene), the provirus is found integrated adjacent to the chicken c-*myc* locus and greatly augments its expression [86–88]. The inserted provirus frequently separates exon 1 from exons 2 and 3 and is in the same transcriptional orientation as the c-*myc* gene. Thus, the long terminal repeat (LTR) of the provirus can act as a substitute promoter for the disrupted c-*myc* gene [86–89]. Occasionally, the provirus inserts downstream of or in the opposite transcriptional orientation to c-*myc*, and the LTR therefore cannot act as a promoter for c-*myc*. In these cases, the enhancer in the retroviral LTR presumably augments expression by enhancing the activity of c-*myc* or cryptic promoters [89,90]. Proviral insertional activation of c-*myc* is not limited to chicken bursal lymphomas and is found in certain rodent T-cell lymphomas. A variety of rodent retroviruses that do not carry oncogenes induce T-cell lymphomas and leukemias in susceptible strains of mice and rats. Examination of these tumors reveals that a significant proportion have proviral integrations adjacent to c-*myc* and augmented c-*myc* expression [91–94]. In contrast to the ALV-induced bursal lymphomas, however, retroviral integration is usually in the opposite transcriptional orientation to c-*myc*, and the augmentation of c-*myc* expression in these rodent T-cell lymphomas is achieved by enhancement rather than promoter insertion.

In human Burkitt's lymphoma (BL) and murine plasmacytomas (MPC), charactersitic translocations occur [95] that involve the chromosomes bearing the various immunoblobulin gene loci and the c-*myc* locus. In BL the classic t(8;14) and in MPC the characteristic t(12;15) translocations bring the c-*myc* locus (on human chromosome 8 and murine chromosome 15) into the vicinity of the immunoglobulin heavy-chain (IgH) locus (on human chromosome 14 and murine chromosome 12) [96–102]. In 10–15% of BL and MPC, variant translocations, t(2;8) or t(8;22) in BL and t(6;15) in MPC, are found. In these cases, one of the immunoglobulin light chain loci (Igϰ is located on human chromosome 2 and murine chromosome 6, and Igλ is located on human chromosome 22) becomes translocated to the chromosome bearing c-*myc* [103–110]. The consequence of these various translocations is to bring together, in relatively close proximity, the c-*myc* locus and the allelically excluded (i.e., nonproductively rearranged) immunoblobulin locus. Exceptions to this rule occur in certain variant BL translocations [107–108] and in most variant MPC translocations [109,110] where the breakpoint is within the Igϰ locus but far away from the c-*myc* locus; in many examples, the translocation occurs more than 72 kb away from the c-*myc* locus [108,110]. The configuration when IgH and c-*myc* loci are juxtaposed is head-to-head, i.e., the 5' end of c-*myc* is fused to the 5' end of IgH, but the configuration when light chain loci and c-*myc* are joined is head-to-tail, i.e., a portion of the chromosome 3' to c-*myc* is fused to the 5' end of Igϰ or Igλ [103,104,106,111]. In many of these tumors, expression of the translocated c-*myc* allele is increased [99,100] and not susceptible to normal transcriptional regulatory control mechanisms, while the nontranslocated allele is silent [101,112,113]. In either the head-to-head or head-to-tail configuration, the Ig promoter is not in a position to direct transcription of c-*myc*, and other explanations must be sought for the mechanism of activation of c-*myc* by these translocation events. Proposed explanations include the following: 1) c-*myc* expression could be enhanced by the Ig enhancer; 2) separation of exon 1 of c-*myc* from exons 2 and 3, or more subtle alterations in promoter usage brought about by the translocation event, may release the main coding exons from regulatory influences exerted by or on exon 1; 3) somatic mutations within the translocated c-*myc* coding domain may reveal its transforming potential; and 4) somatic mutations outside the coding domain could affect expression.

1. A state of augmented c-*myc* expression could arise by bringing the c-*myc* locus under the influence of the Ig heavy chain enhancer as a result of translocation [114,115]. However, tumor c-*myc* mRNA levels, although elevated with respect to resting B-cells, are frequently not markedly elevated compared to normal proliferating B-cells [116], and the heavy chain

enhancer is usually on the reciprocal translocated chromosome and is not available to the c-*myc* gene [116,117].

2. Aberrant c-*myc* mRNAs are frequently found in these tumors, because exon 1, which has been postulated to have a regulatory influence upon c-*myc* expression [118], can be separated from the rest of the c-*myc* gene after translocation [119,120]. In BL, the translocation breakpoint lies outside of the c-*myc* locus in the endemic form (African-type), whereas it frequently disrupts the 5' region of c-*myc* in the sporadic form (American-type) [120]. In those tumors where the 5' region of c-*myc* has been separated, aberrant transcript arise from cryptic promoters within c-*myc* intron 1 that become activated [116,122,123] and can be more stable than normal c-*myc* mRNA [58–60]. Furthermore, now that optional coding sequences have been found in exon 1 [30], its separation from exons 2 and 3 no longer permits the synthesis of one specie of c-Myc, which may be significant since functional or regulatory differences between the two species of c-Myc may exist. In those tumors that have undergone translocation outside of the c-*myc* locus, i.e., have not decapitated the gene, and retain exon 1 sequences in the mRNAs generated, there is a shift in the usage of the normal c-*myc* P1 and P2 promoters compared to other tumors where there has been no c-*myc* translocation [121], and this may alter expression of the gene at either the RNA [121] or protein [31] level.

3. An altered c-*myc* coding domain exists in the active c-*myc* allele of two Burkitt's lymphomas [124,125] and could conceivably produce a c-Myc with activated transforming potential. However, other translocated, active c-*myc* alleles have been sequenced and were not found to contain any coding mutations [16,31] which, therefore, cannot be necessary for c-*myc* activation.

4. In those BL tumors where translocation has left the c-*myc* locus grossly intact, small mutations frequently have been revealed in the sequence of exon 1 and intron 1 by nucleotide sequencing and detailed restriction mapping [120,126,127]. The structure of this region of c-*myc* is important for attenuating or terminating the transcription of downstream sequences [34,53,54], and these noncoding sequence alterations in the BL alleles may abrogate such control. In fact, many BL cells lose this mechanism for regulating c-*myc* expression [51].

c-*myc* activation by chromosomal translocation occurs in other types of tumors besides BL and MPC. In immunocytomas of rats, the characteristic t(6;7) translocation [128] juxtaposes the rat c-*myc* and IgH loci [129]. Some human T-cell malignancies have been found to contain a t(8;14) translocation, and molecular analysis reveals that this juxtaposes the c-*myc* locus with the T-cell receptor α-chain locus which resides on chromosome 14 [130–132]. In other examples, such as hereditary renal cell carcinoma associated with translocations involving chromosome 8, c-*myc* has been shown to be translocated to an as yet undefined genetic locus [133].

Gene amplification is the third genetic abnormality found to affect the c-*myc* locus in tumor cells. First described in HL60 human promyelocytic leukemia cells [134,135], c-*myc* amplification has been found subsequently in COLO 320 human neuroendocrine tumor cells [136] and in SEWA murine osteosarcoma cells [137]. In many of these tumors, characteristic cytogenetic abnormalities such as *double minutes* (small chromosomes without centromeres), homogeneously staining chromosomal regions, and C-bandless chromosomes exist, and the amplified copies of c-*myc* are found to reside in these aberrant chromosomal regions [136,137]. The only type of tumor in which c-*myc* amplification is found in more than sporadic cases [138] is human small-cell lung carcinoma (SCLC), where in vitro large-cell variants frequently have this abnormality [139]. The consequence of c-*myc* gene amplification is overexpression, but unlike c-*myc* activation by proviral insertion and chromosomal translocation, the amplified c-*myc* genes may be susceptible to normal regulatory influences [34,49] and should not be assumed to be deregulated.

The pathogenic significance of these changes involving the c-*myc* gene has been proven experimentally. Overexpressed c-*myc* genes that encode normal c-Myc can cooperate with activated *ras* oncogenes to cotransform normal rodent embryonic cells in culture [140,141]. Nontumorigenic human B-lymphoblastoid cell lines immortalized by Epstein–Barr virus in vitro can be made tumorigenic by introduction of an overexpressed c-*myc* gene [142]. Perhaps the most convincing evidence for a role of these altered c-*myc* alleles in tumorigenesis comes from transgenic mice experiments. Mice bearing c-*myc* transgenes under the transcriptional control of the mouse mammary tumor virus transcriptional regulatory element (expression of which is induced by steroid hormones) were found to develop mammary carcinomas during pregnancy or lactation [143] and other tumors [144]. Mice bearing a c-*myc* transgene under the transcriptional influence of the immunoglobulin heavy chain enhancer consistently developed B-cell lymphomas [145–147]. The conclusion drawn from all these transgenic mice experiments is that aberrant expression of the c-*myc* gene strongly predisposes to the subsequent appearance of neoplasia in susceptable tissues. However, c-*myc* cannot act alone to produce malignancy. In vitro transformation of rat embryo cells by c-*myc* requires a cooperating oncogene (an activated *ras* gene [140,141]), and tumorigenic conversion of B-cells by c-*myc* requires an antecedent event (EBV infection and immortalization [142]). Even in vivo transformation by an aberrantly regulated c-*myc* transgene only results in the delayed appearance of monoclonal tumors arising out of polyclonal tissue hyperplasia [146]. These results imply that, although aberrant c-*myc* expression is necessary for the tumors to develop, it is by itself not sufficient for tumorigenesis, and additional events, presumably the introduction or activation of other oncogenes [148], are needed before overt malignancy develops.

The effect of c-*myc* activation upon cells is often subtle, and morphological changes frequently do not occur. It was found that introduction of activated c-*myc* genes into rat fibroblast cells [149] or mouse neural precursor cells [150] resulted in immortalization of the cells. The immortalized cells appeared normal, and the immortalized neural precursor cells could be induced to differentiate like their mortal counterparts [150]. Some fibroblast cell lines transfected with activated c-*myc* genes were little changed morphologically but became tumorigenic and were able to grow in lower concentrations of serum compared to control cells [151]. On the other hand, certain cells derived from rat fibroblast cells lines showed morphologic and growth characteristic changes (e.g., focus formation and growth in soft agar) when an overexpressed c-*myc* gene was introduced [84]. The degree of c-*myc* overexpression may affect the transformed behavior of cells; higher levels of c-*myc* amplification and overexpression correlated positively with tumorigenicity in two tumor cell lines [152,153]. The contribution of aberrant c-*myc* expression to cell transformation in vivo is more difficult to ascertain. The experience with transgenic mice bearing *myc* coupled to the IgH enhancer indicates that enforced c-*myc* expression induced a prelymphomatous state characterized by polyclonal expansion of the pre-B-cell compartment and reduced numbers of mature B-cells. Such a condition indicates that the cells are in a state that favors proliferation over maturation [146].

Unlike the members of the *ras* family of oncoproteins, mutations in c-Myc need not be present for transforming activity, and normal c-Myc has demonstrated oncogenic potential [16,31,141,154]. Augmented expression or disruption of normally regulated expression appears to underlie its oncogenic activation. This does not preclude the possibility that alterations of c-Myc by mutations may potentiate its transforming capabilities. Mutations that lead to amino acid substitutions are found in the activated c-*myc* alleles of bursal lymphomas [155] and Burkitt's lymphomas [124,125]. Furthermore, all four retroviral v-*myc* genes (from MC29, MH2, OK10, and CM2) contain mutations (compared to chicken c-*myc*) that result in amino acid substitutions [5–10,156]. One of these substitutions results in the replacement of a threonine at amino acid 61 of chicken c-Myc (which is conserved at the equivalent position of human, mouse, and trout c-Myc [156], by alanine in MH2 and OK10 v-Myc and by methionine in MC29 v-Myc [156]. Such a change seems unlikely to have occurred by chance, and indeed a study showed that the presence of methionine instead of threonine at amino acid 61 significantly increased the in vitro transforming potential of *myc* [157]. Thus, coding mutations in a c-*myc* gene may enhance its transforming potential, but in contrast to *ras* genes, no available evidence suggests that *myc* transforming potential can be activated by qualitative changes in the encoded protein, in the absence of additional changes that affect expression.

Normal function

Despite extensive investigation, the function of the c-*myc* gene remains mysterious, and there is no clear insight into c-Myc's molecular activities in cells. Studies on the normal pattern of c-*myc* expression during cell growth and differentiation give the general impression that its expression is necessary for cell proliferation and that decreased expression may play a role in regulating cell differentiation. The cellular consequences of introducing constitutively expressed c-myc genes and of inhibiting c-*myc* expression confirm these impressions. Unfortunately, these generic phenotypes have neither clarified the specifics of c-*myc* effect on cellular processes nor the biochemical basis of c-Myc action, and c-Myc still retains its mystery.

The correlation of c-*myc* expression with cell proliferation was first noted when c-*myc* expression was found to increase in cells after exposure to the appropriate mitogen, prior to the onset of DNA synthesis [158]. Since that seminal observation, the same correlation has been found in many other cell types [159,160] and in in vivo situations of rapid growth stimulation [161]. Since c-*myc* expression is but one component of a complex response to mitogen exposure [162] the significance of these changes were uncertain until more direct evidence showed that the growth requirement of fibroblasts for platelet-derived growth factor was diminished by introduction of a constitutively expressed c-*myc* gene [163] or by microinjection of bacterially synthesized c-*myc* protein [164]. More recently, treatment of T-lymphocytes with antisense *myc* oligonucleotides was used to inhibit mitogen-induced production of c-Myc and prevented the cells from entering S phase, but not progression from G_0 and G_1 [165]. These studies logically lead one to ask whether c-*myc* expression occurs only at specific phases of the cell cycle, e.g., G1, when the cells are preparing to synthesize DNA and proliferate. This has been addressed by cell elutriation studies that showed c-*myc* mRNA and protein levels, although transiently increased following mitogen stimulation, to be constant throughout the cell cycle and even maintained in density-arrested cells [166,167]. The studies described have led to suggestions that c-Myc is an intracellular growth-competence factor that is necessary but not sufficient for cell proliferation.

Cell differentiation frequently is accompanied by cessation of proliferation, and c-*myc* expression decreases in many cell types induced to differentiate in vitro. Thus, HL60 human promyelocytic leukemia cells [49], Daudi Burkitt's lymphoma cells [64,65], F9 murine teratocarcinoma cells [66,67], U937 histiocytic lymphoma cells [168], Friend murine erythroleukemia (MEL) cells [169], TT human medullary thyroid carcinoma cells [170], various rodent myogenic cell lines [171,172], and 3T3-L1 preadipocytes [173] all respond to appropriate inducing agents by decreasing their expression of c-*myc*, ceasing to grow and developing differentiated characteristics appropriate for their cell lineage. Nevertheless, some cell types that terminally differentiate do so without decreasing their expression of c-*myc* [174]. A significant role for the decrease in c-*myc* expression accompanying differentiation has been demonstrated in MEL cells, which have a complex pattern of c-*myc* mRNA response to the differentiating agent DMSO [169]: levels reach a nadir within one to two hours of DMSO exposure, return to pretreatment levels over the next 12–18 hours and then gradually decline again over the ensuing 24–48 hours. Transfection of overexpressed c-*myc* genes resulted in failure of the transfected cells to differentiate normally [175–177], although one study presented puzzling and somewhat contradictory findings [178]. The data from these studies led to the conclusion that the decline in c-*myc* expression, and in particular the early trough of mRNA levels, is essential for EML cells to differentiate normally. A more recent study found that c-Myc levels in MEL cells remain approximately constant throughout the first 12 hours after DMSO treatment despite the marked decrease in mRNA levels during the same period, and this maintenance of c-Myc levels can be explained partly by the increased stability of the protein [179]. These results clearly cast some doubts on the role played by the early decrease in c-*myc* mRNA levels during MEL cell differentiation and the interpretation of the results of the earlier transfection studies. Perhaps the answer lies in the greater importance to differentiation of the sustained late decrease in MEL cell c-*myc* mRNA [169] and protein [179] levels, as has been suggested by the recent study of MEL cells transfected with recombinant c-*myc* genes whose expression can be temporally manipulated [180]. In other experimental systems, constitutive c-*myc* expression from transfected genes has been shown to prevent 3T3-L1 preadipocyte [173] and F9 [181] differentiation. The results of these studies suggest that diminished c-*myc* expression is necessary for differentiation to occur in selected cell types.

It is less clear whether diminished c-*myc* expression is sufficient to trigger differentiation. Transfection of plasmids producing antisense *myc* RNA [182] or treatment with antisense *myc* oligonucleotides decreased HL60 cell proliferation and induced differentiation [183]. Transfection of MEL cells with plasmids that produce antisense *myc* transcripts affected growth of MEL cells and accelerated and enhanced their differentiation in response to DMSO, but did not by itself induce differentiation [184]. A similar experiment performed on F9 cells did not yield long-lived clones of transfected cells, but seemed to induce the appearance of one marker of F9 differentiation [181].

The mechanism by which c-Myc affects cell proliferation and differentiation is unknown. Because of its nuclear location, attention has focused on its possible participation in the regulation of DNA synthesis and transcription. Direct involvement of c-Myc in DNA synthesis was suggested initially by the demonstration that DNA replicative synthesis in isolated nuclei was inhibited by anti-Myc antibodies [185]. However, it was later discovered that inhibition by the anti-Myc antibody preparations used was due to a contaminant and that other antibody preparations did not have this activity [186]. Another report suggested that anti-Myc antibodies inhibited cellular and in vitro replication of a plasmid containing putative mammalian autonomously replicating sequences (ARS) and that c-Myc preferentially bound to DNA containing ARS [187]. These provocative findings need to be confirmed. Even if c-Myc does not participate directly in DNA synthesis, it could participate indirectly and regulate the process. Evidence suggesting that this might be the case is provided by experiments showing that induction of expression of a transfected c-*myc* gene under the transcriptional control of the mouse mammary tumor virus LTR in NIH 3T3 cells was associated with increased DNA replicative synthesis [188]. Another study found that the ability of SV40-based plasmids to replicate in human lymphoid cell lines correlated with the level of endogenous c-*myc* expression and that transfection of a constitutively expressed c-*myc* gene into poorly permissive cells rendered them much more permissive for viral replication [189]. A similar study found that limited replication of transfected plasmids containing the SV40 origin of replication could occur in the absence of SV40 large T-antigen in human cells expressing high levels of c-Myc [190]. These studies all suggest that c-Myc plays a permissive role in DNA replication.

c-Myc may exert its influence on cellular processes by modulating the expression of other genes, and there is evidence that it may have such effects. Transient cotransfection of a c-*myc* gene increased expression from the human and Drosophila heat shock protein (hsp) 70 promoters [191,192] and the adenovirus E4 promoter [193] and decreased expression from the murine metallothionein I promoter [192]. The study of the activation of the E4 promoter by c-*myc* is additionally interesting, because transfection of a c-*myc* plasmid capable of synthesizing only the AUG-initiated (shorter) protein did not result in *trans*-activation, whereas transfection of a c-*myc* plasmid that can synthesize both the AUG-initiated and the non-AUG-initiated (longer) protein resulted in *trans*-activation [193]. These results suggest that the longer c-Myc may have activities or capabilities not possessed by the shorter c-Myc. Since there is some evidence that the levels of the two forms of c-Myc may be differentially regulated [179], one can contemplate the regulatory intricacies permitted by expression of the c-*myc* gene.

Evidence that c-*myc* actually regulates or influences expression of endogenous cellular genes is somewhat limited. In untransfected osteogenic sarcoma cell lines and murine fibroblast cell lines transfected with a plasmid that overexpresses c-*myc*, a correlation was reported between the expression of 1,25-dihydroxyvitamin D_3 receptor protein and *myc* expression [194]. Induced expression of a stably transfected c-*myc* gene under the control of the mouse mammary tumor virus LTR is associated with increased levels of histone H4 mRNA [188]. Similar experiments performed with c-*myc* under the transcriptional control of the Drosophila hsp70 promoter found that two anonymous genes, previously identified as serum-inducible, were induced with c-*myc* expression [195]. Perhaps the most convincing demonstration that c-*myc* expression can influence the expression of other cellular genes is found in a study of human melanomas [196]. An inverse correlation was discovered between c-*myc* and HLA class I gene expression in a panel of melanoma cell lines. Transfection of a c-*myc* expression plasmid into a line expressing low levels of c-*myc* (and high levels of HLA class I mRNA) resulted in independent transfectants that expressed c-*myc* at various levels. Clones with high-level c-*myc* expression showed decreased β2-microglobulin mRNA and HLA class I mRNA and cell surface protein expression, suggesting that expression of these genes became down-regulated (196). However, none of the studies outlined above provide evidence for whether expression of the modulated genes is directly or indirectly affected by c-*myc* expression. The only study that tried to address this issue used genes that fused the majority of the c-*myc* gene to a portion of the bacterial *lexA* gene that encodes the DNA binding domain of the LexA repressor, producing LexA-c-Myc fusion proteins in yeast. When the LexA-c-Myc fusion protein was assayed for its ability to activate transcription of sequences downstream of a LexA operator, it was found to have measurable but weak activity, especially when compared to a LexA-c-Fos fusion which was very active [197]. Thus, although c-Myc may affect the expression of other cellular genes (which would not be surprising), it is far from clear how it does so, and little evidence supports a direct role of c-Myc in transcription.

The difficulties encountered in experimentally deciphering the molecular activities of c-Myc have led to speculations on c-Myc function based on structure and resemblance to other non-structural nuclear proteins:

1. A degree of homology was detected among v-Myc, v-Myb, and adenovirus Ela oncoproteins several years ago [198]. Myc's resemblance to Ela is potentially revealing, since the latter is relatively well characterized and has been shown to activate and suppress the expression of other genes, including endogenous cellular genes (reviewed in [199]). Subsequently, *myc* gene expression has been shown to affect usage of the hsp70 and metallothionein transcriptional control elements in transient cotransfection experiments [191,192].
2. A peptide region encoded by c-*myc* exon 3 strongly resembles segments contained in several other nuclear proteins, such as mammalian MyoD [200], Drosophila *daughterless* protein [201], and *achaete-scute* complex proteins [202], and more weakly resembles a segment of v-Jun [203]. These proteins are believed to regulate the expression of other cellular genes and thereby control differentiation and/or cell transformation. Analysis of human c-Myc indicates that this region of the protein is essential for tranforming activity [84].
3. The C-terminal portion of c-Myc (and N-Myc) contains several leucine residues that conform to the *leucine zipper* motif initially described in the enhancer binding protein, C/EBP, but also found in c-Fos and c-Jun [204,205]. This motif is made up of leucine residues spaced at intervals of every seventh amino acid (heptad repeat) in protein regions predicted to be α-helical; some of the amino acids between the hydrophobic leucine residues are hydrophilic and frequently basic [205]. Such a peptide is postulated to align the hydrophobic leucine side chains along one face of the α-helix and the hydrophilic residues along the opposite face and to favor interdigitation of the leucine side chains of different molecules to produce dimers. The formation of dimers by this mechanism is postulated to be necessary for the DNA-binding and biological activities of the proteins that possess leucine zippers. In fact, mutational analysis has shown that integrity of this portion of c-Myc is essential for the intact molecule

to oligomerize in vitro [81] and for transforming activity [84], but it is not necessary for c-Myc to bind sequence-nonspecific DNA in vitro (C.V. Dang and W.M.F. Lee, unpublished observations). Evidence for the relevance of the results of these in vitro studies to the oligomeric and functional state of c-Myc in cells has already been discussed.

4. An evolutionarily conserved region of c-Myc that contains several acidic residues followed by IleAspVal and that spans the junction encoded by exons 2 and 3 is remarkably similar to a portion of the Drosophila *engrailed* protein, which is a regulatory protein required for proper segmentation of the developing fruit fly [206]. This portion of c-Myc is part of a region that is not essential for rat embryo cell cotransforming activity, but is important for its ability to transform established rat fibroblasts [84]. It also corrsponds to the region of the MC29 *gag-myc* protein that is deleted in MC29 mutants that transform chick embryo fibroblasts but no longer retain the ability to transform bone marrow macrophage cells [207,208]. These speculations based on structural similarities obviously are limited by the lack of detailed information concerning the function and activities of the other nuclear proteins being compared.

N-*myc*

N-*myc* was initially found as a gene with restricted homology to c-*myc* that is frequently amplified and overexpressed in human neuroblastoma cells [209, 210]. The N-*myc* genes of humans [211,212] and of mice [213] have been cloned and found to have three exons with an organization similar to c-*myc*. The first exon contains AUGs, but all the potential reading frames are closed by termination codons, and it is assumed to be noncoding [211–213]. Thus, the coding domain appears to reside exclusively within N-*myc* exons 2 and 3, although the recent discovery of a non-AUG codon initiating translation in c-*myc* exon 1 [30] cautions that a similar situation also might exist in N-*myc*. The region of c-*myc* and N-*myc* homology that was used to detect the presence of N-*myc* resides in exon 2 of both genes [209]. In fact, however, nucleotide sequencing reveals that only two relatively short segments of exon 2 are highly conserved at the nucleotide level between the two genes; other regions of lesser nucleotide homology exist but are scattered throughout the rest of the coding domain [211–213].

The first exon of N-*myc* bears little homology to the corresponding exon of c-*myc* [211,212], but its functional importance is suggested by the conservation of exon 1 sequences between the mouse and human N-*myc* genes [211,213]. Three AUG codons are present within a short distance of each other at the 5' end of the long ORF encompassed by exons 2 and 3 of both the human and mouse N-*myc* genes; the AUG used for authentic translation initiation is not known, but the corresponding proteins are predicted to differ by a maximum of only 11 amino acids, with the longest being 462 amino acids long [211–213]. The coding domain is followed by a long 3' UTR that contains AU-rich regions and the AUUUA motif that is found in many mRNAs with rapid turnover rates [61]. N-*myc* mRNA is approximately 3.2kb long [210], although larger species can be seen and may represent splicing precursors or intermediates [214]. N-*myc* mRNA is very heterogeneous at its 5' end, which indicates the presence of multiple start sites for transcription [211]. The upstream region of N-*myc* differs from c-*myc* in that classic TATA motifs do not exist, and GC-rich regions, which are usually associated with heterogeneous initiation, are found in their place [211].

The predicted structure of N-Myc resembles that of c-Myc, with regions of homology dispersed by regions of total disparity [211–213]. Aside from portions of the protein encoded by the regions of strong nucleotide homology in exon 2, the most striking resemblance lies in the C-terminal quarter of the proteins, where very long stretches of amino acid identity and conservation are found [211,212]. This region of the protein is where c-Myc is most susceptible to mutational inactivation of transforming potential [84] and where a leucine zipper motif is located [81,205]. In regions such as this, the familial relationship between N-*myc* and c-*myc* is more apparent at the protein level than it is at the nucleotide level.

N-Myc has been identified in cells immunologically, and like c-Myc, is a labile nuclear phosphoprotein that binds DNA in vitro. It also migrates as a doublet after SDS-polyacrylamide gel electrophoresis with apparent molecular weights of 65 and 67 kDa [215–217]; N-Myc's calculated molecular weight is approximately 50 kDa, and this disparity is reminiscent of c-Myc. Both species of N-Myc are phosphorylated and do not display a precursor/product relationship [216]. It remains to be seen whether N-terminal heterogeneity accounts for the two N-Myc species as it does for c-Myc [30].

N-*myc* is not expressed in most adult cell types and organs examined, but is expressed widely in embryos and neonatal animals [218,219]. This restricted pattern of expression contrasts with the widespread expression of c-*myc* in both developing and adult animals. Some of the highest levels of N-*myc* expression are to be found in embryonic and neonatal neural tissues, and lower levels persist in these tissues into adult life [218,219]; the kidney and testis are nonneural organs in which low but detectable N-*myc* expression occurs in adults [219]. These findings suggest that N-*myc* expression is developmentally regulated in many tissue types or organs. This is substantiated by an examination of N-*myc* expression in B-lymphoid cells, where it is found in pre-B-cells but not in mature B-cells or plasma cells. This stage-specific expression of N-*myc* in differentiating B-cells contrasts with c-*myc* expression, which is present at all stages of B-cell development, and indicates that cellular regulation of N-*myc* expression is clearly different from that of c-*myc* [218]. These findings probably account for N-*myc*'s restricted expression among tumors and tumor cell lines; it has been found only in neuroblastomas [209, 210], teratocarcinoma cell lines [219,220], retinoblastomas [221], some SCLC [222], hepatoblastomas, medulloblastomas, and Wilm's tumors [223]. All of these tumors are either embryonic in origin and/or derived from neural or neuroendocrine cells. Given that N-*myc* expression is found in many fetal tissues and that it can be found (sometimes consistently) in many of these tumors whether or not gene amplification has occurred [209,210,221–223], it seems likely that N-*myc* expression in these neoplasms, in the absence of gene amplification, does not represent abnormal or activated oncogene expression, but rather is a normal characteristic of the constituent cells.

The significance of N-*myc* expression in relation to the malignant phenotype becomes more apparent in tumors where amplification and overexpression of the gene is found. The great majority of neuroblastoma cell lines [209, 224,225] and many fresh tumor specimens (38% of tumors from untreated patients) [226,227] exhibit N-*myc* amplification and overexpression. A very strong correlation can be drawn between gene amplification and advanced clinical stage of disease: few if any tumors from patients with stage I or II disease have amplified N-*myc*, whereas 50% of tumors from patients with stage III or IV disease have amplification [226,227]. The presence of N-*myc* amplification in the preponderance of neuroblastoma cell lines can be explained by the fact that it is correlated with the ease with which fresh neuroblastoma tumor cells adapt to in vitro cultivation [226]. These data suggest that N-*myc* overexpression contributes to neuroblastoma tumor progression and spread [224,226,227]. Experimental demonstration that this is the case and some insight into possible mechanisms come from studies of major histocompatibility (MHC) class I antigen and N-*myc* expression in neuroblastomas. In human neuroblastoma cell lines, an inverse correlation was shown to exist between the level of N-*myc* amplification and expression and the level of MHC class I gene expression [228]. A causal relationship was demonstrated by transfecting N-*myc* genes into rat neuroblastoma cells that express low levels of endogenous N-*myc* and high levels of MHC class I genes: transfected colonies varied in their expression of the transfected N-*myc* gene, and an inverse correlation was found between N-*myc* and MHC class I gene expression among the different transfectants [228]. When tested in vivo, transfected cells with high levels of N-*myc* expression grew and metastasized much more quickly, although differences in in vitro growth characteristics were more difficult to appreciate [228]. Thus, high levels of N-*myc* expression down-regulate MHC class I gene expression and enhance tumor growth and spread in animals.

N-*myc* activation in tumors always appears to occur by gene amplification. In situ hybridization studies has localized the amplified copies of the gene in neuroblastoma cells to marker chromosomes with homogeneously staining regions or double minute chromosomes, confirming the view that these chromosomal aberrations harbor pathogenetically significant amplified segments of the genome [229]. When amplified N-*myc* is found in tumor cells, it frequently occurs on chromosomes other than the pair that harbor normal N-*myc* genes (short arm of human chromosome 2 [229]), implying that translocation events must also have occurred [210,229]. Activation of N-*myc* by chromosomal translocation without concomitant gene amplification has not been described.

Even though the role played by N-*myc* in the pathogenesis of neuroblastomas is more likely to be during the spread of the tumor rather than in initial transformation events, the N-*myc* gene has demonstrated transforming potential in cultured cells. When placed under the transcriptional control of strong promoters and enhancers, the N-*myc* gene can cooperate with an activated *ras* gene and cotransform early-passage rat embryonic cells [230,231]. In the absence of a cooperating *ras* oncogene, activated N-*myc* genes induce transformation of certain established rat fibroblasts [232]. In these studies, both the N-*myc* gene cloned from normal cells (and encoding the normal protein) and from neuroblastoma tumor cells have the same effect, indicating that activation of its transforming potential only requires augmentation of expression [230].

The physiologic role played by N-*myc* in those cells where it is normally expressed is uncertain. However, a role during cell differentiation is suggested by the finding that a decrease in N-*myc* expression accompanies retinoic acid-induced differentiation of F9 teratocarcinoma [220] and neuroblastoma [233] cells. The significance of these changes remains to be shown.

L-*myc*

This member of the *myc* family of genes was first identified as an amplified and overexpressed gene in certain SCLC lines with homology to, but distinct from, both c-*myc* and N-*myc* [234]. Thus far, the human [235,236] and murine [237] L-*myc* genes have been cloned and analyzed, and a human L-myc pseudogene identified [235]. The human gene is located on the short arm of chromosome 1 and displays restriction fragment length polymorphism after Eco R1 digestion [234]. L-*myc* resembles c- and N-*myc* in being organized into three exons [235–237], but there is a complexity at the L-*myc* mRNA level that has not been described for the other two genes (see figure 2 for a summary for the ensuing discussion). A complicated pattern of L-*myc* transcription termination and alternative splicing has been detected in human SCLC cells by hybridization analysis and cDNA cloning [236]. The mRNAs produced include

1. Transcripts that terminate in exon 3, splice out introns 1 and 2 and fuse exons 1, 2, and 3 to produce a 3.6-kb mRNA (*long-form* mRNA);
2. Transcripts that terminate in exon 3, splice out intron 2, but retain intron 1 (which is only about 360 bp long) to produce a 3.9-kb mRNA (*long-form* mRNA); and
3. A set of transcripts that terminate at one of three potential polyadenylation signals within intron 2 to produce transcripts that lack any exon 3 sequence. These mRNAs are heterogeneous in size, but cluster around 2.2 kb (*short-forms*). Among other things, their size depends on whether they retain intron 1.

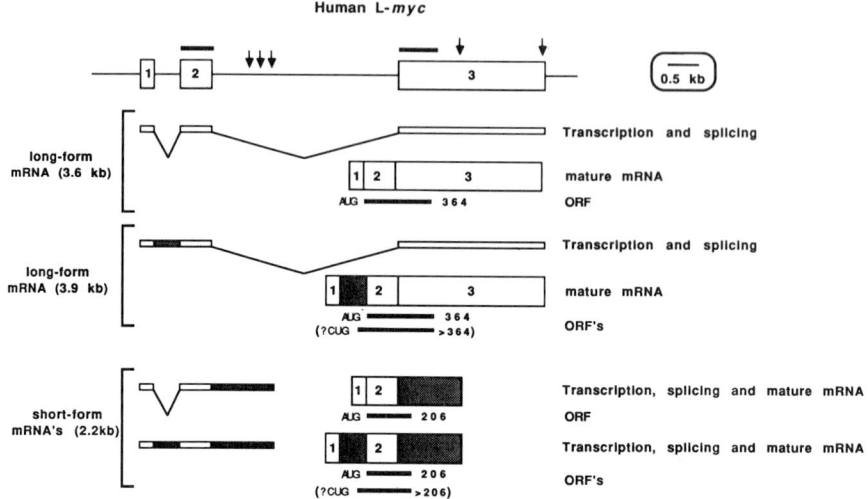

Figure 2. The human L-*myc* gene, alternative mRNA processing, and open reading frames. The human L-*myc* gene is drawn at the top with the three exons indicated by boxes and numbered. Potential transcription termination (polyadenylation) signals are indicated by arrows, and the extent of the major open reading frame (ORF) is indicated by the dark lines above the exons. Below are shown the two types of primary transcripts (determined by the transcription termination site used) and the alternative splicing patterns (determined by the presence or absence of intron 1). The mature mRNAs generated by this complex pattern of mRNA processing and their ORFs are indicated. The shaded boxes in the drawings of the mature mRNAs indicate segments derived from L-*myc* 'intron' sequences. This figure is adapted from data presented in [236].

Long-form transcripts (1) and (2) differ only by the presence of intron 1, and both have the same long ORF that initiates at an AUG at the 5' end of exon 2, is encompassed by exons 2 and 3, and encodes a 364-amino-acid protein resembling c- and N-Myc. In contrast, short-form transcripts will produce a 206-amino-acid L-*myc* protein containing exon 2 encoded sequences and 41 novel C-terminal residues [236].

A meaningful comparison of the regulation of L-*myc* gene expression with that of c- and N-*myc* is difficult to achieve, because few cells express all three genes. SCLC is the only type of cell to do so, albeit usually in different tumors and cell lines. An examination of those SCLC cells that express different members of the *myc* family of genes [52] reveals that the presence of L-*myc* expression is determined at the level of transcription attenuation and not by transcription initiation. Thus, SCLC cells that have no L-*myc* mRNA show transcription of exon 1 sequences but marked attenuation of transcription between exon 1 and 2, whereas those that express L-*myc* mRNA have lost the block to transcript elongation. This contrasts with SCLC expression of c-*myc*, which appears to be regulated both at the level of transcription initiation and elongation, and with SCLC expression of N-*myc*, which is regulated only at the level of transcription initiation [52].

Immunologic detection of proteins produced by L-*myc* [238] reveals the presence in SCLC cells of a protein doublet with apparent molecular weights of 60 and 66 kDa. As is the case for the other *myc* oncoproteins, these sizes exceed the calculated molecular weights of the anticipated protein. The proteins are nuclear phosphoproteins with half-lives of about two hours, which is significantly longer than the half-life of c-Myc. Furthermore, these pulse-chase experiments do not indicate a precursor–product relationship between the two proteins in the doublet. In vitro translation studies have been used to help assign proteins to particular L-*myc* mRNAs, and indicate that the 3.9-kb L-*myc* mRNA produces both the 60- and 66-kDA proteins, whereas the 3.6-kb mRNA only produces the 60-kDa form. In vitro translation of a 2.2-kb short-form mRNA that includes intron 1 yields peptides of 32 and 37 kDa, which however are not detected in cells. Thus, the 66-kDa protein is seen only when transcripts containing intron 1 are used as template, and the 60-kDa protein is produced whether or not intron 1 sequences are present. These results suggest that the 60-kDa protein initiates from the AUG at the 5' end of exon 2 and the 66-kDa protein initiates from within intron 1. Since no in-frame AUGs exist in L-*myc* intron 1, and possibility arises that, as in the case of c-*myc* [30], non-AUG initiation codons are used; indeed, inframe CUGs (the alternate initiation codon used in c-*myc* [30] exist in L-*myc* intron 1, a short distance 5' to the exon 2 AUG. This potential use of different initiation codons combined with a pattern of alternate mRNA termination and splicing indicates that cellular regulation of L-*myc* expression is probably complex and proceeds at many different levels.

The amino acid sequence of L-Myc (translated from the long-form mRNAs) is predicted to resemble those of c-Myc and N-Myc in several regions of the protein and to diverge in the intervening regions [235–237]. The *myc* homology boxes in exon 2 [209], and the regions of strong peptide homology in the C-terminal portion of the proteins are conserved in L-*myc*. There are regions conserved between c- and N-Myc that are not present in L- Myc, and regions conserved between N- and L-Myc that are not present in c-Myc; it is relatively unusual to find sequences conserved between c- and L-Myc that are absent in N-Myc. This comparison suggests that the L-*myc* gene is more closely related (evolutionarily or functionally) to N-*myc* than it is to c-*myc*, but the kinship among the three genes and proteins is quite evident. Translation of the L-*myc* short-form mRNAs (for which there is no evidence in vivo) is predicted to produce a much shorter protein that shares exon 2 encoded homology but contains 41 novel C-terminal amino acids that bear no obvious relationship to those encoded by exon 3 [236].

L-*myc* expression in tissues and cells is even more restricted than N-*myc* expression [218]. Expression at significant levels is found in the brain, kidney, and lung of embryos and neonatal mice, but only in the lung of adult mice. Interestingly, the level of pulmonary L-*myc* expression does not diminish with maturation of the animal. This restricted pattern of normal expression correlates with the apparently restricted expression of L-*myc* in tumors. To date, L-*myc* expression in neoplastic cells has been described only in certain SCLC tumors and cell lines [234]. It should not be surprising if, in the future, other tumors of embryonic or neural origin were found to express this gene. The L-*myc* gene can be expressed in SCLC cells whether or not it has been amplified [234], and the presence of expression in individual SCLC cell lines appears to be dictated by the presence or absence of L-*myc* transcription attenuation [52]. The only described abnormality that affects L-*myc* in SCLS is gene amplification. Although this frequently results in augmented gene expression, the significance of the latter remains unclear because SCLC cell lines bearing L-*myc* amplification, unlike those that bear c-*myc* amplification [139], do not have variant morphologies, retain many differentiated features, and grow slowly [236]. The two EcoRI restriction fragment length polymorphic L-*myc* alleles are present in SCLC tumors and cell lines in proportion to their frequency in the normal population, which indicates that neither is more predisposed to amplification nor preferentially associated with this type of malignancy [234].

Despite the uncertainty associated with L-*myc*'s contribution to the malignant phenotype in SCLC, its oncogenic potential has been demonstrated in vitro [235,239]. Cotransfection of a plasmid that expressed the 3.9-kb L-*myc* mRNA with a mutant *ras* gene results in the transformation of rat embryo cells. By comparison with c-*myc* and N-*myc*, however, the cotransforming activity of L-*myc* is low, and the L-*myc*/*ras* cotransformed cells take longer to form foci and do not always become established cell lines. The apparently weaker transforming potential of L-*myc* may be determined to some extent by the cellular target of transformation, since established rat fibroblasts are transformed by L-*myc* and c-*myc* with comparable efficiencies [239].

B-*myc* and other members of the *myc* family of genes

Other genes within the mammalian genome have been identified and cloned by virtue of their homology to c-, N-, or L-*myc*. B-*myc* is a gene isolated from a rat genomic library using a mouse c-*myc* cDNA probe [240]. Both by restriction analysis and rat chromosome localization, it was shown to be distinct from the rat homologs of any of the three previously characterized members of the *myc* family [240,241]. Partial nucleotide sequence data have been reported and clearly reveal a strong resemblance, both at the nucleotide and protein level, between B-*myc* and part of c-*myc* exon 2. The B-*myc* gene is transcribed and produces a single 1.3-kb mRNA that is found in a wide variety of tissues from fetal and adult rats; the highest level of expression is found in the brain [240].

The existence of two other genes with *myc* family homology, termed R-*myc* and P-*myc*, has been reported in cursory fashion [242]. Both genes were identified initially and cloned using a L-*myc* exon 3 probe. An LTR-activated R-*myc* gene reportedly possesses rat embryo cell cotransforming activity.

Summary

Several members of the *myc* family of proto-oncogenes have been described, and some (c-, N-, and L-*myc*) have been characterized in considerable detail. They are united by a common gene structure and nucleotide homologies that were used to identify some of them initially. Their protein products also have scattered regions of amino acid identity or homology. Although the cellular activities of the various proteins are unknown, some members may play a role in regulating cell growth and differentiation. They share the ability to cooperate with an activated *ras* gene and cotransform embryonic rodent cells. In naturally occurring tumors, the members of the *myc* family of oncogenes appear to be activated by genetic changes (proviral insertion, chromosomal translocation, and gene amplification) that augment or otherwise disrupt normally regulated expression.

The members of this family of genes differ markedly in their tissue specificity and developmental regulation of expression. This may account in part for the frequent appearance of activated c-*myc* genes in a wide variety of neoplasms and the limited appearance of activated N- and L-*myc* genes in tumors of embryonic or neural origin. The c-*myc* gene may be activated in tumors by a variety of mechanisms, whereas N- and L-*myc* appear to be activated only by gene amplification. Regulation of expression of the different *myc* genes also appears to occur by different mechanisms. Finally, the products of the different genes differ in many regions of the protein, and this divergence probably reflects their specific and individual functions.

References

1. Vennstrom B, Sheiness D, Zabielski J, Bishop JM: Isolation and characterization of c-*myc*, a cellular homolog of the oncogene (v-*myc*) of avian myelocytomatosis virus strain 29. J Virol 42:773–779, 1982.
2. Watson DK, Reddy EP, Duesberg PH, Papas TS: Nucleotide sequence analysis of the chicken c-*myc* gene reveals homologous and unique coding regions by comparison with the transforming gene of avian myelocytomatosis virus MC29, δ*gag-myc*. Proc Natl Acad Sci USA 80:2146–2150, 1983.
3. Vennstrom B, Moscovici C, Goodman HM, Bishop JM: Molecular cloning of the avian myelocytomatosis virus genome and recovery of infectious virus by transfection of chicken cells. J Virol 39:625–631, 1981.
4. Robins T, Bister K, Garon C, Papas T, Duesberg P: Structural relationship between a normal chicken DNA locus and the transforming gene of the avian acute leukemia virus MC29. J Virol 41:635–642, 1982.
5. Alitalo K, Bishop JM, Smith DH, Chen EY, Colby WW, Levinson AD: Levinson Nucleotide sequence of the v-*myc* oncogene of avian retrovirus MC29. Proc Natl Acad Sci USA 80:100–104, 1983.
6. Reddy EP, Reynolds RK, Watson DK, Schultz RA, Lautenberger J, Papas TS: Nucleotide sequence analysis of the proviral genome of avian myelocytomatosis virus (MC29). Proc Natl Acad Sci USA 80:2500–2504, 1983.
7. Kan, NC, Flordellis CS, Garon CF, Duesberg PH, Papas TS: Avian carcinoma virus MH2

contains a transformation-specific sequence, *mht*, and shares the *myc* sequence with MC29, CMII and OK10 viruses. Proc Natl Acad Sci USA 80:6566–6570, 1983.
8. Kan NC, Flordellis CS, Mark GE, Duesberg PH, Papas TS Nucleotide sequence of avian carcinoma virus MH2: two potential *onc* genes, one related to avian virus MC29 and the other related to murine sarcoma virus 3611. Proc Natl Acad Sci USA 81:3000–3004, 1984.
9. Hayflick J, Seeburg PH, Ohlsson R, Pfeifer-Ohlsson S, Watson D, Papas T, Duesberg PH: Nucleotide sequence of two overlapping *myc*-related genes in avian carcinoma virus OK10 and their relationship to the *myc* genes of other viruses and the cell. Proc Natl Acad Sci USA 82:2718–2722, 1985.
10. Walther N, Jansen HW, Trachmann C, Bister K: Nulceotide sequence of the CMII v-*myc* allele. Virology 154:219–223, 1986.
11. Graf T, Beug H: Avian leukemia viruses: interaction with their target cells in vivo and in vitro. Biochim Biophys Acta 516:269–299, 1978.
12. Sheiness D, Bishop JM: DNA and RNA from uninfected vertebrate cells contain nucleotide sequences related to the putative transforming gene of avian myelocytomatosis virus. J Virol 31:514–521, 1979.
13. Dalla-Favera R, Gelmann EP, Martinotti S, Franchini G, Papas TS, Gallo RC, Wong-Staal F: Cloning and characterization of different human sequences related to the *onc* gene (v-*myc*) of avian myelocytomatosis virus (MC29). Proc Natl Acad Sci USA 79:6497–6501, 1982.
14. Colby WW, Chen EY, Smith DH, Levinson AD: Identification and nucleotide sequence of a human locus homologous to the v-*myc* oncogene of avian myelocytomatosis virus MC29. Nature (London) 301:722–725, 1983.
15. Watson DK, Psallidopoulos MC, Samuel KP, Dalla-Favera R, Papas TS: Nucleotide sequence analysis of human c-*myc* locus, chicken homologue, and myelocytomatosis virus MC29 transforming gene reveals a highly conserved gene product. Proc Natl Acad Sci USA 80:3642–3645, 1983.
16. Stanton L, Fahrlander PD, Tesser PM, Marcu KB: Nucleotide sequence comparison of normal and translocated murine c-*myc* genes. Nature (London) 310:423–425, 1984.
17. Steffen D: Proviruses are adjacent to c-*myc* in some murine leukemia virus-induced lymphomas. Proc Natl Acad Sci USA 81:2097–2101, 1984.
18. Hayashi K, Makino R, Kawamura H, Arisawal A, Yoneda K: (1987). Characterization of rat c-*myc* and adjacent regions. Nucleic Acids Res 15:6419–6436, 1987.
19. Neil JC, Hughes D, McFarlane R, Wilkie N, Onions DE, Lees G, Jarrett O: Transduction and rearrangement of the *myc* gene by feline leukaemia virus in naturally occurring T-cell leukaemias. Nature (London) 308:814–820, 1984.
20. Stewart MA, Forrest D, McFarlane R, Onions D, Wilkie N, Neil JC: Conservation of the c-*myc* coding sequence in transduced feline v-*myc* genes. Virology 154:121–134, 1986.
21. Katzir N, Rechavi G, Cohen JB, Unger T, Simoni F, Segal S, Cohen D, Givol D: 'Retroposon' insertion into the cellular oncogene c-*myc* in canine transmissible venereal tumor. Proc Natl Acad Sci USA 82:1054–1058, 1985.
22. King MW, Roberts JM, Eisenman RN: Expression of the c-*myc* proto-oncogene during development of *Xenopus laevis*. Mol Cell Biol 6:4499–4508, 1986.
23. Taylor MV, Gusse M, Evan, GI, Dathan N, Mechali M: *Xenopus myc* proto-oncogene during development: expression as a stable maternal mRNA uncoupled from cell division. EMBO J 5:3563–3570, 1986.
24. Godeau F, Persson H, Gray HE, Pradee AB: c-*myc* expression is dissociated from DNA synthesis and cell division in *Xenopus* oocyte and early embryonic development. EMBO J 5:3571–3577, 1986.
25. Van Beneden RJ, Watson DK, Chen TT, Lautenberger JA, Papas TS: Cellular *myc* (c-*myc*) in fish (rainbow trout): Its relationship to other vertebrate *myc* genes and to the transforming genes of the MC29 family of viruses. Proc Natl Acad Sci USA 83:3698–3702, 1986.
26. Watt R, Stanton LW, Marcu KB, Gallo RC, Croce CM Rovera G: Nucleotide sequence of

cloned cDNA of human c-*myc* oncogene. Nature (London) 303:725–728, 1983.
27. Hamlyn PH, Rabbitts TH: Translocation joins c-*myc* and immunoglobulin γ1 genes in a Burkitt lymphoma revealing a third exon in the c-*myc* oncogene. Nature 304:135–139, 1983.
28. Watt R, Nishikura K, Sorrentino J, ar-Rushdi A, Croce CM, Rovera G: The structure and nucleotide sequence of the 5' end of the human c-*myc* oncogene. Proc Natl Acad Sci USA 80:6307–6311, 1983.
29. Shih C-K, Linial M, Goodenow MM, Hayward WS: Nucleotide sequence 5' of the chicken c-*myc* coding region: Localization of a noncoding exon that is absent from *myc* transcripts in most avian leukosis virus-induced lymphomas. Proc Natl Acad Sci USA 81:4697–4701, 1984.
30. Hann SR, King MW, Bentley DL, Anderson CW, Eisenman RN: A non-AUG translational initiation in c-*myc* exon 1 generates a N-terminally distinct whose synthesis is disrupted in Burkitt's lymphomas. Cell 52:185–195, 1988.
31. Battey J, Moulding C, Taub R, Murphy W, Stewart T, Potter H, Lenoir G, Leder P: The human c-*myc* oncogene: Structural consequences of translocation into the IgH locus in Burkitt lymphoma. Cell 34:779–787, 1983.
32. Bentley DL, Groudine M: Novel promoter upstream of the human c-*myc* gene and regulation of c-*myc* expression in B-cell lymphomas. Mol Cell Biol 6:3481–3489, 1986.
33. Ray D, Meneceur P, Tavitian A, Robert-Lezenes J: Presence of a c-*myc* transcript initiated in intron 1 in Friend erythroleukemia cells and in other murine cell types with no evidence of c-*myc* gene rearrangement. Mol Cell Biol 7:940–945, 1987.
34. Bentley DL, Groudine M: A block to elongation is largely responsible for decreased transcription of c-*myc* in differentiated HL60 cells. Nature (London) 321:702–706, 1986.
35. Gazin C, de Dinechin SD, Hampe A, Masson J-M, Martin P, Stehelin D, Galibert F: Nucleotide sequence of the human c-*myc* locus: provocative open reading frame within the first exon. EMBO J 3:383–387, 1984.
36. Gazin C, Rigolet M, Briand JP, Van Regenmortel MHV, Galibert F: Immunochemical detection of proteins related to the human c-*myc* exon 1. EMBO J 5:2241–2250, 1986.
37. Remmers EF, Yang J-Q, Marcu KB: A negative transcriptional control element located upstream of the murine c-*myc* gene. EMBO J 5:899–904, 1986.
38. Yang J-Q, Remmers EF, Marcu KB: The first exon of the c-*myc* proto-oncogene contains a novel positive control element. EMBO J 5:3553–3562, 1986.
39. Lipp M, Schilling R, Wiest S, Laux G, Bornkamm G: Target sequences for cis-acting regulation within the dual promoter of the human c-*myc* gene. Mol Cell Biol 7:1393–1400, 1987.
40. Hay N, Bishop JM, Levens D: Regulatory elements that modulate expression of human c-*myc*. Genes Devel 1:659–671, 1987.
41. Greenberg ME, Ziff EB: Stimulation of 3T3 cells induces transcription of the c-*fos* proto-ocncogene. Nature (London) 311:433–438, 1984.
42. Dean M, Levine RA, Ran W, Kindy MS, Sonenshein GE, Campisi J: Regulation of c-*myc* transcription and mRNA abundance by serum growth factors and cell contact. J Biol Chem 261:9161–9166, 1986.
43. Levine RA, McCormack JE, Buckler A, Sonenshein GE, Transcriptional and post-transcriptional control of c-*myc* gene expression in WEHI 231 cells. Mol Cell Biol 6:4112–4116, 1986.
44. Mechti N, Piechaczyk M, Blanchard J-M, Marty L, Bonnieu A, Jeanteur P, Lebleu B: Transcriptional and post-transcriptional regulation of c-*myc* expression during the differentiation of murine erythroleukemia Friend cells. Nucleic Acids Res 14:9653–9666, 1986.
45. Chung J, Sussman DJ, Zeller R, Leder P: The c-*myc* gene encodes superimposed RNA polymerases II and III promoters. Cell 51:1001–1008, 1987.
46. Eick D, Bornkamm GW: Transcriptional arrest within the first exon is a fast control mechanism in c-*myc* gene expression. Nucleic Acids Res 14:8331–8346, 1987.
47. Nepveu A, Marcu KB: Intragenic pausing and anti-sense transcription within the murine c-

myc locus. EMBO J 5:2859–2865, 1986.
48. Kindy MS, McCormack JE, Buckler AJ, Levine RA, Sonenshein GE: Independent regulation of transcription of the two strands of the c-*myc* gene. Mol Cell Biol 7:2857–2862, 1987.
49. Reitsma PH, Rothberg PG, Astrin SM, Trial J, Bar-Shavit Z, Hall A, Teitelbaum SL, Kahn AJ: Regulation of *myc* gene expression in HL-60 leukemia cells by a vitamin D metabolite. Nature (London) 306:492–494, 1983.
50. Grosso LE, Pitot HC: Transcriptional regulation of c-*myc* during chemically induced differentiation of HL60 cultures. Cancer Res 45:847–850, 1985.
51. Cesarman E, Dalla-Favera R, Bentley D, Groudine M: Mutations in the first exon are associated with altered transcription of c-*myc* in Burkitt's lymphoma. Science 238:1272–1275, 1987.
52. Krystal G, Birrer M, Way J, Nau M, Sausville E, Thompson C, Minna J, Battey J: Multiple mechanisms for transcriptional regulation of the *myc* gene family in small-cell lung cancer. Mol Cell Biol 8:3373–3381, 1988.
53. Bentley DL, Groudine M: Sequence requirements for premature termination of transcription in the human c-*myc* gene. Cell 53:245–256, 1988.
54. Kerppola TK, Kane CM: Intrinsic sites of transcription termination and pausing in the c-*myc* gene. Mol Cell Biol 8:4389–4394, 1988.
55. Siebenlist U, Bressler P, Kelly K: Two distinct mechanisms of transcriptional control operate on c-*myc* during differentiation of HL60 cells. Mol Cell Biol 8:867–874, 1988.
56. Dani C, Blanchard JM, Piechaczyk M, El Sabouty S, Marty L, Jeanteur P: Extreme instability of *myc* mRNA in normal and transformed human cells. Proc Natl Acad Sci USA 81:7046–7050.
57. Jones TR, Cole MD: Rapid cytoplasmic turnover of c-*myc* mRNA: Requirement of the 3' untranslated sequences. Mol Cell Biol 7:4513–4521, 1987.
58. Piechaczyk M, Yang J-Q, Blanchard J-M, Jeanteur P, Marcu KB: Posttranscriptional mechanisms are responsible for accumulation of truncated c-*myc* RNAs in murine plasma cell tumors. Cell 42:589–597, 1985.
59. Eick D, Piechaczyk M, Henglein B, Blanchard J-M, Traub B, Kofler E, Wiest S, Lenoir GM, Bornkamm GW: Aberrant c-*myc* mRNAs of Burkitt's lymphoma have longer half-lives. EMBO J 4:3717–3725, 1985.
60. Rabbitts PH, Forster A, Stinson MA, Rabbitts TH: Truncation of exon 1 from the c-*myc* gene results in prolonged c-*myc* mRNA stability. EMBO J 4:3727–3733, 1985.
61. Shaw G, Kamen R: A conserved AU sequence from the 3' untranslated region of GM-CSF mRNA mediates selective mRNA degradation. Cell 46:659–667, 1986.
62. Swartwout SG, Preisler H, Guan W, Kinniburgh AJ: Relatively stable population of c-*myc* RNA that lacks long poly(A). Mol Cell Biol 7:2052–2058, 1987.
63. Blanchard J-M, Piechaczyk M, Dani C, Chambard J-C, Franchi A, Pouyssegur J, Jeanteur P: c-*myc* is transcribed at high rate in G0-arrested fibroblasts and is post-transcriptionally regulated in response to growth factors. Nature (London) 317:443–445, 1985.
64. Knight E Jr, Anton ED, Fahey D, Friedland BK, Jonak GJ: Interferon regulates c-*myc* gene expression in Daudi cells at the post-transcriptional level. Proc Natl Acad Sci USA 82:1151–1154, 1985.
65. Dani C, Mechti N, Piechaczyk M, Lebleu B, Jeanteur P, Blanchard J-M: Increased rate of degradation of c-*myc* mRNA in interferon-treated Daudi cells. Proc Natl Acad Sci USA 82:4896–4899, 1985.
66. Dony C, Kessel M, Gruss P: Post-transcriptional control of *myc* and *p53* expression during differentiation of the embryonal carcinoma cell line F9. Nature (London) 317:637–639, 1985.
67. Dean M, Levine RA, Campisi J: c-*myc* regulation during retinoci acid-induced differentiation of F9 cells is post-transcriptional and associated with growth arrest. Mol Cell Biol 6:518–524, 1986.
68. Saito H, Hayday AC, Wiman K, Hayward WS, Tonegawa S: Activation of the c-*myc* gene

by translocation: a model for translational control. Proc Natl Acad Sci USA 80:7476–7480, 1983.
69. Darveau A, Pelletier J, Sonenberg N: Differential efficiencies of in vitro translation of mouse c-*myc* transcripts differing in the 5' untranslated region. Proc Natl Acad Sci USA 82:2315–2319, 1985.
70. Nilsen TW, Maroney PA: Translational efficiency of cMyc mRNA in Burkitt lymphoma cells. Mol Cell Biol 4:2235–2238, 1984.
71. Butnick NZ, Miyamoto C, Chizzonite R, Cullen BR, Ju G, Skalka AM: Regulation of the human c-*myc* gene: 5' noncoding sequences do not affect translation. Mol Cell Biol 5: 3009–3016, 1985.
72. Hann SR, Abrams HD, Rorschneider LR, Eisenman RN: Proteins encoded by the v-*myc* and c-*myc* oncogenes: identification and localization in acute leukemia virus transformants and bursal lymphoma cell line. Cell 34:789–798, 1983.
73. Hann SR, Eisenman RN: Proteins encoded by the human c-*myc* oncogene: differential expression in neoplastic cells. Mol Cell Biol 4:2486–2497, 1984.
74. Ramsay G, Evan GI, Bishop JM: The protein encoded by the human proto-oncogene c-*myc*. Proc Natl Acad Sci USA 81:7742–7746, 1984.
75. Alitalo K, Ramsay G, Bishop JM, Ohlsson S, Colby WW, Levinson AD: Identification of nuclear proteins encoded by viral and cellular *myc* oncogenes. Nature 306:274–277, 1983.
76. Persson H, Leder P: Nuclear localisation and DNA binding properties of a protein expressed by human c-*myc* oncogene. Science 225:718–720, 1984.
77. Watt RA, Schatzman AM, Rosenberg M: Expression and characterization of the human c-*myc* DNA-binding protein. Mol Cell Biol 5:448–456, 1985.
78. Spector DL, Watt RA, Sullivan NF: The v- and c-*myc* oncogene proteins co-localize in situ with small nuclear ribonucleoprotein particles. Oncogene 1:5–12, 1987.
79. Eisenman, RN, Tachibana CY, Abrams HD, Hann SR: v-*myc* and c-*myc* encoded proteins are associated with the nuclear matrix. Mol Cell Biol 4:114–126, 1985.
80. Evan GI, Hancock DC: Studies on the interaction of the human c-*myc* protein with cell nuclei: p62$^{c\text{-}myc}$ as a member of a discrete subset of nuclear proteins. Cell 43:253–261, 1985.
81. Dang CV, McGuire MA, Buckmire M, Lee WMF: Involvement of the 'leucine zipper' region in the oligomerization and transforming activity of human c-*myc* protein. Nature (London) 337:664–666, 1989.
82. Bader JP, Ray DA: MC29 virus-coded protein occurs as monomers and dimers in transformed cells. J Virol 53:509–514, 1985.
83. Sarid J, Halazonetis TD, Murphy W, Leder P: Evolutionary conserved regions of the human c-*myc* protein can be uncoupled from transforming activity. Proc Natl Acad Sci USA 84:170–173, 1987.
84. Stone J, de Lange T, Ramsay G, Jokobovits E, Bishop JM, Vermus HE, Lee WMF: Definition of regions in human c-*myc* that are involved in transformation and nuclear localization. Mol Cell Biol 7:1697–1709, 1987.
85. Dang CV, Lee WMF: Identification of the human c-*myc* protein nuclear translocation signal. Mol Cell Biol 8:4048–4054, 1988.
86. Hayward WS, Neel BG, Astrin SM: ALV-induced lymphoid leukosis: activation of a cellular *onc* gene by promoter insertion. Nature (London) 290:475–480, 1981.
87. Payne GS, Bishop JM, Varmus HE: Mutliple arrangements of viral DNA and an activated host oncogene (c-*myc*) in bursal lymphomas. Nature (London) 295:209–214, 1982.
88. Fung YKT, Fadly AM, Crittenden LB, Kung H-J: On the mechanism of retrovirus-induced avian lymphoid leukosis: deletion and integration of the provirus. Proc Natl Acad Sci USA 78:3418–3422, 1981.
89. Robinson HL, Gagnon GC: Patterns of proviral insertion and deletion in avian leukosis virus-induced lymphomas. Mol Cell Biol 6:28–36, 1986.
90. Linial M, Groudine M: Transcription of three c-*myc* clones is enhanced in chicken bursal lymphoma cell lines. Proc Natl Acad Sci USA 82:53–57, 1985.
91. Li Y, Holland CA, Hartley JW, Hopkins N: Viral integrations near c-*myc* in 10–20% of

MCF247-induced AKR lymphomas. Proc Natl Acad Sci USA 81:6808–6811, 1984.
92. Corcoran LM, Adams JM, Dunn AR, Cory S: Murine T lymphomas in which the cellular *myc* oncogene has been activated by retroviral insertion. Cell 37:113–122, 1984.
93. Steffen D: proviruses are adjacent to c-*myc* in some murine leukemia virus-induced lymphomas. Proc Natl Acad Sci USA 81:2097–2101, 1984.
94. Selten G, Cuypers HT, Zijlstra M, Melief C, Berns A: Involvement of c-*myc* in MuLV-induced T cell lymphomas in mice: frequency and mechanism of activation. EMBO J 3:3215–3222, 1984.
95. Klein G: The role of gene dosage and genetic transpositions in carcinogenesis. Nature (London) 294:313–318, 1981.
96. Shen-Ong GLC, Keath EJ, Piccoli SP, Cole MD: Novel *myc* oncogene RNA from abortive immunoglobulin-gene recombination in mouse plasmacytomas. Cell 31:443–452, 1982.
97. Taub R, Kirsch I, Morton C, Lenoir G, Swan D, Tronick S, Aaronson S, Leder P: Translocation of the c-*myc* gene into the immunoglobulin heavy chain locus in human Burkitt lymphoma and murine plasmacytoma cells. Proc Natl Acad Sci USA 79:7837–7841, 1982.
98. Crews S, Barth R, Hood L, Prehn J, Calame K: Mouse c-*myc* oncogene is located on chrombosome 15 and translocated to chromosome 12 in plasmacytomas. Science 218:1319–1321, 1982.
99. Marcu KB, Harris LJ, Stanton LW, Erikson J, Watt R, Croce CM: Transcriptionally active c-*myc* oncogene is contained within NIARD, a DNA sequence associated with chromosome translocations in B cell neoplasia. Proc Natl Acad Sci USA 80:519–524, 1983.
100. Erikson J, ar-Rushdi A, Drwing HL, Nowell PC, Croce CM: Transcriptional activation of the translocated c-*myc* oncogene in Burkitt lymphoma. Proc Natl Acad Sci USA 80: 820–824, 1983.
101. Adams J, Gerondakis S, Webb E, Corcoran LM, Cory S: Cellular *myc* oncogene is altered by chromosome translocation to the immunoglobulin locus in murine plasmacytomas and is rearranged similarly in human Burkitt lymphoma. Proc Natl Acad Sci USA 80:1982–1986, 1983.
102. Erikson J, Miller DA, Miller OJ, Abcarian PW, Skurla RM, Mushinski JF, Croce CM: The c-*myc* oncogene is translocated to the involved chromosome 12 in mouse plasmacytoma. Proc Natl Acad Sci USA 82:4212–4216, 1985.
103. Erikson J, Nishikura K, ar-Rushdi A, Finan J, Emanuel B, Lenoir G, Nowell PC, Croce CM: Translocation of an immunoglobulin ϰ locus to a region 3′ of an unrearranged c-*myc* oncogene enhances c-*myc* transcription. Proc Natl Acad Sci USA 80:7581–7585, 1983.
104. Croce CM, Thierfelder W, Erikson J, Nishikura K, Finan J, Lenoir GM, Nowell PC: Transcriptional activation of an unrearranged and untranslocated c-*myc* oncogene by translocation of a C_λ locus in Burkitt lymphoma cells. Proc Natl Acad Sci USA 80:6922–6926, 1983.
105. Davis M, Malcolm S, Rabbitts TH: Chromosome translocation can occur on either side of the c-*myc* oncogene in Burkitt lymphoma cells. Nature 308:286–288, 1984.
106. Hollis GF, Mitchell KF, Battey J, Potter H, Taub RA, Lenoir G, Leder P: A variant translocation places the λ immunoglobulin genes 3′ to the c-*myc* oncogene in Burkitt lymphoma. Nature 307:752–755, 1984.
107. Taub R, Moulding C, Battey J, Latt S, Lenoir GM, Tantravahi U, Tu Z, Leder P: A novel alteration in the structure of an activated c-*myc* gene in a variant t(2;8) Burkitt lymphoma. Cell 37:511–520, 1984.
108. Graham M, Adams JM: Chromosome 8 breakpoint far 3′ of the c-*myc* oncogene in a Burkitt's lymphoma 2;8 variant translocation is equivalent to the murine *pvt*-1 locus. EMBO J 5:2845–2851, 1986.
109. Webb E, Adams JM Cory S: Variant (6;15) translocation in a murine plasmacytoma occurs near an immunoglobulin ϰ gene but far from the *myc* oncogene. Nature 312:777–779, 1984.
110. Cory S, Graham M, Webb E, Corcoran L, Adams JM: Variant (6;15) translocations in murine plasmacytomas involve a chromosome 15 locus at least 72 kb from the c-*myc*

oncogene. EMBO J4:675–681, 1985.
111. Banerjee, Wiener F, Spira J, Babonits M, Nilsson M-G, Sumegi J, Klein G: Mapping of the c-*myc*, *pvt*-1 and immunoglobulin kappa genes in relation to the mouse plasmacytoma-associated variant (6;15) translocation breakpoint. EMBO J 4:3183–3188, 1985.
112. Nishikura K, ar-Rushdi A, Erikson J, Watt R, Rovera G, Croce CM: Differential expression of the normal and of the translocated human c-*myc* oncogenes in B cells. Proc Natl Acad Sci USA 80:4822–4826, 1983.
113. ar-Rushdi A, Nishikura K, Erikson J, Watt R, Rovera G, Croce CM: Differential expression of the translocated and the untranslocated c-*myc* oncogenes in Burkitt lymphoma. Science 222:390–393, 1983.
114. Hayday AC, Gillies SD, Saito H, Wood C, Wiman K, Hayward WS, Tonegawa S: Activation of a translocated human c-*myc* gene by an enhancer in the immunoglobulin heavy-chain locus. Nature (London) 307:334–340, 1984.
115. Corcoran LM, Cory S, Adams JM: Transposition of the immunoglobulin heavy chain enhancer to the *myc* oncogene in a murine plasmacytoma. Cell 40:71–79, 1985.
116. Keath EJ, Kelekar A, Cole MD: Transcriptional activation of the translocated c-*myc* oncogene in mouse plasmacytomas: similar RNA levels in tumor and proliferating normal cells. Cell 37:521–528, 1984.
117. Rabbits TH, Forster A, Baer R, Hamlyn PH: Transcription enhancer identified near the human Cμ immunoglobulin heavy chain gene is unavailable to the translocated c-*myc* gene in a Burkitt lymphoma. Nature (London) 306:806–809, 1983.
118. Leder P, Battey J, Lenoir G, Moulding C, Murphy W: Translocations among the antibody genes in human cancer. Science 222:765–771, 1983.
119. Cory S, Gerondakis S, Adams JM: Interchromosomal recombination of the cellular oncogene c-*myc* with the immunoglobulin heavy chain locus in murine plasmacytomas is a reciprocal exchange. EMBO J 2:697–704, 1983.
120. Pelicci P-G, Knowles DM II, Magrath I, Dalla-Favera R: Chromosomal breakpoints and structural alterations of the c-*myc* locus differ in endemic and sporadic forms of Burkitt lymphoma. Proc Natl Acad Sci USA 83:2984–2988, 1986.
121. Yang J-Q, Rauer SR, Mushinski JF, Marcu KB: Chromosomal translocations clustered 5' of the murine c-*myc* gene qualitatively affect promoter usage: implications for the site of normal c-*myc* regulation. EMBO J 4:1441–1447, 1985.
122. Calabi F, Neuberger MS: Chromosome translocation activates heterogeneously initiated, bipolar transcription of a mouse c-*myc* gene. EMBO J 4:667–674, 1985.
123. Prehn J, Mercola M, Calame K: Translocation affects normal c-*myc* promoter usage and activates fifteen cryptic c-*myc* transcription starts in M603. Nucleic Acids Res 12:8987–9007, 1984.
124. Rabbitts TH, Hamlyn PH, Baer R: Altered nucleotide sequences of a translocated c-*myc* gene in Burkitt lumphoma. Nature 306:760–765, 1983.
125. Showe LC, Ballantine M, Nishikura K, Erikson J, Kaji H, Croce CM: Cloning and sequencing of a c-*myc* oncogene in a Burkitt's lymphoma cell line that is translocated to a germ line alpha switch region. Mol Cell Biol 5:501–509, 1985.
126. Rabbitts TH, Forster A, Hamlyn PH, Baer R: Effect of somatic mutations within translocated c-*myc* genes in Burkitt lymphoma. Nature 309:592–597, 1984.
127. Taub R, Moulding C, Battey J, Murphy W, Vasicek T, Leder P: Activation and somatic mutation of the translocated c-*myc* gene in Burkitt lymphoma cells. Cell 36:339–348, 1984.
128. Sumegi J, Spira J, Bazin H, Szpirer J, Levan G, Klein G: Rat c-*myc* oncogene is located on chromosome 7 and rearranges in immunocytomas with a t(6;7) translocation. Nature (London) 306:497–499, 1983.
129. Pear WS, Wahlstrom G, Nelson SF, Axelson H, Szeles A, Wiener F, Bazin H, Klein G, Sumegi J: 6;7 translocation in spontaneously arising rat immunocytomas: Evidence for c-*myc* breakpoint clustering and correlation between isotypic expression and the c-*myc* target. Mol Cell Biol 8:441–451, 1988.
130. Shima EA, Le Beau MM, McKeithan TW, Minowada J, Showe LC, Mak TW, Minden

MD, Rowley JD, Diaz MO: Gene encoding the α chain of the T-cell receptor is moved immediately downstream of c-*myc* in a chromosomal 8;14 translocation in a cell line from a human T-cell leukemia. Proc Natl Acad Sci USA 83:3439–3443, 1986.
131. Erikson J, Finger L, Sun L, ar-Rushdi A, Nishikura K, Minowada J, Finan J, Emanuel BS, Nowell PC, Croce CM: Deregulation of c-*myc* by translocation of the α-locus of the T-cell receptor in T-cell leukemias. Science 232:884–886, 1986.
132. McKeithan TW, Shima EA, Le Beau MM, Minowada J, Rowley JD, Diaz MO: Molecular cloning of the breakpoint junction of a human chromosomal 8;14 translocation involving the T-cell receptor α chain gene and sequences on the 3′ side of *MYC*. Proc Natl Acad Sci USA 83:6636–6640, 1986.
133. Drabkin HA, Bradley C, Hart I, Bleskan J, Li FP, Patterson D: Translocation of c-*myc* in the hereditary renal cell carcinoma associated with a t(3;8) (p14.2;q24.13) chromosomal translocation. Proc Natl Acad Sci USA 82:6980–6984, 1985.
134. Collins S, Groudine M: Amplification of endogenous *myc* related DNA sequences in human myeloid leukaemia cell line. Nature (London) 298:679–681, 1982.
135. Dalla-Favera R, Wong-Staal F, Gallo RC: *onc* Gene amplification in promyelocytic leukaemia cell line HL60 and primary leukaemic cells in the same patient. Nature (London) 299:61–63, 1982.
136. Alitalo K, Schwab M, Lin CC, Varmus HE, Bishop JM: Homogeneously staining chromosomal regions contain amplified copies of an abundantly expressed cellular oncogene (c-*myc*) in malignant neuroendocrine cells from a human colon carcinoma. Proc Natl Acad Sci USA 80:1707–1711, 1983.
137. Schwab M, Ramsay G, Alitalo K, Varmus HE, Bishop JM, Martinsson T, Levan G, Levan A: Amplification and enhanced expression of the c-*myc* oncogene in mouse SEWA tumour cells. Nature (London) 315:345–347, 1985.
138. Yokota J, Tsunetsugu-Yokota Y, Battifora H, LeFevre C, Cline MJ: Alterations of *myc*, *myb* and *ras*^{Ha} proto-oncogenes in cancers are frequent and show clinical correlation. Science 231:261–264, 1986.
139. Little CD, Nau MM, Carney DN, Gazdar AF, Minna JD: Amplification and expression of the c-*myc* oncogene in human lung cancer cell lines. Nature 306:194–196, 1983.
140. Land H, Parada LF, Weinberg RA: Tumorigenic conversion of primary embryo fibroblasts requires at least two cooperating oncogenes. Nature (London) 304:596–602, 1983.
141. Lee WMF, Schwab M, Westaway D, Varmus HE: Augmented expression of normal c-*myc* is sufficient for cotransformation of rat embryo cells with a mutant *ras* gene. Mol Cell Biol 5:3345–3356, 1985.
142. Lombardi L, Mewcomb EW, Dalla-Favera R: Pathogenesis of Burkitt lymphoma: expression of an activated c-*myc* oncogene causes the tumorigenic conversion of EBV-infected human B-lymphocytes. Cell 49:161–170, 1987.
143. Stewart TA, Pattengale PK, Leder P: Spontaneous mammary adenocarcinomas in transgenic mice that carry and express MTV/*myc* fusion genes. Cell 38:627–637, 1984.
144. Leder A, Pattengale PK, Kuo A, Stewart TA, Leder P: Consequences of widespread deregulation of the c-*myc* gene in transgenic mice: multiple neoplasms and normal development. Cell 45:485–495, 1986.
145. Adams JM, Harris AW, Pinkert CA, Corcoran LM, Alexander WS, Cory S, Palmiter RD, Brinster RL: The c-*myc* oncogene driven by immunoglobulin enhancers induces lymphoid malignancies in transgenic mice. Nature (London) 318:533–538, 1985.
146. Langdon WY, Harris AW, Cory S, Adams JM: The c-*myc* oncogene perturbs B lymphocyte development in Eμ-*myc* transgenic mice. Cell 47:11–18, 1986.
147. Suda Y, Aizawa S, Hirai S, Inoue T, Furuta Y, Suzuki M, Hirohashi S, Ikawa Y: Driven by the same Ig enhancer and SV40 T promoter *ras* induced lung adenomatous tumors, *myc* induced pre-B cell lymphomas and SV40 large T gene a variety of tumors in transgenic mice. EMBO J 6:4055–4065, 1987.
148. Sinn E, Muller W, Pattengale P, Tepler I, Wallace R, Leder P: Coexpression of MMTV/ v-Ha-*ras* and MMTV/c-*myc* genes in transgenic mice: synergistic action of oncogenes in

vivo. Cell 49:465–475, 1987.
149. Mougneau E, Lemieux L, Rassoulzadegan M, Cuzin F: Biological activities of v-*myc* and rearranged c-*myc* oncogenes in rat fibroblast cells in culture. Proc Natl Acad Sci USA 81:5758–5762, 1984.
150. Bartlett PF, Reid HH, Bailey KA, Bernard O: Immortalization of mouse neural precursor cells by the c-*myc* oncogene. Proc Natl Acad Sci USA 85:3255–3259, 1988.
151. Keath EJ, Caimi PG, Cole MD: Fibroblast lines expressing activated c-*myc* oncogenes are tumorigenic in nude mice and syngeneic animals. Cell 39:339–348, 1984.
152. Lavialle C, Modjtahedi N, Cassingena R, Brison O: High c-*myc* amplification level contributes to the tumorigenic phenotype of the human breast carcinoma cell line SW 613-S. Oncogene 3:335–339, 1988.
153. Martinsson T, Stahl F, Pollwein P, Wenzel A, Levan A, Schwab M, Levan G: Tumorigenicity of SEWA murine cells correlates with degree of c-*myc* amplification. Oncogene 3:437–441, 1988.
154. Hahn M, Hayward WS: Absence of missense mutations in activated c-*myc* genes in avian leukosis virus-induced B-cell lymphomas. Mol Cell Biol 8:2659–2663, 1988.
155. Westaway D, Pain G, Varmus HE: Proviral deletions and oncogene base-substitutions in insetionally mutagenized c-*myc* alleles may contribute to the progression of avian bursal tumors. Proc Natl Acad Sci USA 81:843–847, 1984.
156. Papas TS, Leutenberger JA: Sequence curiosity in v-*myc* oncogene. Nature (London) 318:237, 1985.
157. Frykberg L, Graf T, Vennstrom B: The transforming activity of the chicken c-*myc* gene can be potentiated by mutations. Oncogene 1:415–421, 1987.
158. Kelly K, Cochran BH, Stiles CD, Leder P: Cell-specific regulation of the c-*myc* gene by lymphocyte mitogens and platelet-derived growth factor. Cell 35:603–610, 1983.
159. Lacy J, Sarkar SN, Summers WC: Induction of c-*myc* expression in human B lymphocytes by B-cell growth factor and anti-immunoglobulin. Proc Natl Acad Sci USA 83:1458–1462, 1986.
160. Conscience J-F, Verrier B, Martin G: Interleukin-3-dependent expression of the c-*myc* and c-*fos* proto-oncogenes in hematopoietic cell lines. EMBO J 5:317–323, 1986.
161. Makino R, Hayashi K, Sugimura T: c-*myc* transcript is induced in rat liver at a very early stage of regeneration or by cycloheximide treatment. Nature (London) 310:697–698, 1984.
162. Muller R, Bravo R, Burckhardt J, Curran T: Induction of c-*fos* gene and protein by growth factors precedes activation of c-*myc*. Nature (London) 312:716–720, 1984.
163. Armelin HA, Armelin MCS, Kelly K, Stewart T, Leder P, Cochran BH, Stiles CD: Functional role for c-*myc* in mitogenic response to platelet-derived growth factor. Nature (London) 310:655–660, 1984.
164. Kaczmarek, Hyland JK, Watt R, Rosenberg M, Baserga R: Microinjected c-*myc* as a competence factor. Science 228:1313–1314, 1985.
165. Heikkila R, Schwab G, Wickstrom E, Loke SL, Pluznik DH, Watt R, Neckers LM: A c-*myc* antisense oligodeoxynucleotide inhibits entry into S phase but not progress from G_0 to G_1. Nature (London) 328:445–449, 1987.
166. Thompson CB, Challoner PB, Neiman PE, Groudine M: Levels of c-*myc* oncogene mRNA are invariant throughout the cell cycle. Nature (London) 314:363–366, 1985.
167. Hann SR, Thompson CB, Eisenman RN: c-*myc* oncogene protein synthesis is independent of the cell cycle in human and avian cells. Nature (London) 314:366–369, 1985.
168. Einat M, Resnitzky D, Kimchi A: Close link between reduction of c-*myc* expression by interferon and G0/G1 arrest. Nature (London) 313:597–600, 1985.
169. Lachman H, Skoultchi A: Expression of c-*myc* changes during differentiation of mouse erythroleukemia cells. Nature (London) 310:592–594, 1984.
170. de Bustros A, Baylin SB, Berger CL, Roos BA, Leong SS, Nelkin BD: Phorbol esters increase calcitonin gene transcription and decrease c-*myc* mRNA levels in cultured human medullary thyroid carcinoma. J Biol Chem 260:98–104, 1985.
171. Sejersen T, Suemegi J, Gingertz NR: Density-dependent arrest of DNA relication is

accompanied by decreased levels of c-*myc* mRNA in myogenic but not in differentiation-defective myoblasts. J Cell Physiol 125:465–470, 1985.
172. Endo T, Nadal-Ginard B: Transcriptional and posttranscriptional control of c-*myc* during myoenesis: its mRNA remains inducible in differentiated cells and does not suppress the differentiated phenotype. Mol Cell Biol 6:1412–141, 1986.
173. Freytag SO: Enforced expression of the c-*myc* oncogene inhibits cell differentiation by precluding entry into a distinct predifferentiation state in G_0/G_1. Mol Cell Biol 8:1614–1624, 1988.
174. Dotto GP, Gilman MZ, Maruyama M, Weinberg RA: c-*myc* and c-*fos* expression in differentiating mouse primary keratinocytes. EMBO J 5:2853–2857, 1986.
175. Coppola JA, Cole MD: Constitutive c-*myc* oncogene expression blocks mouse erythroleukaemia cell differentiation but not commitment. Nature (London) 320:760–763, 1986.
176. Dmitrovsky E, Kuehl WM, Hollis GF, Kirsch IR, Bender TP, Segal S: Expression of a transfected human c-*myc* oncogene inhibits differentiation of a mouse erythroleukaemia cell line. Nature (London) 322:748–750, 1986.
177. Prochownik EV, Kukowska J: Deregulated expression of c-*myc* by murine erythroleukaemia cells prevent differentiation. Nature (London) 322:848–850, 1986.
178. Lachman HM, Cheng G, Skoultchi AI: Transfection of mouse erythroleukemia cells with *myc* sequences changes the rate of induced commitment to differentiate. Proc Natl Acad Sci USA 83:6480–6484, 1986.
179. Wingrove TG, Watt R, Keng P, Macara IG: Stabilization of *myc* proto-oncogene proteins during Friend murine erythroleukemia cell differentiation. J Biol Chem 263:8918–8924, 1988.
180. Kume TU, Takada S, Obinata M: Probability that the commitment of murine erythroleukemia cell differentiation is determined by the c-*myc* level. J Mol Biol 202:779–786, 1988.
181. Griepp A, Westphal H: Antisense *Myc* sequences induce differentiation of F9 cells. Proc Natl Acad Sci USA 85:6806–6810, 1988.
182. Yokoyama K, Imamoto F: Transcriptional control of the endogenous MYC protooncogene by antisense RNA. Proc Natl Acad Sci USA 84:7363–7367, 1987.
183. Holt JT, Redner RL, Nienhuis AW: An oligomer complementary to c-*myc* mRNA inhibits proliferation of HL-60 promyelocytic cells and induces differentiation. Mol Cell Biol 8:963–973, 1988.
184. Prochownik EV, Kukowska J, Rodgers C: c-*myc* antisense transcripts accelerate differentiation and inhibit G_1 progression in murine erythroleukemia cells. Mol Cell Biol 8:3683–3695, 1988.
185. Studzinski GP, Brelvi ZS, Feldman SC, Watt RA: Participation of c-*myc* protein in DNA synthesis of human cells. Science 234:467–470, 1986.
186. Gutierrez C, Guo Z-S, Farrell-Towt J, Ju G, DePamphilis ML: c-*myc* protein and DNA replication: Separation of c-*myc* antibodies from an inhibitor of DNA synthesis. Mol Cell Biol 7:4597–4598, 1987.
187. Iguchi-Ariga SMM, Itani T, Kiji Y, Ariga H: Possible function of the c-*myc* product: promotion of cellular DNA replication. EMBO J 6:2365–2371, 1987.
188. Cavalieri F, Goldfarb M: Growth factor-deprived BALB/c 3T3 murine fibroblasts can enter the S phase after induction of c-*myc* gene expression. Mol Cell Biol 7:3554–3560, 1987.
189. Classon M, Henriksson M, Sumegi J, Klein G, Hammaskjold M-L: Elevated c-*myc* expression facilitates the replication of SV40 DNA in human lymphoma cells. Nature (London) 330:272–275, 1987.
190. Iguchi-Ariga SMM, Itani T, Yamaguchi M, Ariga H: c-*myc* protein can be substituted for SV40 T antigen in SV40 DNA replication. Nucleic Acids Res 15:4889–4899, 1987.
191. Kingston RE, Baldwin AS Jr, Sharp PA: Regulation of heat shock protein 70 gene expression by c-*myc*. Nature 312:280–282, 1984.
192. Kaddurah-Daouk R, Greene JM, Baldwin AS Jr, Kingston RE: Activation and repression of mammalian gene expression by the c-*myc* protein. Genes Devel 1:347–357, 1987.
193. Onclercq R, Gilardi P, Lavenu A, Cremisi C: c-*myc* products trans-activate the adenovirus

E4 promoter in EC stem cells by using the same target sequence as E1A products. J Virol 62:4533–4537, 1988.
194. Manolagas SC, Provvedini DM, Murray EJ, Murray SS, Tsonis PA, Spandidos DA: Association between the expression of the c-*myc* oncogene mRNA and the expression of the receptor protein for 1,25-dihydroxyvitamin D_3. Proc Natl Acad Sci USA 84:856–860, 1987.
195. Schweinfest CW, Fujiwara S, Lau LF, Papas TS: c-*myc* can induce expression of G0/G1 transition genes. Mol Cell Biol 8:3080–3087, 1988.
196. Versteeg R, Noordermeer IA, Kruse-Wolters M, Ruiter DJ, Schrier PI: c-*myc* down-regulates class I HLA expression in human melanomas. EMBO J 7:1023–1029, 1988.
197. Lech K, Anderson K, Brent R: DNA-bound Fos proteins activate transcription in yeast. Cell 52:179–186, 1988.
198. Ralston R, Bishop JM: The protein products of the *myc* and *myb* oncogenes and adenovirus E1a are structurally related. Nature (London) 306:803–805, 1983.
199. Kingston RE, Baldwin AS, Sharp PA: Transcriptional control by oncogenes. Cell 41:3–5, 1985.
200. Davis RL, Weintraub H, Lasser AB: Expression of a single transfected cDNA converts fibroblasts to myoblasts. Cell 51:987–1000, 1987.
201. Caudy M, Vassin H, Brand M, Tuma R, Jan LY, Jan YN: *daughterless*, a Drosophila gene essential for both neurogenesis and sex determination, has sequence similarities to *myc* and *achaete-scute* complex. Cell 55:1061–1067, 1988.
202. Villares R, Cabrera CV: The *achaete-scute* gene complex of D. melanogaster: conserved domains in a subset of genes required for neurogenesis and their homology to *myc*. Cell 50:415–424, 1987.
203. Vogt PK, Bos TJ, Doolittle RF: Homology between the DNA-binding domain of the GCN4 regulatory protein of yeast and the carboxy-terminal region of a protein coded for by the oncogene *jun*. Proc Natl Acad Sci USA 84:3316–3319, 1987.
204. Landschulz WH, Johnson PF, Adashi EY, Graves BJ, McKnight SL: Isolation of a recombinant copy of the gene encoding C/EBP. Genes Devel 2:786–800, 1988.
205. Landschulz WH, Johnson PF, McKnight SL: The lecine zipper: a hypothetical structure common to a new class of DNA binding proteins. Science 240:1789–1794, 1988.
206. Kassis JA, Poole SJ, Wright DK, O'Farrell PH: Sequence conservation in the protein coding and intron regions of the *engrailed* transcription unit. EMBO J 5:3583–3589, 1986.
207. Ramsay GR, Hayman MJ: Isolation and biochemical characterization of partially transformation-defective mutants of avian myelocytomatosis virus strain MC29: localization of the mutation of the *myc* domain of the 110,000-dalton *gag-myc* polyprotein. J Virol 41:745–753, 1982.
208. Bister K, Trachman C, Jansen HW, Schroeer B, and Patschinsky T: Structure of mutant and wild-type MC-29 v-*myc* alleles and biochemical properties of their protein products. Oncogene 1:97–109, 1987.
209. Schwab M, Alitalo K, Klempnauer K-H, Varmus HE, Bishop JM, Gilbert F, Brodeur G, Goldstein M, Trent J: Amplified DNA with limited homology to the *myc* cellular oncogene is shared by human neuroblastoma cell lines and a neuroblastoma tumor. Nature (London) 305:245–248, 1983.
210. Kohl NE, Kanda W, Schreck RR, Bruns G, Latt SA, Gilbert F, Alt FW: Transposition and amplification of oncogene-related sequences in human neuroblastomas. Cell 35:359–367, 1983.
211. Kohl NE, Legouy E, DePinho RA, Nisen PD, Smith RK, Gee CE, Alt FW: Human N-*myc* is closely related in organization and nucleotide sequence to c-*myc*. Nature (London) 319:73–77, 1986.
212. Stanton LW, Schwab M, Bishop JM: Nucleotide sequence of the human N-*myc* gene. Proc Natl Acad Sci USA 83:1772–1776, 1986.
213. DePinho RA, Legouy E, Feldman LB, Kohl NE, Yancopoulos GD, Alt FW: Structure and expression of the murine N-*myc* gene. Proc Natl Acad Sci USA 83:1827–1831, 1986.

214. Nau MM, Burke BJ, Carney DN, Gazdar AF, Battey JF, Sausville EA, Minna JD: Human small-cell lung cancers show amplification and expression of the N-*myc* gene. Proc Natl Acad Sci USA 83:1092–1096, 1986.
215. Slamon DJ, Boone TC, Seeger RC, Keith DE, Chazin V, Lee HC, Souza LM: Identification and characterization of the protein encoded by the human N-*myc* oncogene. Science 232:768–772, 1986.
216. Ramsay G, Stanton L, Schwab M, Bishop JM: The human proto-oncogene N-*myc* encodes nuclear proteins that bind DNA. Mol Cell Biol 6:4450–4457, 1986.
217. Ikegaki N, Bukovsky J, Kennett RH: Identification and characterization of the NMYC gene product in human neuroblastoma cells by monoclonal antibodies with defined specificities. Proc Natl Acad Sci USA 83:5929–5933, 1986.
218. Zimmerman KA, Yancopoulos GD, Collum RG, Smith RK, Kohl NE, Denis KA, Nau MM, Witte ON, Toran-Allerand D, Gee CE, Alt FW: Differential expression of *myc* family genes during murine development. Nature 319:780–783, 1986.
219. Jakobovits A, Schwab M, Bishop JM, Martin G: Expression of N-*myc* in teratocarcinoma cells and mouse embryos. Nature 318:188–191, 1985.
220. Sejersen T, Rahm M, Szabo G, Ingvarsson S, Sumegi J: Similarities and differences in the regulation of N-*myc* and c-*myc* genes in murine embryonal carcinoma cells. Exp Cell Res 172:304–317, 1987.
221. Lee W-H, Murphree AL, Benedict WF: Expression and amplification of the N-*myc* gene in primary retinoblastoma. Nature (London) 309:458–460, 1984.
222. Nau MM, Brooks BJ Jr, Carney DN, Gazdar AF, Battey JF, Sausville EA, Minna JD: Human small-cell lung cancers show amplification and expression of the N-*myc* gene. Proc Natl Acad Sci USA 83:1092–1096, 1986.
223. Nisen PD, Zimmerman KA, Cotter SV, Gilbert F, Alt FW: Enhanced expression of the N-*myc* gene in Wilm's tumors. Cancer Res 46:6217–6222, 1986.
224. Schwab M, Ellison J, Busch M, Rosenau W, Varmus HE, Bishop JM: Enhanced expression of the human gene N-*myc* consequent to amplification of DNA may contribute to malignant progression of neuroblastoma. Proc Natl Acad Sci USA 81:4940–4944, 1984.
225. Kohl NE, Gee CE, Alt FW: Activated expression of the N-*myc* gene in human neuroblastomas and related tumors. Science 226:1335–1337, 1984.
226. Brodeur GM, Seeger RC, Schwab M, Vermus HE, Bishop JM: Amplification of N-*myc* in untreated human neuroblastomas correlates with advanced stage disease. Science 224:1121–1124, 1984.
227. Seeger RC, Brodeur GM, Sather H, Dalton A, Siegel SE, Wong KY, Hammond D: Association of multiple copies of the N-*myc* oncogene with rapid progression of neuroblastomas. N Engl J Med 313:1111–1116, 1985.
228. Bernards R, Dessain SK, Weinberg RA: N-*myc* amplification causes down-modulation of MHC class I antigen expression in neuroblastoma. Cell 47:667–674, 1986.
229. Schwab M, Varmus HE, Bishop JM, Grzeschik K-H, Naylor SL, Sakaguchi AY, Brodeur G, Trent J: Chromosome localization in normal human cells and neuroblastomas of a gene related to c-*myc*. Nature (London) 308:288–291.
230. Schwab M, Varmus HE, Bishop JM: Human N-*myc* gene contributes to neoplastic transformation of mammalian cells in culture. Nature 316:160–162, 1985.
231. Yancopoulos GD, Nisen PD, Tesfaye A, Kohl NE, Goldfarb MP, Alt FW: N-*myc* can cooperate with *ras* to transform normal cells in culture. Proc Natl Acad Sci USA 82:5455–5459, 1985.
232. Small MB, Hay N, Schwab M, Bishop JM: Neoplastic transformation by the human N-*myc* gene. Mol Cell Biol 7:1638–1645, 1987.
233. Thiele CJ, Reynolds CP, Israel MA: Decreased expression of N-*myc* precedes retinoic acid-induced morphological differentiation of human neuroblastoma. Nature (London) 313:404–406, 1985.
234. Nau MM, Brooks BJ, Battey J, Sausville E, Gazdar AF, Kirsch IR, McBride OW, Bertness V, Hollis GF, Minna JD: L-*myc*, a new *myc*-related gene amplified and expressed in human

small cell lung cancer. Nature (London) 318:69–73, 1985.
235. DePinho RA, Hatton KS, Tesfaye A, Yancopoulos GD, Alt FW: The human *myc* gene family: structure and activity of L-*myc* and an L-*myc* pseudogene. Genes Devel 1:1311–1326, 1987.
236. Kaye F, Battey J, Nau M, Brooks B, Seifter E, De Greve J, Birrer M, Sausville E, Minna J: Structure and expression of the human L-*myc* gene reveal a complex pattern of alternative mRNA processing. Mol Cell Biol 8:186–195, 1988.
237. Legouy E, De Pinho R, Zimmerman K, Collum R, Yancopoulos G, Mitsock L, Kriz R, Alt FW: Structure and expression of the murine L-*myc* gene. EMBO J 6:3359–3366, 1987.
238. De Greve J, Battey J, Fedorko J, Birrer M, Evan G, Kaye F, Sausville E, Minna J: The human L-*myc* gene encodes multiple nuclear phosphoproteins from alternatively processed mRNAs. Mol Cell Biol 8:4381–4388, 1988.
239. Birrer MJ, Segal S, De Greve JS, Kaye F, Sausville EA, Minna JD: L-*myc* cooperates with *ras* to transform primary rat embryo fibroblasts. Mol Cell Biol 8:2668–2673, 1988.
240. Ingvarsson S, Asker C, Axelson H, Klein G, Sumegi J: Structure and expression of B-*myc*, a new member of the *myc* gene family. Mol Cell Biol 8:3168–3174, 1988.
241. Ingvarsson S, Asker C, Wirschubsky Z, Szpirer J, Levan G, Klein G, Sumegi J: Mapping of L*myc* and N*myc* to rat chromosomes 5 and 6. Somat Cell Mol Genet 13:335–339, 1987.
242. DePinho R, Mitsock L, Hatton K, Ferrier P, Zimmerman K, Legouy E, Tesfaye A, Collum R, Yancopoulos G, Nisen P, Kriz R, Alt F: Myc family of cellular oncogenes. J Cell Biochem 33:257–266, 1987.

4. The *ras* family of oncogenes

Channing J. Der

The first evidence implicating a role for the cellular *ras* genes in oncogenesis came from studies of the highly oncogenic RNA tumor viruses [1–4]. The cellular *ras* genes were first identified to be the cellular counterparts to the viral genes responsible for the oncogenic properties of Harvey (v-H-*ras*) and Kirsten (v-K-*ras*) murine sarcoma viruses [5,6]. Further interest in the role of cellular *ras* genes in carcinogenesis exploded in 1982, when the first human transforming genes were identified as activated cellular counterparts of viral *ras* genes [7–9]. Over the past six years, an enormous research effort has centered on characterizing the biochemistry and biology of these potential human oncogenes. Of the 40 or so cellular oncogenes that have been identified to date, the cellular *ras* genes have demonstrated the strongest association with human carcinogenesis. The frequent identification of activated *ras* genes in a wide variety of human neoplasms has provided strong circumstantial evidence for the role of these genes in the malignant process. Consequently, it is generally believed that determining the mechanism of action of *ras* will contribute significantly to our understanding of the molecular mechanisms of human carcinogenesis.

Although studies on cellular *ras* genes have centered on defining their role in human carcinogenesis, elucidating the importance of these genes in normal cellular physiology will also be of equal importance. Supporting a crucial role for these genes in normal cells is the observed strong evolutionary conservation of *ras* structure and function, and their expression in virtually every cell type. Furthermore, with the identification of an increasing number of *ras*-related genes, it appears that *ras* may represent only one branch of a larger gene family of *ras*-related proteins.

Several recent reviews have provided comprehensive overviews of the experimental developments in the various areas of *ras* research [10–12]. This chapter centers on studies concerning the structure and biochemistry of the *ras* and *ras*-related proteins, with the specific aim of defining the differences between the normal and oncogenic forms of *ras*. This review is not intended to be comprehensive, but rather, to summarize representative data reflecting our current understanding of the mechanisms of oncogenesis by *ras* proteins.

Benz, C. and Liu, E., (eds.), Oncogenes. © *1989 Kluwer Academic Publishers.*
ISBN 0-7923-0237-0. All rights reserved.

Primary structure

Human ras *genes*

The human *ras* gene family is comprised of at least three distinct members, represented by H-*ras*, K-*ras*, and N-*ras*. Two structurally distinct H-*ras* genes (H-*ras*-1 and H-*ras*-2) and K-*ras* genes (K-*ras*-1 and K-*ras*-2) have been identified [13,14], while only one N-*ras* gene has been detected [15–17]. H-*ras*-1, K-*ras*-2, and N-*ras* represent the functional *ras* genes, with two pseudogenes, H-*ras*-2 and K-*ras*-1 [13,14], also present in the human genome. Although their exon–intron splice junctions correspond identically in the three genes, the sizes of the respective intron sequences are highly variable. While the entire functional H-*ras*-1 genomic sequence is found within a 6-kb segment [18], the genomic structure of N-*ras* spans approximately 20 kb [16,17], and of K-*ras*-2 greater than 45 kb of DNA [14,21]. Each of the three functional *ras* genes encodes for highly related proteins of approximately 21,000 daltons, designated p21s [19,20]. The H-*ras*-1 and N-*ras* genes encode 189-amino-acid proteins, while the K-*ras*-2 encodes either a 189-(4A) or 188-(4B) amino-acid version, due to the use of two alternative fourth exons [14,21,22]. While the 4A version of the rat K-*ras*-2 gene corresponds to the transduced sequences in the viral K-*ras* genome, the 4B version appears to be the predominant transcript in human cells [21,23]. In nonvirally transformed cells, the exon 4B is used preferentially, such that 99% of all K-*ras*-2 transcripts contain exon 4B sequences. Both K-*ras* 4A and 4B genes can generate transforming forms of the p21 protein.

The chromosomal location of each *ras* gene has been determined [24–29, 235]. H-*ras*-1 has been assigned to the short arm of human chromosome 11 (11p15.1-p15.5), while K-*ras*-2 has been assigned to chromosome 12 (12p12.1), and N-*ras* assigned to the short arm of chromosome 1 (1p22-p32). The chromosomal location of the H-*ras*-2 pseudogene has been assigned to the X chromosome, and the K-*ras*-1 pseudogene to chromosome 6 (6p12-p23). While chromosomal rearrangements in the region of the *ras* genes have been observed in certain human tumors [30,31], no evidence for the specific deletion or rearrangement of internal *ras* sequences has been documented. Although several studies have suggested the correlation of specific rare allelic forms of H-*ras* with increased risk of developing human malignancy [32,33], other studies have found no relationship [35,36,273].

The three different *ras* proteins are approximately 85% homologous at the amino acid level (figure 1). The degree of homology is not uniform, and the primary amino acid sequences can be characterized by four domains. The first domain comprises amino acids 1–85 of each *ras* protein and is the most highly conserved; the three different *ras* proteins are identical in this domain. The second most conserved (85% homology) *ras* region is consists of the next 80 amino acids. The remaining stretch of 19–20 amino acids, up to the consensus Cys-A-A-X (where A is any aliphatic amino acid) carboxyl-

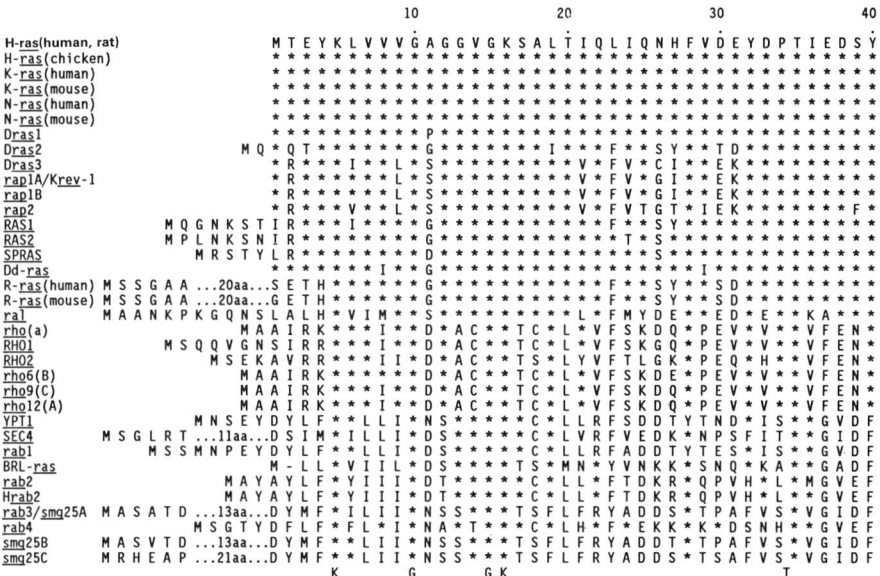

Figure 1. Amino acid sequence comparison of *ras* and *ras*-related proteins. Amino acids identical to the human H-*ras* protein are designated by an asterisk. Numbers correspond to amino acid positions in the human *ras* proteins. Amino acid residues present in all proteins are designated at the bottom. Single-letter abbreviations for the amino acid residues are as follows: A, alanine; C, cysteine; D, aspartic acid; E, glutamic acid; F, phenylalanine; G, glycine; H, histidine; I, isoleucine; K, lysine; L, leucine; M, methionine; N, asparagine; P, proline; Q, glutamine; R, arginine; S, serine; T, threonine; V, valine; W, tryptophan; Y, tyrosine.

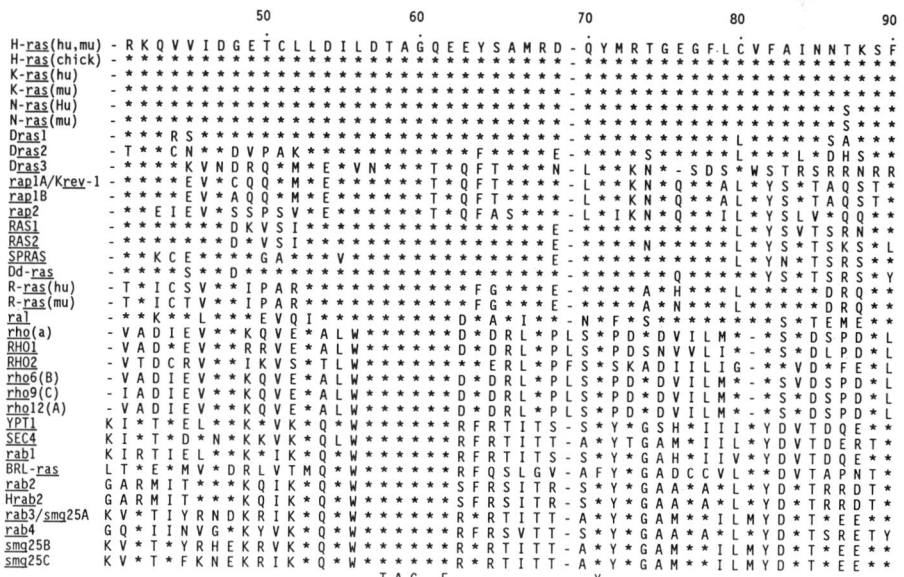

Figure 1 (cont.)

```
                                            100                 110                 120
H-ras(hu,mu)    E D I H Q Y - - - - - R E Q I K R V K D S D D V P M V L V G N K C D L A - - - - - - - - - - - - - A R T
H-ras(chick)    * * * * * * - - - - - * * * * * * * * * * * * * * * * * * * * * * * * P - - - - - - - - - - - - - * * *
K-ras(hu)       * * * * H * - - - - - * * * * * * * * * * E * * * * * * * * * * * * * P - - - - - - - - - - - - - S * *
K-ras(mu)       * * * * H * - - - - - * * * * * * * * * * E * * * * * * * * * * * * * P - - - - - - - - - - - - - S * *
N-ras(hu)       A * * N L * - - - - - * * * * * * * * * * * * * * * * * * * * * * * * P - - - - - - - - - - - - - T * *
N-ras(mu)       A * * N L * - - - - - * * * * * * * * * * * * * * * * * * * * * * * * P - - - - - - - - - - - - - T * *
Dras1           * * * G T * - - - - - * * * * * H * * * A E E * * * * * A * * * * * * * - - - - - - - - - - - - - S W N
Dras2           D E * P K F - - - - - Q R * * L * * * * R * E F * * L M * * * * * * * K - - - - - - - - - - - - - H Q Q
Dras3           L T * C R T - - - - - * * * * L * * * * T * * * * * * * * * * * * * * E - - - - - - - - - - - - - E * V
rap1A/Krev-1    N * L Q D L - - - - - * * * * L * * * * T E * * * * I * * * * * * * * E D - - - - - - - - - - - - E * V
rap1B           N * L Q D L - - - - - * * * * L * * * * T * * * * * I * * * * * * * * E D - - - - - - - - - - - - E * V
rap2            Q * * K P M - - - - - * D * * I * * * R Y E K * * V I * * * * * V * * E S - - - - - - - - - - - - E * E
RAS1            D E L L S * - - - - - Y Q * * Q * * * * * * Y I * V * V * * * * L * * E - - - - - - - - - - - - - N E R
RAS2            D E L M T * - - - - - Y Q * * L * * * * T * Y * * I * V * * * * S * * E - - - - - - - - - - - - - N E K
SPRAS           D E * S T F - - - - - Y Q * * L * * * * K * T F * V * * * A * * * * * E - - - - - - - - - - - - - * E R
Dd-ras          D E * A S F - - - - - * * * * L * * * * K * R * * L I * * * * * A * * D - - - - - - - - - - - - - H E R
R-ras(hu)       N E V G K L - - - - - F T * * L * * * * R * * F * V * * * * * * A * * E S - - - - - - - - - - - - Q * Q
R-ras(mu)       N E V G K L - - - - - F T * * L * * * * R * * F * I * * * * * * A * * E N - - - - - - - - - - - - Q * Q
ral             A A T A D F - - - - - * * * * L * * * E D E N * * F L * * * * * S * * E D - - - - - - - - - - - - K * Q
rho(a)          * N * P E K - - - - - W T P E V * - H F C P N * * I I * * * * * K * * R N D E S T K R E L M K M K Q E P
RHO1            * N V Q E K - - - - - W I A E V L - H F C Q G * * I I * * * C * V * * R N D P Q T I E Q L R Q E G Q Q P
RHO2            I N A R T K - - - - - W A D E A L - R Y C P * A * I * * * * L * K * * R Q E A H F K E N A T - - - D E M
rho6(B)         * N * P E K - - - - - W V P E V K - H F C P N * * I I * * A * * K * * R S D E H V R T E L A R M K Q E P
rho9(C)         * N * P E K - - - - - W T P E V K - H F C P N * * I I * * * * * K * * R Q D E H T R R E L A K M K Q E P
rho12(A)        * N * P E K - - - - - W T P E V K - H F C P N * * I I * * * * * K * * R N D E H T R R E L A K M K Q E P
YPT1            N G V K M W - - - - - L Q E * D * Y A T * T - * L K L * * * * * * * * K D - - - - - - - - - - - - K * V
SEC4            T N * K * W - - - - - F K T V N E H A N D E - A Q L L * * * * * S * M E I - - - - - - - - - - - - T * V
rab1            N N V K * W - - - - - L Q E * D * Y A S E - N * N K L * * * * * * * * T T - - - - - - - - - - - - K K V
BRL-ras         K T L D S W R D E F L I Q A S P * - D P E - N F P F * V L * * * I * * E N - - - - - - - - - - - - R Q V
rab2            N H L T T W - - - - - L * D A R Q H S N * - N M V I M * I * * * S * * E S - - - - - - - - - - - - R * E
Hrab2           N H L T T W - - - - - L * D A R Q H S N * - N M V I M * I * * * S * * E S - - - - - - - - - - - - R * E
rab3/smg25A     N A V Q D W - - - - - S T * * * T Y S W D - N A Q V L * * * * * * * M E D - - - - - - - - - - - - E * V
rab4            N A L T N W - - - - - L T D A R M L A S Q - N I V I I * C * * * K * * D A - - - - - - - - - - - - D * E
smg25B          N A V Q D W - - - - - A T * * * T Y S W D - N A Q V I * * * * * * * M E E - - - - - - - - - - - - E * V
smg25C          N A V Q D W - - - - - S T * * * T Y S W D - N A Q V I * * * * * * * M E D - - - - - - - - - - - - E * V
                                                                              K   D
```

Figure 1 (cont.)

```
                            130                     140                 150                 160                     170
H-ras(hu,mu)    V E S R Q - A Q D L A R S Y - G I - P Y I E T S A K T R Q G V E D A F Y T L V - R E I R Q H - K L R K
H-ras(chick)    * * T * * - * * * * * * * * - * * - * * * * * * * * * * * * * * * * * * * * * - * * * * * * - * * * *
K-rasA(hu)      * D T K * - * * * * * * * * - * * - * F * * * * * * * * * R * * * * * * * * * - * * * * * Y - R * K *
K-rasA(mu)      * D T K * - * * E * * * * * - * * - * F * * * * * * * * * R * * * * * * * * * - * * * * * Y - R * K *
K-rasB(hu)      * D T K * - * * * * * * * * - * * - * F * * * * * * * * * * * * D * * * * * * - * * * * K * - * E K M
K-rasB(mu)      * D T K * - * * E * * * * * - * * - * F * * * * * * * * * * * * D * * * * * * - * * * * K * - * E K M
N-ras(hu)       * D T K * - * H E * * K * * - * * - * F * * * * * * * * * * * * * * * * * * * - * * * * * Y - R M K *
N-ras(mu)       * D T K * - * H E * * K * * - * * - * F * * * * * * * * * * * * * * * * * * * - * * * * * Y - R * K *
Dras1           * N N E * - * R E V * K Q * - * * - * * * * * * * * * * M * * * D * * * * * * - * * * * K * - * D N *
Dras2           Q V * L E E * * N T S * N L - M * - * * * * C * * * L * V N * D Q * * H E * * - * I V * K F - Q I A E
Dras3           * G K E L - G K N * * T Q F - N C - A F M * * * * * A K V N * N * I * * D W S G * S T * S R - P R * -
rap1A/Krev-1    * G K E * - G * N * * * Q W C N C - A F L * S * * * S K I N * N E I * * D * * R Q I N * K T - P V E -
rap1B           * G K E * - G * N * * * Q W N N C - A F L * S * * * S K I N * N E I * * D * * R Q I N * K T - P V P -
rap2            * S * S E - G R A * * E E W - * C - * F M * * * * * S K T M * D E L * A E I * R Q M N Y A A - Q P D -
RAS1            Q V * Y E D G L R * * K Q L - N A - * F L * * * * * Q A I N * D E * * * S * I - * L V * D D - G G K Y
RAS2            Q V * Y * D G L N M * K Q M - N A - * F L * * * * * Q A I N * * E * * * * * A - * L V * D E - G G K Y
SPRAS           * V * * R E G E Q * * K * M - H C - L * V * * * * * L * L N * * E * * * S * * - * T * * R Y - N K S E
Dd-ras          Q V * V N E G * E * * K D S - L S - - F H * S * * * S * I N * * E * * * S * * - * * * * K E - L K G D
R-ras(hu)       * P R S E - * S A F G A * H - H V - A * F * A * * * L * L N * D E * * E Q * * - * A V * K Y - Q E Q E
R-ras(mu)       * L R S E - * S S F S A * H - H M - T * F * A * * * L * L N * D E * * E Q * * - * A V * K Y - Q E Q E
ral             * S V E E - * K N R * D Q W - N V - N * V * * * * * * * A N * D K V * F D * M - * * * * A R - * M E D
rho(a)          * R P E D - G R A M * E K I - N A Y S * L * C * * * * K E * * R * V * E * A T - * A A L * V - * K - -
RHO1            * T * Q E - G * S V * D Q I - * A T G * Y * C * * * * G Y * * R E V * E A A T - * A S L M G - * S K T
RHO2            * P I E D - * K Q V * * A I - * A K K * M * C * * L * G E * * D * V * E V A T - * T S L L M - * K - -
rho6(B)         * R T D D - G R A M * V R I - Q A Y D * L * C * * * * K E * * R E V * E * A T - * A A L * K - R Y - -
rho9(C)         * R * E E - G R * M * N R I - S A F G * L * C * * * * K E * * R E V * E M A T - * A G L * V - R K - -
rho12(A)        * K P E E - G R * M * N R I - * A F G * M * C * * * * K D * * R E V * E M A T - * A A L * A - R R - -
YPT1            * * Y D V - * K E F * D A N - K M - * F L * * * * L D S T N * * * * * L * M A - * Q * K * S M S Q Q N
SEC4            * T A D * - G E A * * K Q L - * * - * F * * S * * * N D D N * N E I * F * * A - K L * Q E K I D S N *
rab1            * D Y T T - * K E F * D * L - * * - * F L * * * * * N A T N * * Q S * M * M A - A * * K K R - M G P G
BRL-ras         A T - K R - * * A W C Y * K N N * - * * F * * * * * E A I N * * Q A * Q T I A - R N A L K Q - E T E V
rab2            * K K E E - G E A F * * E H - * L - I F M * * * * * * A S N * * E * * I N T A - K * * Y E K - I Q E G
Hrab2           * K K E E - G E A F * * E H - * L - I F M * * * * * * A S N * * E * * I N T A - K * * Y E K - I Q E G
rab3/smg25A     * S * E R - G R Q * * D H L - * F - E F F * A * * * D N I N * K Q T * E R * * - D V * C E K - M S E S
rab4            * T F L E - * S R F * Q E N - E L - M F L * * * * L * G E N * * E * * M Q C A - * K * L N K - I E S G
smg25B          * P T E K - G R L * * E Q L - * F - D F F * A * * * E N I S * R Q * * E R * * - D A * C D K - M S D T
smg25C          I S T E R - G * H * G E Q L - * F - E F F * * * * * D N I N * K Q T * E R * * - D I * C D K - M S E S
                                                              S A         V       F
```

Figure 1 (cont.)

```
                                      180                          189
H-ras(hu,mu)    L N P - - P D E S G P G C M S C K      - - - - - - C V L S
H-ras(chick)    * * * - - * * * * * * * * N * *        - - - - - - * * I *
K-rasA(hu)      I S K - - E E K T P G C V K I K *      - - - - - * * I I M
K-rasA(mu)      I S K - - E E K T P G C V K I K *      - - - - - - * * I M
K-rasB(hu)      S K D - - G K K K K K K S K - T *      - - - - - - * * I M
K-rasB(mu)      S K D - - G K K K K K K S R - T R      - - - - - - * T V M
N-ras(hu)       * * S - - S * D G T Q * * * G L P      - - - - - - * * V M
N-ras(mu)       * * S - - S * D G T Q * * * G S P      - - - - - - * * * M
Dras1           G R R - - G R K M N K P N C R F *      - - - - - - * K M L
Dras2           R P F - - I E Q D Y K K K G K R *      - - - - - - * C * M
Dras3           - * R - - R S R K V - - - - - - P      - - - - - - * * * L
rap1A/Krev-1    - K K - - K P K K K - - - - - - S      - - - - - - * L * L
rap1B           - G K - - A R K K S - - - - - - S      - - - - - - * L Q L
rap2            - K D - - D P C C S - - - - - - A      - - - - - - * N I Q
RAS1            N S M - - N R Q L D N T N E I R D  (106 aa)  Y S G G C * I I C
RAS2            N K T - - L T * N D N S K Q T S Q  (109 aa)  G S G G C * I I *
SPRAS           E K G - - F Q N K Q A V Q I A Q V   (19 aa)  V S T K C * * I C
Dd-ras          Q S S - - G K A Q K K K K Q - - -            - - - - - * L I L
R-ras(hu)       * P * - - S P P * A * R K K G G G            - - - C P * * * L
R-ras(mu)       * P * - - S P P * A * R K K D G G            - - - C P * * * L
ral             S K E K N G K K K R - K S L - A *            R I R E R * C I L
rho(a)          - - - - - - - - - - - K K K G G              - - - - - - * * V L
RHO1            N G K - - A K K N T T E K K K K *            - - - - - - * * * L
RHO2            - - - - - - - - - - - E P G A N C            - - - - - * I I L
rho6(B)         - - - - - - - - - - - G S Q N G              - C I N C * K V L
rho9(C)         - - - - - - - - - - - N K R R R              - - - - G * P I L
rho12(A)        - - - - - - - - - - - K K K S G              - - - - - * L V L
YPT1            * * E - - T T Q K K E D K G N V N    (8 aa)  T G G G C *
SEC4            * V G - - V G N G K E - - G N I S    (8 aa)  S K S N C *
rab1            - - - - A T A G G A E K S N - V *    (8 aa)  S G G G C *
BRL-ras         - - - - E L Y N E F P - E P - I *   (10 aa)  A E S C S *
rab2            V F D I N N E A N * I K I G - P Q   (16 aa)  A G G G C *
Hrab2           V F D I N N E A N * I K I G - P Q   (16 aa)  A G G G C *
rab3/smg25A     * D T A D * A V T * A K Q G - P Q    (8 aa)  H Q D C A *
rab4            E L D P E R M G * * I Q Y G - D A   (15 aa)  A Q E C G *
smg25           * D T - D * S L L * T S K N - T R    (8 aa)  Q Q N C S *
smg25C          * E T - D * A I T A A K Q N - T R    (8 aa)  Q P N C G *
                                                                        C
```

Figure 1 (cont.)

terminus sequence present in all three *ras* proteins, is highly variable among the three members.

Other eukaryotic ras *genes*

The *ras* genes have been highly conserved in vertebrate evolution, with homologous genes identified in all species analyzed. In addition to man, *ras* genes have been found in mouse, rat, mink, hamster, turkey, bat, cat, dog, horse, monkey, chicken, and goldfish [19,37,38]. The goldfish K-*ras* gene [38] encodes a protein that shares approximately 96% homology with human K-*ras* (4A). This degree of conservation in vertebrate evolution is similar to that observed for the histone 4B protein, suggesting that conservation of *ras* primary structure is important for function.

Highly related *ras* sequences have also been identified in a range of invertebrate species (figure 1). Three *ras* homologues, Dras1, Dras2 and Dras3, have been identified in the fruit fly *Drosophila melanogaster* [39–41], in both the budding yeast *Saccharomyces cerevisiae* (*RAS1* and *RAS2*) [42,43] and the fission yeast *Schizosaccharomyces pombe* (*SPRAS*) [44], the slime mold *Dictyostelium discoideum* (Ddras) [45] and in the mollusk *Aplysia* (Apl-*ras*) [46]. While the invertebrate *ras* genes typically encode proteins of similar size to the mammalian *ras* proteins, the *S. cerevisiae RAS1* and *RAS2* genes code for proteins of 40 kDa (309 amino acids) and 41 kDa (322 amino acids), respectively. The larger size of these two yeast *ras* proteins is accounted for

Table 1. Properties of ras-related proteins

Gene	Origin	Residues	Isolation	% Homology[a]
ral	Simian	206	Oligomers (57–63)[b]	49
rho				
rho (a)	Aplysia	192	Fortuitous	33
rho6 (B)	Human	196	rho(a)	30
rho9 (C)	Human	193	rho(a)	31
rho12 (A)	Human	193	rho(a)	31
RHO1	Yeast	209	rho(a)	32
RHO2	Yeast	192	rho(a)	30
YPT1-related				
rab1	Rat	205	Oligomers (57–63)[b]	32
rab2	Rat	212	Oligomers (57–63)[b]	30
rab3	Rat	220	Oligomers (57–63)[b]	29
rab4	Rat	213	Oligomers (57–63)[b]	29
smg25A	Bovine	220	Oligomers[c]	29
smg25B	Bovine	219	Oligomers[c]	30
smg25C	Bovine	227	Oligomers[c]	29
Hrab2	Human	212	Fortuitous	30
YPT1	Yeast	206	Fortuitous	34
SEC4	Yeast	215	Genetic analysis	29
BRL-ras	Rat	201	Fortuitous	28
R-ras				
	Human	218	v-H-ras	55
	Mouse	218	R-ras(human)	55
Dras-related				
rap1A/Krev-1	Human	184	Dras3, suppression	51
rap1B	Human	184	rap1A	51
rap2	Human	183	Dras3	43
Dras1	Drosophila	189	v-H-ras	75
Dras2	Drosophila	190	v-H-ras	56
Dras3	Drosophia	182	v-H-ras	48

[a] Degree of amino acid homology with human H-ras (see figure 1).
[b] Synthetic DNA oligonucleotides corresponding to H-ras amino acid residues 57–63.
[c] Synthetic DNA oligonucleotides corresponding to deduced amino acid sequences from purified proteins.

by the presence of seven extra amino acids at the amino terminus and the presence of a larger carboxyl-terminal region of the proteins [42,43].

Overall, the invertebrate ras proteins share significant amino acid sequence homology with the mammalian proteins, with greater than 80% homology to the highly conserved amino-terminal sequences of human ras (table 1). The homology is decreased significantly in the second, less conserved domain, with essentially no homology with the ras hypervariable domain. Finally, all invertebrate ras proteins possess the conserved carboxyl terminal Cys-A-A-X sequence.

ras-*related genes*

A number of eukaryotic genes encoding proteins that show limited sequence homology to the ras genes have now been identified (figure 1, table 1). This growing number of *ras*-related genes suggests that *ras* genes may represent just one branch of a larger *ras* superfamily.

A number of yeast and mammalian genes, designated *YPT1*- related, have now been isolated. The *YPT1* (originally designated *YP2*) gene was first found in an open reading frame between the actin and tubulin genes of the yeast *S. cerevisiae* [47]. Subsequently, synthetic oligonucleotide probes, corresponding to the well-conserved amino acid sequence of human *ras* residues 57–63, have been used to isolate four *YPT1*-related genes (*rab*1, 2, 3, and 4) from a rat-brain library [48]. These four genes, encoding 205–220 amino acid proteins that share from 37%–75% amino acid homology with *YPT1*, share approximately 30% homology with *ras* proteins [48,49]. The *rab*1 encoded protein shares 75% homology with *YPT1*, and is the mammalian homologue of this yeast gene. Furthermore, utilizing the yeast *YPT1* coding sequence as a probe, the mouse homologue of *rab*1 was isolated [50]. The mouse and rat *rab*1 genes, as well as an isolated human *rab*1 gene [48], encode identical proteins. *SEC4* represents another yeast protein that may be included in the *YPT1* family. The gene encodes a 23.5-kDa protein product that shares 47.5% homology with *YPT1* and 32% homology with *ras* proteins [51].

The *Aplysia rho* gene represents the second *ras*-related gene that was identified, and was isolated fortuitously in library screening using a human chorionogonadotropin DNA sequence probe [52]. The *rho* gene was first identified in the marine mollusc *Aplysia californica*, designated *rho*, for *ras*-homologous gene. At least two *rho* genes have also been identified in yeast (*RHO1* and *RHO2*) [53], and three in humans (*rho* A, B, and C) [52,54,55]. Similar to the *ras* genes, the *rho* proteins from yeast, molluscs, and humans share greater than 70% homology, indicating that this family of proteins is as well conserved in evolution as the *ras* proteins. Like the *ras* proteins, *rho* proteins are approximately 21 kDa (192–209 amino acids), and they share approximately 30% homology with the *ras* proteins.

Synthetic oligonucleotide probes corresponding to a sequence of seven amino acids strictly conserved in all *ras* proteins, and the two *ras*-related proteins, *YPT1* and *rho*, were used to search for additional members of the *ras* gene family [56]. From these studies, the *ral* gene was isolated from a simian B-lymphocyte cDNA library. The *ral* gene encodes a 206-amino-acid protein of expected molecular weight of 23.5 kDa that shares greater than 50% homology with the *ras* proteins.

The R-*ras* gene was isolated from human DNA by low-stringency hybridization with a viral H-*ras* probe, and a strongly homologous R-*ras* gene has also been isolated from mouse DNA [57]. The major difference between the 218-amino-acid R-*ras* encoded protein and *ras* proteins is an additional 26-amino-acid extension at the amino terminus of R-*ras*. Overall, R-*ras* displays 55% homology with the H-*ras* protein. R-*ras* has been mapped to human chromosome 19.

Utilizing the *Drosophila Dras3* gene as a probe for low-stringency screening of a human cDNA library, two additional *ras*-related genes have been isolated and sequenced [58]. Designated *rap*1A and *rap*2, these homologs of the *Drosophila* gene encode 183–184-amino-acid proteins that are approximately 50% homologous to the human *ras* proteins. A third human member, *rap*1B, was subsequently isolated using the human *rap*1A as a probe [58,59]. The proteins encoded by *rap*1A and 1B share 95% homology. Employing a biological selection procedure for human genes that possess *ras*-suppressing activity, the *rap*1A gene was independently identified by Noda and coworkers [60,61]. Designated Krev-1, the predicted coding sequence of this gene was found to be identical to the bovine *rap*1A encoded protein. Similarly to the *ras* genes, the Krev-1/*rap*1A gene is also well conserved evolutionarily.

Overall, analysis of the *ras*-related genes reveals an evolutionary conservation similar to that observed between *ras* genes. Thus, these *ras*-related genes are also likely to represent genes important in normal cell physiology.

Mechanisms of activation

Nucleotide sequence comparisons of activated *ras* genes with their normal counterparts have identified *ras* activation to be a consequence of single point mutations in the coding sequences (table 2). Activated *ras* genes isolated from tumors are most commonly activated by substitutions at positions 12 [62–64] or 61 [65], and less frequently by mutations at position 13 [66]. In vitro mutagenesis studies have determined that substitutions at positions 59, 63, 116, 117, and 119 will also activate H-*ras* transforming potential [67–70].

Further analysis of the nature of substitutions sufficient for activation has demonstrated that 18 of the possible 19 substitutions for the glycine at position 12 will activate H-*ras* [71]. This suggests that glycine may confer a crucial conformation of the normal *ras* protein that is disrupted by any substitution, except proline. Consistent with this possibility are the observations that the deletion of the glycine-12 or the insertion of additional amino acids (two or four) between amino acid positions 11 and 12 will also enhance H-*ras* transforming potential [72]. A similar analysis at position 61 demonstrated that the substitution of the normal glutamine with 15 different amino acids activated H-*ras* transforming potencies [73]. Only a proline or glutamic acid substitution resulted in *ras* proteins with no enhanced transforming ability. The diverse variety of lesions that will activate *ras* transforming activity suggests that these activating lesions may be disrupting a property of the normal *ras* protein. Alternatively, these activating lesions may induce a disruption of the conformation of the *ras* protein, resulting in the constitutive expression of an otherwise regulated activity of the normal protein.

In addition to structural mutations that activate *ras* transforming activity, experimental overexpression of normal *ras* protein has also been shown to fully transform NIH 3T3 mouse fibroblasts. Either the expression of cellular *ras* from a strong viral promoter [74], or the transfection of greater than 30 copies per cell [272], is sufficient to induce malignant transformation of NIH

Table 2. Amino acid substitutions that activate human ras proteins

Position	12	13	59	61	63	116	117	119
Sequence	Gly	Gly	Ala	Gln	Glu	Asn	Lys	Asp
In vivo	Val Arg Asp Cys Ala Ser Phe	Asp Val Arg		Arg His Leu Lys				
In vitro	Ala Asn Gln Glu His Ile Leu Lys Met Phe Ser Thr Trp Tyr	Ser	Thr	Val Ala Cys Asn Ile Met Thr Tyr Trp Phe Gly	Lys	His Ile	Glu Arg	His Glu Ala Asn

Table 3. Oncogenic murine retroviruses containing ras oncogenes

Virus	Pathology	Gene	Origin
Harvey-MSV	Sarcomas, erythroleukemia	H-ras	Rat
Kirsten-MSV	Sarcomas, erythroleukemia	K-ras	Rat
Rasheed-MSV	Sarcomas	H-ras	Rat
BALB-MSV	Sarcomas, erythroleukemia	H-ras	Mouse
AF-1	Sarcomas, malignant histiocytosis	H-ras	Mouse
NC.C58 MSV-1	Sarcomas, erythroleukemia	H-ras	Mouse
NC.C58 MSV-2	Sarcomas, erythroleukemia	H-ras	Mouse

3T3 cells. Microinjection of high levels of normal H-*ras* protein into NIH 3T3 cells will also induce morphologic transformation [76]. However, there appears to be a qualitative difference between the normal and activated *ras* proteins, since overexpression of the normal gene appears not to be completely sufficient to fully transform Rat-1 fibroblasts [80]. The level of expression of an oncogenic *ras* protein is also important and can further potentiate transforming activity [73,77–80].

Biochemical properties of *ras* proteins

The cellular *ras* proteins bind guanine nucleotides (GTP and GDP) with high affinity, possess a low intrinsic GTPase activity, interact with a GTPase activating protein (GAP), and are localized to the inner surface of the plasma membrane. Amino acid sequence comparisons have identified significant, but limited, homologies between the *ras* proteins and other guanine nucleotide-binding proteins, including elongation factors of protein synthesis (EF-Tu and EF-G) and members of the signal-transducing G protein family (figure 2). Since *ras* proteins share both structural and functional characteristics with these regulatory G proteins, it has been proposed that *ras* biological activity may be similarly regulated by guanine nucleotide binding and may function in signal transduction [81–83].

The G proteins are a family of GTP-binding regulatory proteins that serve as intermediaries in transmembrane signaling pathways to transmit signals generated by ligand interactions with specific cell surface receptors into changes in cellular metabolism [84]. Located on the cytoplasmic side of plasma membranes, each G protein is a heterodimer that consists of three different subunits, α (39–52 kDa), β (35–36 kDa), and γ (8–10 kDa). The α subunits, which bind and hydrolyze guainine nucleotides, are distinct for each G protein family member. Common β and γ subunits are probably shared among some α subunits to form the specific oligomers.

G protein function is regulated cyclically by guanine nucleotide association. The association of GTP with the α subunit activates the G protein, with the subsequent regulation of the activity of its appropriate effector. The hydrolysis of GTP to GDP and P_i cycles the protein to its inactive state. One such example is the hormone-regulated adenylate cyclase system, which has been studied in great detail. Two G proteins, G_s and G_i, stimulate and inhibit, respectively, adenylate cyclase activity. The breakdown of phosphatidylinositol by phospholipase C is controlled by the putative G protein, G_p. Other guanine nucleotide-binding proteins that are considered members of the same gene family include transducin, which stimulates a retinal cyclic GMP phosphodiesterase, and G_o, a GTP-binding protein of brain with a still unknown function [85].

In this section, the experimental studies addressing the biochemical properties of the *ras* proteins will be summarized, and discussed with regard to the present model for *ras* function based on their similarity to the G proteins [85–88].

Functional domains

Extensive studies utilizing site-specific antibodies and the generation of *ras* structural mutants have defined specific regions of the *ras* protein important for both *ras* biochemistry and biology. A general profile of the functional domains of the *ras* proteins is shown in figure 3, and experimental data are described below.

GTPase activity and the GTPase activating protein (GAP). Since structural mutations are responsible for the activation of *ras* transforming activity, an

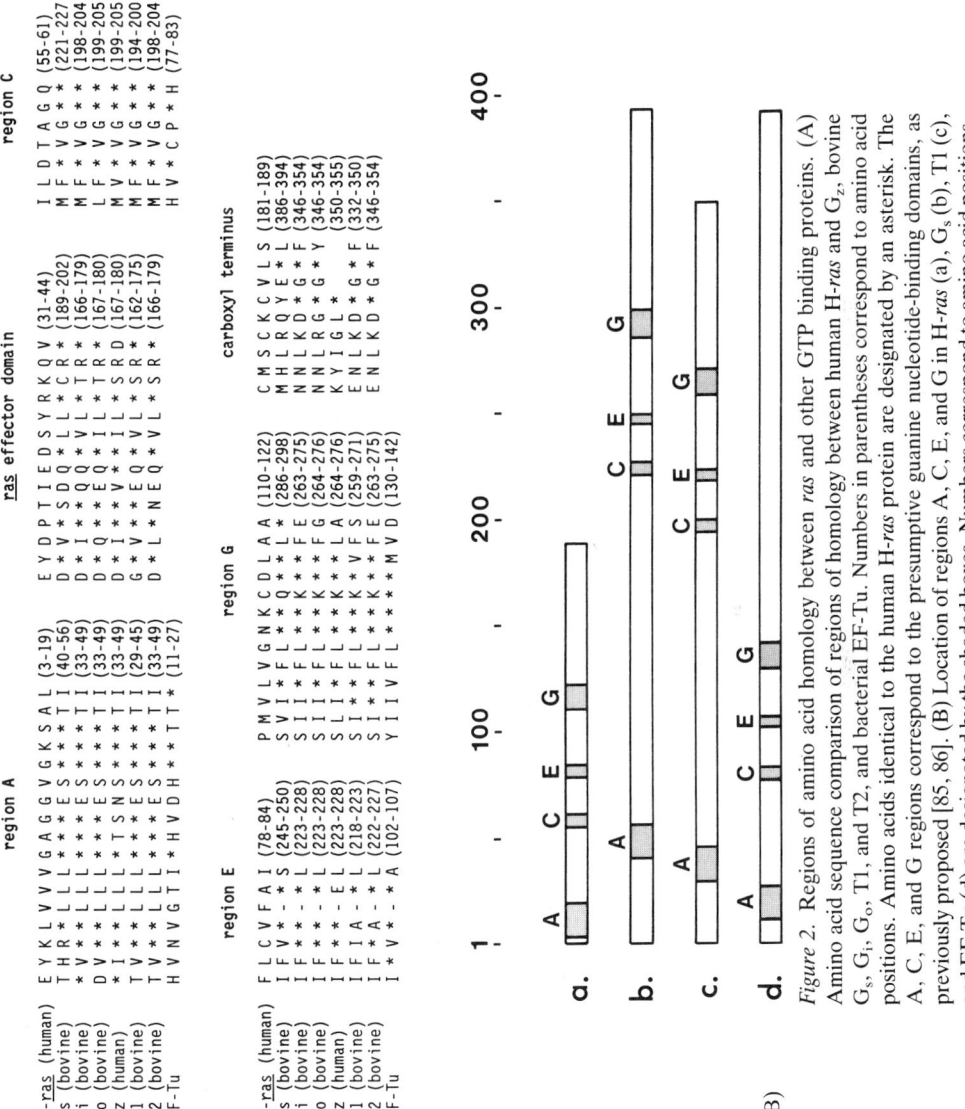

Figure 2. Regions of amino acid homology between *ras* and other GTP binding proteins. (A) Amino acid sequence comparison of regions of homology between human H-*ras* and G_z, bovine G_s, G_i, G_o, T1, and T2, and bacterial EF-Tu. Numbers in parentheses correspond to amino acid positions. Amino acids identical to the human H-*ras* protein are designated by an asterisk. The A, C, E, and G regions correspond to the presumptive guanine nucleotide-binding domains, as previously proposed [85, 86]. (B) Location of regions A, C, E, and G in H-*ras* (a), G_s (b), T1 (c), and EF-Tu (d) are designated by the shaded boxes. Numbers correspond to amino acid positions.

important goal has been to elucidate the functional alterations due to these activating lesions. Biochemical comparisons of the normal *ras* proteins with their activated counterparts have demonstrated that lesions at 12 or 61 do not alter the subcellular localization, posttranslational modification, or in vitro guanine nucleotide-binding affinities and specificities of *ras* proteins [89]. Subsequent to these studies, investigations in several laboratories determined that activating substitutions at positions 12 or 61 significantly reduced the rate of GTP hydrolysis catalyzed by these activated proteins [73,90–94]. By analogy to the G proteins, these observations have led to the speculation that the mechanism of mutational activation of *ras* genes is inhibition of GTP hydrolysis, thereby inhibiting the physiological deactivation of *ras* proteins (figure 3).

Although a reduced in vitro GTPase activity is typically associated with activating lesions in *ras*, exceptions to this correlation have been observed [73,95,96]. In one study, site-directed mutagenesis was employed to introduce mutations encoding 17 different amino acids at codon 61 of the human H-*ras* protein [73]. Fifteen of these substitutions increased H-*ras* transforming activity; two mutants, encoding proline and glutamic acid, displayed transforming activities similar to the normal gene. Overall, these mutants vary over 1000-fold in transforming potency. However, all 17 different mutant proteins displayed equivalently reduced rates of GTP hydrolysis, 8- to 10-fold lower than the normal protein. There was no quantitative correlation between reduction in GTPase activity and transformation, indicating that reduced GTP hydrolysis is not sufficient to activate *ras* transforming potential. In a study by Trahey et al., two fully transforming N-*ras* mutant proteins still retained 12%–43% of wild-type GTPase activity [95]. Finally, substitution of a threonine for the alanine normally present at position 59 results in full transforming activity, without a corresponding reduction in GTPase activity [96]. Altogether, these results suggest that additional

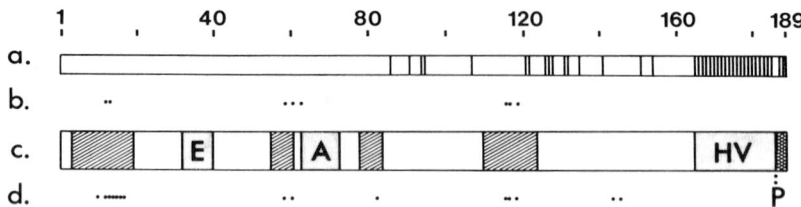

Figure 3. Functional domains of human *ras* proteins. (a) Amino acid conservation among human H-, K-, and N-*ras* proteins; variable amino acid residues are designated by the black lines. Numbers correspond to amino acid positions, (b) Amino acid residues where substitutions activate *ras* transforming potential, (c) Location of domains A, C, E, and G conserved among GTP-binding proteins (hatched boxes), the effector domain (E), the antibody neutralizing domain (A), the hypervariable domain (HV), and the membrane-binding domain (cross-hatched box). The palmitic acid (P) is believed to be covalently attached to the cysteine at position 186, (d) Amino acid residues where substitutions alter *ras* guanine nucleotide binding and hydrolysis activities.

biochemical alterations responsible for *ras* transforming activity remain to be identified.

The observed discrepancies between *ras* transforming activity and intrinsic GTPase activity have been partially reconciled with the identification of a cytoplasmic GTPase activating protein (GAP) that stimulates the GTPase activities of normal H-*ras* and N-*ras* proteins (>100-fold) but does not affect their activated counterparts [97]. The net result would be to favor the GDP-bound form of the normal protein, while the oncogenic forms would persist in the active, GTP-bound form of the protein.

GAP is a monomeric polypeptide with an apparent molecular weight of 125,000-daltons, and lacks an intrinsic GTPase activity [98,99]. A second form of the protein, encoding a predicted 116,000-dalton protein, appears to be generated by a differential splicing mechanism [135]. GAP appears to be widely expressed in cells of higher eukaryotes, including human, bovine, hamster, rat, mouse, frog, and insect cells (*Spodoptera fragipedra*) [97,98,100]. Interestingly, no GAP activity was detected in either of two yeast strains, *S. cerevisiae* or *S. pombe*. GAP activity is present in both normal and transformed cells. GAP activity is detectable in most tissues, with the highest concentrations in testes and brain [100]. The levels of GAP activity in BALB/c 3T3 mouse fibroblasts was proportional to cell density, with lower levels in actively growing cells than in density-arrested cells, suggesting that GAP is involved in the regulation of cell proliferation [101].

The predicted amino acid sequences of both bovine [98] and human [135] GAP possess several regions of interesting homology with other known proteins. First, there is a low degree of homology between the entire GAP sequence and residues in the noncatalytic domain of adenylate cyclase. Second, there are two regions with strong homology between the N-terminus of GAP and the SH2 region conserved among the nonreceptor tyrosine kinases (designated B and C), such as *crk*, and the phospholipase C-148. The possible regulatory role of the SH2 domain suggests that GAP, the nonreceptor tyrosine kinases, and PLC-148 may share some common regulatory mechanism [281].

In competition assays using purified GAP, GAP interacts preferentially with the active GTP complexes of both normal and oncogenic H-*ras* proteins compared with the inactive GDP-*ras* complexes [98]. Consequently, the ability of GAP to interact with oncogenic forms of *ras* suggests that the lack of GTPase stimulation is due to the lack of intrinsic *ras* GTPase activity. Finally, since GAP displays a stronger association with the GTP-bound form, the absence of GTPase stimulation of oncogenic *ras* would result in a constitutive association between GAP and *ras*. The association of GAP with the normal protein would be expected to be transient, and regulated by the nucleotide state of the protein.

At present, it is not known whether GAP acts upstream or downstream of *ras*. If GAP operates upstream of *ras*, it would function as a negative regulator of *ras* activity by catalyzing the cycling of the protein from the active

GTP-bound form, to the inactive GDP-bound form. If GAP operates in a downstream fashion, then GAP would be the target of the active GTP-bound *ras* complex. The interaction of GAP with the normal protein would be transient whereas, in the absence of any inducible GTPase activity, the association with oncogenic proteins would be prolonged. In the downstream scheme, GAP would function in a manner analogous to the bacterial elongation factor, EF-Tu. The interaction of EF-Tu with its target molecule, the ribosome, also stimulates its GTPase activity [145,152].

Evidence that GAP may serve as the downstream effector target for *ras* function was derived from experiments characterizing the ability of GAP to stimulate structural mutants of normal *ras*. Single amino acid substitutions in the *ras* effector domain that abolish transforming activity were also observed to prevent GAP stimulation [99,103]. In contrast, a substitution at position 39 that did not impair transforming activity also did not prevent GAP stimulation, suggesting a good relationship between GAP interaction and *ras* transforming activity.

Guanine nucleotide binding. Amino acid sequence comparisons between *ras* proteins, bacterial elongation factors, and other guanine nucleotide-binding proteins have identified four principal domains of homology [85–88]. These regions correspond to human *ras* residues 3–19 (region A), 56–61 (region C), 78–84 (region E), and 110–122 (region G). These regions of homology are collinear among the different GTP-binding proteins (figure 2 and 3). Because of the diverse functions of these proteins, these short stretches of homology are likely to correspond to domains involved in the binding and hydrolysis of GTP. The importance of these regions in guanine nucleotide interactions have now been established by both site-directed modification of specific residues in these four domains and by functional assays employing in vitro random mutagenesis approaches. As described above, mutations at residues 12 or 61 alter the intrinsic GTPase activities [73, 90–94]. Single amino acid substitutions in regions A (residues 10, 13–17), C (residue 59), and E (residues 116, 117, 119), as well as others (residues 83, 144, and 146) alter the GDP and/or GTP binding affinities [68–70, 104–106, 269]. The decreased equilibrium binding affinities are typically a consequence of an increased dissociation rate for the bound nucleotide, resulting in an increased rate of nucleotide exchange [70,96,106,107,270]. Thus, both regions A and C influence the binding and hydrolysis of GTP. Substitutions in residues 116–119 (region E), corresponding to the consensus NKXD guanine nucleotide-binding sequence present in all GTP-binding proteins, do not affect hydrolysis, but result in both reduced binding affinities and enhanced exchange rates. Although the domain including *ras* residues 144 and 146 is not significantly homologous to other GTP-binding proteins, this domain is believed to be involved in the formation of the nucleotide-binding pocket [108,109].

The importance of GTP binding for *ras* biological activity has been evaluated by several approaches that have resulted in conflicting conclusions.

Initial studies with anti-*ras* antibodies suggested that GTP binding is necessary for *ras* transforming activity. A monoclonal antibody (designated anti-p21ser) that was directed against epitopes located within the amino terminal region around *ras* residue 12 inhibited GTP/GDP binding by purified *ras* proteins [110]. Conversely, the ability of these antibodies to bind to *ras* proteins was inhibited by preincubation with GTP or GDP. These results, together with the observation that microinjection of this antibody into *ras*-transformed cells causes a transient reversion to the normal phenotype, suggested that guanine nucleotide binding is essential for the transforming function of *ras* [111]. Similarly, studies utilizing the Y13-259 monoclonal antibody [20], which recognizes the *ras* region corresponding to amino acids between 63–73, also demonstrated blocking of GTP binding [112], and microinjection of this antibody was capable of blocking *ras* activity [113,114]. However, a second study utilizing the same monoclonal antibody did not observe any inhibition of GTP-binding activity of *ras* protein [115]. The importance for GTP binding in *ras* biological activity was further suggested by the construction of deletion mutants of viral H-*ras* that lacked both guanine nucleotide-binding and transforming activities [116,117].

In contrast to the antibody studies, several structure–function studies have demonstrated that single amino acid substitutions that result in significant reductions in equilibrium GTP-binding afinities do not compromise H-*ras* focus-forming activities [68,69,104]. In one study, a series of H-*ras* mutants was generated containing amino acid substitutions in a guanine nucleotide-binding consensus sequence, NKXD [85,87,88], which is present in all *ras* proteins and other guanine nucleotide-binding proteins. Overall, significant reductions in GTP-binding affinities (from 10- to 10,000-fold) did not affect the ability of oncogenic H-*ras* to transform rodent fibroblast or epithelial cells [70]. Thus, it appears that the high affinity binding of guanine nucleotides is not essential for *ras* transforming activity, but is presumably still important for the normal function of *ras*. Furthermore, the retention of transforming activity by two *ras* mutants that do not display any detectable GTP binding suggests that the active conformation of the protein can be achieved without any guanine nucleotide association [70,105].

The observation that single amino acid substitutions at positions 116, 117, or 119 in the normal H-*ras* protein activated the transforming activity of an otherwise normal *ras* protein has suggested an alternate mechanisms for *ras* activation [68–70]. In contrast to the activating mutations at positions 12 or 61, which reduce intrinsic *ras* GTPase activity, this alternate mechanism is proposed to be a consequence of the increased exchange rate for bound nucleotide. Since intracellular levels of guanine nucleotides are in the millimolar range [118] and the concentration of GTP is believed to be 20-fold higher than GDP levels (119), an increased exchange rate would favor the formation of the active, GTP-bound form of the protein (figure 3).

Although *ras* proteins activated by mutations in the consensus guanine nucleotide sequence Asn-Lys-X-Asp (NKXD) display efficient focus-forming activity on NIH 3T3 cells, only *ras* proteins activated by mutations at positions 12, 13, or 61 have been observed in tumors. Consequently, the importance of such activating lesions for in vivo *ras* carcinogenesis is unclear. However, in a study assessing a variety of in vitro biological parameters, it was demonstrated that normal H-*ras* proteins activated by altered nucleotide exchange are biologically similar to H-*ras* proteins activated by lesions affecting GTPase activity. These results implicate a role for this alternate mechanism of activation in *ras* carcinogenesis, and demonstrate the important involvement of the NKXD sequence in regulating the biological activity of *ras* proteins. The recent identification of H-*ras* activation in chemically induced mouse hepatomas by mutations at position 117 provides further support for this possibility [120].

Fatty acid acylation and membrane association. Immunofluorescence and electron microscopic immunocytochemistry studies by Willingham et al. [121] have localized *ras* p21 to the inner surface of the plasma membrane. Analysis of MDCK dog cells transformed by viral H-*ras* demonstrated that p21 was confined to the interdigitating microvillus structures and almost absent from desmosomes or gap junctions. Very little p21 was detected in the cytosol, and none was observed in the nucleus, suggesting that the site of *ras* action is at the plasma membrane.

In contrast to the classical localization of membrane-associated proteins, the *ras* proteins do not contain signal sequences and are first synthesized in free cytosolic polysomes as a precursor, pre-p21, with an apparent molecular weight of 23-kDa [122]. After approximately 20 minutes, the *ras* proteins become associated with the plasma membrane, with this mature form exhibiting a faster mobility on SDS polyacrylamide gels. Associated with the transport to the membrane, the *ras* protein becomes palmitylated by the covalent addition via an ester linkage to the SH group of a cysteine residue located at the carboxyl terminus [123–126]. Palmitylation is believed to be partly responsible for the processing to the mature form, since removal of the palmitate from the mature protein does not restore p21 to the precursor size [126]. However, there is evidence from the processing of yeast *RAS* proteins for an intermediate, soluble, nonpalmitylated form of the protein [127]. Consequently, additional posttranslational modifications of *ras* are believed to occur also.

Recently, Clarke et al. [276] have demonstrated the carboxyl methylation of H-*ras* in transformed rat embryo fibroblasts. This methylation also appears to be at the carboxyl terminus of the H-*ras* protein. The additional demonstration of a guanine-nucleotide-dependent carboxyl methylation of 20–23-kDa membrane-associated proteins suggests that this modification may be a general property of *ras* and *ras*-related proteins [129]. Finally, the ability of GTP and nonhydrolyzable GTP analogs, but not GDP, to stimulate this methylation suggests a possible regulatory role for this physiologically reversible modification.

Analysis of the kinetics of *ras* processing in both mammalian and yeast cells have suggested a third possible posttranslational modification step in *ras* development. Recently, Tamanoi et al. [127] have shown that two precursors are involved in the processing of yeast *RAS* proteins. Similarly, a soluble intermediate processed form has also been indicated in mammalian cells [123,126,128]. On the basis of homologies with other acylated proteins such as the fungal mating factors, it has been suggested that acylation may be preceded by removal of the last three amino acids, thus placing the H-*ras* 186-Cys at the carboxyl terminus [127].

The posttranslational addition of palmitate is believed to occur at a cysteine residue near the carboxyl terminus (Cys-186). Mutants of activated *ras* lacking the 186-Cys residue are not palmitylated, are not processed to the faster-migrating mature form, remain in the cytosol, and are unable to induce morphologic transformation of NIH 3T3 cells [124,130]. Consequently, the addition of palmitate appears to be essential for membrane association and transforming activity. Consistent with the role of palmitate for membrane association, it has been shown that complete removal of the palmitate by mild hydroxylamine treatment can release N-*ras* protein from membranes, although removal from the membrane was not quantitative [128]. This observation is consistent with the possibility that modifications other than acylation may also contribute to *ras* membrane interactions.

Further characterization of the dynamics of *ras* protein palmitylation suggest that this lipid modification may also play a regulatory role in *ras* activity [128]. Magee et al. demonstrated that the N-*ras* protein can be acylated hours after synthesis, and that turnover of the palmitate moiety (t1/2 of approximately 20 minutes) is very rapid compared with the lifetime of the protein (t1/2 of approximately 24 hours). Thus, the acylation–deacylation cycling of *ras* may function in modulating the association of *ras* with the membrane in a signal transduction function.

While palmitylation is essential for *ras* function, the specific role of this fatty acid is unclear. A more precise requirement for palmitylation of *ras* has been addressed in studies utilizing a second type of fatty acid acylation [131]. In the case of the *src* oncogene protein, the covalent modification by the addition of a myristic acid appears to serve an analogous function for *src* as palmitic acid does for *ras*. Nonmyristylated variants of viral *src* are defective in both membrane association and transformation [131,277]. Two recent studies have constructed chimeric genes encoding nonpalmitylated *ras* proteins that contain myristic acid at their amino termini, to determine if a different form of lipid modification could restore either membrane association or transforming activity [102,132]. Myristylated, nonpalmitylated forms of oncogenic H-*ras* proteins exhibited both efficient membrane association and full transforming activity. These results demonstrate that membrane association is essential for transformation, but does not specifically require palmitate, since myristate can substitute for this fatty acid. Surprisingly, myristylated forms of normal H-*ras* were also able to transform NIH 3T3 cells

[132]. Since the normal function of *ras* is altered by myristate, palmitate must provide the protein with unique properties that cannot be replaced by myristate. The activation of normal *ras* by myristate may be a consequence of the localization of *ras* to an inappropriate membrane target with which cellular *ras* does not usually associate. Alternatively, since the myristate is a permanent addition to the protein, whereas palmitate is transient, the normal regulatable association of *ras* with the membrane may now be altered.

Putative effector domain. Structure–function studies aimed at defining the *ras* domains essential for function have identified regions that are dispensable and regions that are indispensable for transformation. Of particular interest has been the demonstration that single amino acid substitutions or small deletions in oncogenic *ras* residues 32–40 result in the loss of *ras* transforming activity [133,134]. Additionally, since these substitutions eliminate *ras* biological activity, but do not disrupt *ras* membrane association, guanine nucleotide binding, or intrinsic GTPase activity, this region of *ras* has been proposed to interact with the effector targets of *ras* proteins. Thus, it has been suggested that mutations in this region block *ras* function by preventing its interaction with the putative downstream target(s) for *ras* activity.

The recently identified GAP protein may represent a possible effector target for *ras*. Effector mutations that block *ras* transforming activity also result in the blockage of stimulation by GAP [99,103]. However, it is not clear whether mutations in amino acids 35–40 block GAP activity directly, or indirectly through conformational changes elsewhere in the *ras* protein. Alternatively, substitutions here may be directly blocking GAP stimulation, while indirectly preventing interaction of *ras* with its target substrates. Thus, it remains to be determined whether GAP represents an upstream negative regulator of *ras* function, or is a downstream target for *ras* activity.

Recently, a detailed analysis of the *ras* effector domain was carried out by Stone et al. [134]. A variety of single amino acid substitutions at positions 32–40 were introduced into v-H-*ras*, and were characterized for focus-forming activity on NIH 3T3 cells. These studies identified three classes of codons within this region. Some residues could not be altered, even conservatively, without the loss of transforming function (codons 32 and 35). A second class was residues that retained detectable transforming activity with conservative changes, but lost function with more drastic substitutions (codons 36 and 40). The third group included residues that retained function even with a nonconservative substitution (codon 39). The analysis of GAP stimulation of this series of effector mutants will provide a good assessment of the relationship between this domain and GAP in *ras* function [274].

Neutralizing domain. The rat monoclonal antibody, designated Y13-259 [20], has been a very useful reagent for characterizing *ras* biological activity. Originally generated against the viral H-*ras* p21 protein, the ability of this antibody to recognize each of the three mammalian *ras* proteins [136], as well as the proteins encoded by the yeast *RAS1* and *RAS2* [43,137], *Dictyostelium* Dd-*ras* [138] and *Aplysia* Apl-*ras* [46] genes, suggests that this antibody must bind to a highly conserved domain shared among *ras* proteins. A number of microinjection studies have demonstrated the neutralizing activity of this antibody on *ras* biological activity. Kung et al. [114] demonstrated that the microinjection of Y13-259 reverses the transformed phenotype of *ras*-transformed NIH 3T3 cells. Furthermore, microinjection of this antibody into untransformed NIH cells specifically blocks the serum-induced mitogenic response, suggesting that normal *ras* proteins may function in this capacity in normal cells [113]. Y13-259 also blocks the stimulatory effect of yeast *RAS* on the in vitro yeast adenylate cyclase activity [133].

The Y13-259 antibody recognition sequence has been mapped to *ras* amino acid residues 63–73. Termed the neutralizing domain, the exact importance of this region for *ras* activity is unclear. The observation that single amino acid substitutions in this region that block Y13-259 binding (corresponding to *ras* residues 63-Glu, 65-Ser, 66-Ala, 67-Met, 70-Gln, and 73-Arg) do not abolish *ras* transforming activity suggests that this neutralization is indirect and results either from distortion of the protein or from steric factors [133]. One possible explanation for the neutralizing effect of this antibody is the observation that, while Y13-259 does not block nucleotide binding, it apparently severely hampers nucleotide exchange between bound and exogenous nucleotide [115,139]. This activity may block the reactivation of *ras* by preventing the exchange of GTP for GDP.

Recently, the Y13-259 monoclonal antibody has been shown to block the ability of GAP to stimulate either H-*ras* or N-*ras* GTPase activity [97,103]. However, another monoclonal antibody (Y12-238) [20], which has no neutralizing activity [114], was also capable of blocking GAP stimulation [103]. Consequently, it is likely that this GAP blocking activity may not be the basis for the neutralizing activity of Y13-259.

Dispensable domains for transformation. Amino acid comparisons of the three *ras* proteins have defined four principal *ras* domains. While three of these domains are well conserved among the *ras* proteins, the regions corresponding to the 20 amino acids between residues 165 and 185 are very divergent from each other, and hence, likely to be dispensable for transforming activity. The observation that deletions in this domain of viral H-*ras* do not compromise transforming activity supports this possibility [116].

In addition to the dispensable nature of the hypervariable region, insertion –deletion mutagenesis of the v-H-*ras* protein reveals at least three additional *ras* domains dispensable for transformation [116]. In these studies, dispensable domains corresponding to *ras* residues 64–76, 93–108, and 120–138 were defined. These three regions are within the first 160 amino acids of the *ras* proteins, and are highly conserved among the *ras* proteins from humans to yeast. Among the three human *ras* proteins, 44 to 48 amino acids in these three segments are identical or have conservative changes, while 28 are identical or conserved between yeast and human *ras* proteins. Thus, although these regions represent well-conserved *ras* sequences, they are apparently dispensable for the oncogenic properties of *ras*.

A final region that appears to be dispensable for *ras* transforming activity is the amino-terminus sequence. The observations that the N-terminus of *ras* may be extended an additional length of 4 to 59 amino acids at the N-terminus [140–143], that residues in this region are variable among the different *ras* proteins (figure 1), and that the first four amino acids can be altered without affecting transforming activity [141,142,144] suggest that the transforming function of *ras* is not compromised by variations at the N-terminus. However, substitution of v-H-*ras* residues 2, 3, and 4 did result in a 10-fold reduction in transforming activity, suggesting that this region is not completely dispensable for transforming activity (J. Buss and C. Der, unpublished observations).

The significance of these dispensable domains for *ras* activity remains to be determined. While dispensable for *ras* transforming activity, these domains may still encode *ras* functions essential for the normal functions of *ras*.

ras *conformation*

An important component in understanding the biochemical and biological activities of normal and oncogenic *ras* proteins will be the determination of the three-dimensional structure of the protein. Towards this goal, Kim and co-workers [109] have recently determined the three-dimensional structure of the normal H-*ras* protein (figure 4). Utilizing bacterially expressed H-*ras* protein, the crystal structure of the catalytic domain of normal H-*ras* protein complexed with GDP was determined. While lacking the flexible carboxyl-terminal 18 residues, this *ras* protein still retained the GTP binding and hydrolytic activities of the full-length protein. The protein consists of a six-stranded β sheet, four α helices, and nine connecting loops. The loops are generally exposed at the outer boundaries of the protein, and are designed L1–L9, beginning from the N-terminus.

Four loops are involved in interactions with bound guanosine diphosphate: one with the phosphates (L1), another with the ribose (L2), and two with the guanine base (L7 and L9). Most of the transforming proteins have single amino acid substitutions at one of a few key positions in three of these four loops plus one additional loop. The activating mutations at residues 12 and 13 are localized within loop L1 near the phosphates. Consequently, substitutions in this region may directly affect the binding and hydrolysis of GTP. Activating substitutions at positions 59, 61, and 63 are localized within loop L4, which is not in contact with the phosphate groups of GDP but is in direct contact with loop L1. Consequently, mutations in this region may activate *ras* through indirect conformational changes in loop L1 via reduced GTPase activities [73,107]. Activating mutations at residues 116, 117, and 119 [68–70] are localized in loop L7. Consistent with the formation of the nucleotide

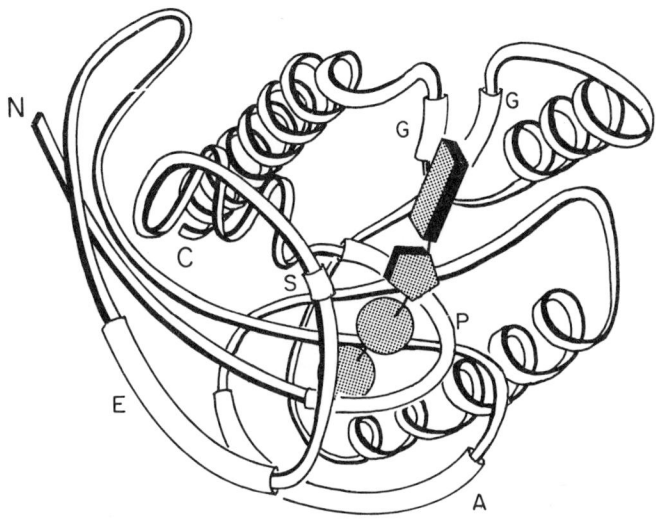

Figure 4. Conformation of the human H-*ras* protein catalytic domain. The backbone structure of human normal H-*ras* protein looking into the GDP-binding pocket. The regions that bind guanine base (G), ribose sugar (S), phosphates (P), and antibody neutralizing (A) and effector (E) regions are indicated by sleeved tubes. This figure is reprinted from [109] with permission.

binding pocket by loops L1, L2, L7, and L9, mutations in loops L1, L7, and L9 reduce the equilibrium binding affinities for GTP (residues 100,102,145, 147 and 148), while mutations in loop L1 also influence GTP hydrolysis rates [90–94].

The biological functions of the remaining five loops and the other exposed regions are at present unknown. However, residues corresponding to the binding site for a neutralizing monoclonal antibody are also located on L4. Thus, the neutralizing effect of antibody binding may result from indirect conformational changes on L1. Another loop (L2) corresponds to the putative effector domain. The region of L2 corresponding to the effector domain is not in direct contact with the GTP binding pocket, and is located in a very well-exposed portion of the protein. The remaining loops may be important for *ras* interaction with membrane receptors, or downstream target molecules.

Prior to the determination of the *ras* crystal structure, *ras* three-dimensional models were proposed based on the crystal structure of another GTP binding protein, the bacterial elongation factor EF-Tu [108,145]. Overall, the *ras* model based on the structure for EF-Tu is very similar to the determined structure, although some differences are observed. Further refinement of both the *ras* and EF-Tu crystal structures will be important to understand the regulation of protein conformation by guanine nucleotides of these two proteins, as well as that of other regulatory GTP binding proteins [85,146].

Together with the structure–function studies of *ras* proteins, the knowledge of the crystal structure will be helpful in defining the functional domains of *ras*, as well as defining additional domains that interact with membrane receptor(s) as well as with *ras* target molecules. Of importance will be the determination of the differences of the full-length versions of the normal and activated forms of *ras*. Additionally, a comparison of the structure of the *ras* proteins in the GTP versus the GDP form will help to decipher the conformation of the active form of the protein. Preliminary characterization of the crystal structures of two oncogenic H-*ras* proteins (12-Val and 61-Leu) reveals little difference from the normal protein, suggesting that the conformational states of the protein may be limited to subtle modifications influencing the guanine nucleotide-binding pocket [109].

Model for ras *function*

Since *ras* proteins share both structural and functional properties with the regulatory G proteins, the present model for *ras* function is based on an analogy to these proteins (figure 5). The *ras* proteins are believed to function as biological switches, serving as intermediaries between membrane receptors and downstream effector targets. The *ras* protein activities are dictated by guanine nucleotides, to modulate extracellular signals to an intracellular effector pathway. A simplified diagram of the present model for *ras* function is shown in figure 5. In this model, *ras* is proposed to exist in an equilibrium between an active, GTP-bound state, and an inactive, GDP-bound state. The normal *ras* protein is believed to exist predominantly in the inactive, GDP-bound form. Only when the appropriate upstream signal, via a presumed

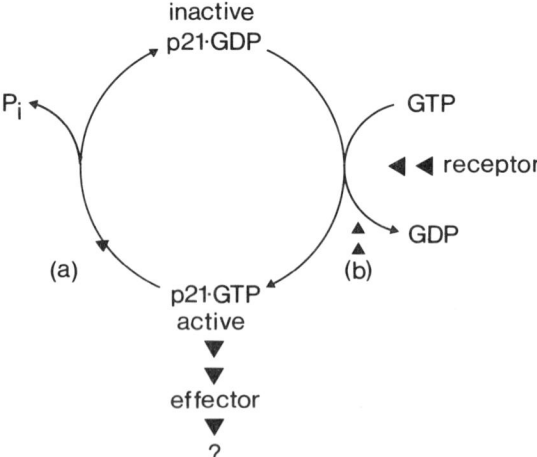

Figure 5. Model for *ras* function. Mutations that activate *ras* transforming activity shift the equilibrium to favor formation of the active, GTP-p21 conformation by either (a) reduced GTPase/GAP activities or (b) enhanced nucleotide exchange rates.

growth-related receptor, stimulates the exchange of GTP for GDP does the *ras* protein enter into the active GTP-bound conformation. While in the active state, *ras* stimulates the transduction of signals to a downstream effector target. Since normal *ras* protein possesses an intrinsic GTPase activity that is stimulatable by cytoplasmic GAP, hydrolysis of bound GTP would result in cycling the *ras* protein back to the inactive, GDP-bound state.

The biochemical basis of *ras* activation is consistent with this model. The observed oncogenic lesions in *ras* typically occur at either positions 12 or 61, resulting in a deficient GTPase activity that is not stimulated by GAP. In this model, the net result of this lesion is the maintenance of the protein in the active, GTP-bound conformation, resulting in a continuous transduction of stimulatory signal to the downstream effector target. An enhanced off-rate for bound guanine nucleotides (via mutations in the NKXD sequence), coupled with a presumed 10- to 20-fold higher intracellular level of GTP versus GDP [119], should result in favoring the active GTP-bound form of the protein. Thus, both altered GTPase activities and altered nucleotide binding can activate *ras* transforming activity presumably by shifting the equilibrium to now favor the active, GTP-bound conformation.

Experimental studies have provided data supporting this model. In vivo nucleotide association analysis has demonstrated that the normal *ras* proteins exist predominantly in the GDP-bound state, while their oncogenic counterparts are associated predominantly with GTP. For example, normal N-*ras* protein microinjected into *Xenopus* oocytes was associated predominantly with GDP, while activated N-*ras* proteins were associated with GTP [97]. Both yeast *RAS1* and *RAS2* proteins were found to be bound entirely to GDP in exponentially growing *S. cerevisiae* cells [147]. Endogenous *ras* p21 expressed in PC12 rat pheochromocytoma cells were also found predominantly in the GDP-bound form, whereas an introduced oncogenic *ras* p21 (12-Val) was present mostly in the GTP-bound state [148]. Field et al. [149] demonstrated that while yeast *RAS2* protein bound to GTP was active in adenylate cyclase stimulation, the GDP-bound form was virtually inactive. Microinjection studies utilizing nonhydrolyzable analogs of GTP have demonstrated that the GTP-bound form of either normal or oncogenic *ras* is the active form [97]. Normal *ras* p21 prebound with a nonhydrolyzable GTP analog effectively induced neurite extension of PC12 cells. In contrast, activated H-*ras* (12-Val) complexed with nonhydrolyzable GDP was entirely inactive [150]. Activation of *ras* by enhanced nucleotide exchange was also observed to favor the GTP-bound form of the protein (G. Patel and C. Der, unpublished observation). Collectively, these observations demonstrate that the relative association of normal or oncogenic *ras* proteins with either GDP or GTP is responsible for their different biological activities.

A third mechanism for *ras* activation is represented by several oncogenic H-*ras* mutants (with substitutions at residues 10 or 116) that display no in vitro GTP binding or in vivo phosphorylation, suggesting that activation can occur in the absence of GTP binding [70,105]. One possible explanation for the transforming nature of these mutants is that these substitutions induce the active conformation of the *ras* protein without GTP binding.

A fourth mechanism of *ras* activation entails overexpression of the normal *ras* protein [74,272]. While this mechanism does not disrupt the equilibrium to favor the active state, the presumed mechanism for transformation by normal *ras* overexpression is to favor the active state by enhancing the absolute levels of the active GTP-bound form of the *ras* protein. Consistent with this possibility is the observation that GAP preferentially interacts with the GTP-bound forms of *ras* protein [98]. Activation of normal *ras* by addition of a myristate may also be a consequence of overexpressing the protein. Since the myristate is a permanent modification [131], whereas palmitate is transient, the myristylated *ras* protein may be chronically associated with the membrane [132].

Properties of ras-*related proteins*

Overall, the *ras*-related proteins share approximately 30%–50% homology with the *ras* proteins, with the strongest regions of homology corresponding to the regions involved in guanine nucleotide binding. This strong degree of homology suggests that *ras* and *ras*-related proteins share both conformational and functional properties. Since the homologies of *ras*-related proteins with *ras* proteins extend beyond the guanine nucleotide binding domains, it is likely that they will also share other functional properties with *ras* proteins. However, some of the *ras*-related protein families possess characteristics that distinguish them from the *ras* proteins. In particular, while a conservation of amino acids corresponding to the *ras* residues involved with oncogenic activation is seen with most of the *ras*-related proteins, some exceptions are observed (figure 1). Whether the *ras*-related proteins could also be similarly activated by amino acid substitutions at these positions remains to be determined. At present, no oncogenic forms of any of the *ras*-related proteins have been identified, a fact that argues against their role as potential cellular oncogenes.

The conservation of at least one cysteine residue near the carboxyl-terminal end of all *ras* and *ras*-related proteins is seen (figure 1). Since most *ras* and *ras*-related proteins share this carboxyl-terminus consensus sequence Cys-A-A-X (CAAX), where A is an aliphatic amino acid and X is any amino acid, it is likely that they are similarly processed by acylation for promoting translocation to the membrane. The yeast *YPT1* protein, which contains two terminal cysteines rather than this consensus sequence, is also palmitylated [279]. Similar to the results seen with *ras* proteins, nonpalmitylated mutants of *YPT1* were both soluble and nonfunctional. The palmitylation of *YPT1* suggests that the CAAX sequence may be required for the other processing steps, including the cleavage of the terminal three amino acids, followed by the palmitylation of the now-terminal cysteine residue. This variation in the structural organization of this domain might reflect a different subcellular localization of these proteins. Supporting this possibility, yeast and mouse *YPT1/rab1* proteins are localized to the Golgi apparatus [151]. Thus, it may be that the different *ras* and *ras*-related proteins share the common property of utilizing GTP binding and hydroylsis to produce two different protein conformations, while regulating a diverse spectrum of functions, some possibly distinct from signal transduction [152].

As shown in the sequence comparisons in figure 1, the *YPT1*-related proteins display the strongest homology with the *ras* proteins in the regions important for binding and hydroysis of guanine nucleotides. However, in contrast to other *ras*-related proteins, these proteins do not have the conserved glycine corresponding to residue 12 of the *ras* proteins. Since essentially all amino acid substitutions of the *ras* 12-Gly result in the activation of transforming activity, these proteins may already be partially activated.

As expected from the strong conservation of amino acids corresponding to those in *ras* involved with guanine nucleotide binding, the recently described *SEC4* gene encodes a GTP-binding protein [153]. However, unlike *ras* proteins, the *SEC4* protein is associated not only with the plasma membrane but also with secretory vesicles. Furthermore, while *SEC4* has the same tandem cysteines at the carboxyl terminus as *YPT1*, there is evidence that this protein may not be posttranslationally modified by palmitate [153]. Similar to *ras* proteins, the *SEC4* protein is initially synthesized as a soluble protein, but it associates with membranes much more rapidly than do the yeast *RAS1* and *RAS2* proteins. These results suggest that posttranslational modifications other than palmitylation can facilitate protein translocation to the membrane.

Bacterially expressed *Aplysia rho* protein displays high-affinity binding of guanine nucleotdes and an intrinsic GTPase activity essentially identical to *ras* protein activities [154]. However, unlike H-*ras*, *rho* protein has an approximately four-fold higher affinity for GDP than for GTP, and nonguanine nucleotides (ATP, CTP, TTP, and UTP) can compete for GTP binding. Recently, a bovine *rho* protein was shown to be a substrate for the botulinum toxin [155,156]. Interestingly, it is well established that diphtheria toxin, cholera toxin, and pertussis toxin can ADP-ribosylate EF-2, G_s, and G_i, respectively, resulting in functional consequences for these G proteins [84]. Whether this covalent modification of *rho* results in a similar functional consequence remains to be determined. The findings that botulinum toxin type D inhibits exocytosis in adrenal chromaffin cells [157], and that microinjection of oncogenic H-*ras* protein results in degranulation of mast cells [158], suggest that mammalian *rho* proteins are part of the machinery associated with exocytosis [159]. However, since the N-*ras* and H-*ras* proteins are not substrates for toxin ribosylation, a role for *ras* proteins in exocytosis is not likely [160].

The p23 R-*ras* encoded protein is palmitylated, is localized to the membrane, binds GTP, and displays a GTPase activity [161]. In contrast to *ras*, a mutant of the R-*ras* (38-Val) protein with a substitution corresponding to an oncogenic substitution in *ras* (12-Val) did not display any transforming activity in rat fibroblasts. The generation of chimeric R-*ras*/H-*ras* proteins suggested that carboxyl-terminal sequences of R-*ras* p23 inhibit the transforming activity of *ras* [162]. This result is consistent with the role of the variable domains in dictating the specific function of each *ras* and *ras*-related protein.

One common feature shared between *ras* proteins and K*rev*-1/*rap* proteins is the sequence similarity of the amino acids corresponding to the effector domain of *ras* (figure 1). This suggests that the *rap* proteins may also be regulated by interaction with GAP. One feature that distinguishes the *rap*/D*ras*3 proteins with the other *ras* and *ras*-related proteins is the presence of a threonine instead of a glutamine at the position corresponding to residue 61 of the *ras* proteins [58]. While this substitution in the human H-*ras* protein results in an oncogenic protein [73], neither D*ras*3 nor *rap*1A display any transforming activity when transfected into NIH 3T3 cells (L. Quilliam, J. Schaeffer, and C. Der, unpublished observations).

While the different *ras*-related proteins are strongly homologous in the domains involved in the binding and hydrolysis of GTP, the complete divergence of sequences in other regions indicate that the different *ras* subgroups may each utilize common functions to achieve different effects. Support for this possibility comes from genetic yeast studies of *RAS*, *RHO*, *YPT1*, and *SEC4*, which suggest that each subgroup of the *ras* superfamily may have distinctly separate functions. Studies with yeast have clearly established that the *RAS1* and *RAS2* genes [258,259], the *YPT1* gene [151,260–262], the *RHO1* gene [263], and the *SEC4* gene [51,153] are essential for cell viability but, in spite of their structural and functional relatedness, fulfill different biological functions in yeast.

Biological and biochemical activities of *ras* expression

ras *and cellular transformation*

In vitro cell studies on the transforming properties of *ras* genes have concentrated on use of the NIH 3T3 mouse fibroblast cell line [163]. Whereas the introduction of normal *ras* results in no phenotypic changes, NIH 3T3 cells harboring an activated *ras* gene are morphologically transformed, form colonies in soft agar, display reduced serum requirements, and form progressive tumors when inoculated into athymic nude mice. Although a striking biological difference between normal and activated *ras* is observed in these cells, these responses may be somewhat misleading, since NIH 3T3 cells are not completely normal, but more closely approximate preneoplastic cells. Furthermore, NIH 3T3 cells will undergo spontaneous transformation at a high frequency. Studies utilizing cells more closely approximating normal cells have demonstrated a more limited transforming potential of activated *ras* genes, and are more consistent with a multistep progression of malignant transformation.

While oncogenic *ras* will induce malignant tranformation of NIH 3T3 cells as well as other established rodent fibroblast cell lines [18,164], a limited transforming potency of *ras* oncogenes is observed in primary rat embryo fibroblasts (designated REF cells) [164–168], as well as in lymphoid cells [169], epithelial cells [170–172], chondrocytes [173], or Schwann cells [174]. Transformation of these cells requires the cooperation of *ras* and other oncogenes, such as those that have been categorized as being immortalizing oncogenes. These are typically nuclear oncogenes such as v-*myc*/c-*myc* [164, 165,169,170], N-*myc* [166,175], adenovirus E1A [168,174], polyoma large T [165], SV40 large T [174], or p53 [173,176,177]. Complete transformation by *ras* can also be complemented by cellular changes induced by radiation treatment [178]. A similar limited transforming function of *ras* is also seen in Balb/MK mouse epidermal keratinocytes. These cells normally require the presence of exogenous epidermal growth factor (EGF) for growth, and high levels of calcium will induce terminal differentiation of these cells [171,172]. The introduction of oncogenic *ras* alleviates the requirement for EGF, and blocks the differentiation response to calcium. However, these cells still fail to form tumors when inoculated into animals. Instead, the addition of the v-*myc* oncogene is required to complement *ras* for complete malignant transformation (C. Der and B. Weissman, unpublished observations).

The limited potential of oncogenic *ras* to transform cells is further demonstrated by their effects on primary human cells. Normal human fibroblasts transfected with activated H-*ras* continue to display normal properties and reach senescence after limited in vitro proliferation [179]. The introduction of viral H-*ras* into normal human bronchial epithelial cells prolongs the in vitro proliferation of these cells, but the majority of cells eventually senesce. However, after extensive time in culture, the outgrowth of a small percentage of tumorigenic cells occurs [180]. Presumably, the prolonged time required for transformation allows the accumulation of additional genetic lesions to complement *ras* activity. Both infection with viral K-*ras* and an Ad12-SV40 hybrid virus was required for malignant transformation of primary human keratinocytes [181].

The requirement for complementing oncogenes to achieve complete transformation of primary REF cells is not absolute, and can be partially bypassed by several mechanisms. Elevated expression of oncogenic *ras* appears to be sufficient for transformation [182], suggesting that increased expression may be functionally equivalent to some activity otherwise provided by a complementing oncogene. The introduction of acitvated *ras* into these cells in a selectable vector, followed by selection for the transfected cell population, allows *ras* transformation in the absence of another cooperating oncogene [167,182]. Apparently, in the absence of selection for the *ras*-transfected cell population, the surrounding normal cells display an inhibitory effect on *ras* transformation. Nevertheless, transformation of primary rodent fibroblast by *ras* requires additional complementary genetic changes to result in full transformation.

ras *and cellular differentiation*

Similar to *ras* action in Balb/MK mouse epidermal keratinocytes, most cells are blocked in their differentiating activities by activated *ras*. For example, mouse skeletal myoblast cells transfected with oncogenic H-*ras* or N-*ras* are blocked in their ability to differentiate into multinucleated myotubes [36]. However, oncogenic H-*ras* did not interfere with the retinoic acid-induced differentiation of the multipotential embryonal carcinoma cell line P19 into neurons, astrocytes, and fibroblast–like cells [184]. In contrast, *ras* oncogenes can induce the terminal differentiation of the PC12 rat pheochromocytoma cell line [182,183]. PC12 cells respond to nerve growth factor by shifting from a chromaffin–like phenotype to a neurite-bearing sympathetic neuron–like phenotype [185]. A similar induction of neurite extensions is also seen with cAMP treatment [186]. However, the *ras*-induced response appears to be independent of cAMP, and more closely parallels the NGF response. The demonstration that microinjection of PC12 cells with anti-*ras* protein monoclonal antibodies inhibits NGF-induced neurite formation suggests that *ras* may participate in a signal transduction pathway used by NGF [187]. A similar induction of differentiation has also been observed in a viral H-*ras*-infected human medullary thyroid carcinoma cell line, which is closely related developmentally to PC12 cells [188]. Thus, while oncogenic *ras* may potentiate the growth properties of one cell type, it may facilitate the differentiation of another cell type.

Suppression of oncogenic ras *activity*

While complementation studies have implicated the cooperative interaction between *ras* and other oncogenes for cellular transformation, there is also evidence that the loss of specific genetic loci can also complement *ras*-induced malignant transformation. Several lines of investigation have suggested the existence of genes that exert a dominant, suppressing activity of *ras* oncogenicity. The generation of somatic cell hybrids between normal fibroblasts and tumorigenic cells that harbor activated *ras* genes results in suppression of the tumorigenic phenotype [189–191]. The nonrandom loss of chromosome 15 is observed in tumors resulting from hamster embryo cells transfected with v-H-*ras* and v-*myc*, consistent with the existence of *ras* suppressor genes [280]. Schaefer et al. [192] have recently reported the detection and cloning of a human DNA fragment that partially reverts the transformed phenotype of H-*ras*-transformed FE-8 rat fibroblasts. In another study, flat revertants of NIH 3T3 cells transformed with viral K-*ras* have been isolated [193]. Since these revertant cells continue to express oncogenic *ras* protein, and cannot be retransformed by the introduction of additional viral K-*ras* sequences, the activation of a cellular suppressor gene has been proposed. Fusion of one revertant cell line with cell lines transformed by other viral oncogenes demonstrated the dominant nature of suppression. Furthermore, the observation that the transforming activity of other oncogenes is also suppressed (v-*fes*, v-*src*), while that of others (v-*mos*, v-*fms*, and v-*sis*) is not, suggests the generality of this suppressing activity.

Noda and colleagues have recently identified and isolated a number of human genes with *ras*-suppressing activity [60]. A human fibroblast cDNA expression library was transfected into viral K-*ras*-transformed NIH 3T3 cells, and flat revertant cell populations were isolated from the transfected cell population. Seven independent flat revertants were isolated, all of which continued to express the oncogenic K-*ras* protein, yet displayed reduced tumorigenic potential. Fusion of the revertant cell lines to viral K-*ras*-transformed NIH 3T3 cells demonstrated the dominant nature of the suppressor activities. In particular, one of these suppressor genes was isolated and sequenced, and was found to encode a *ras*-related protein, designated Krev-1. This *ras*-related protein is identical to the independently identified *rap*1A protein [58]. Transfection of Krev1/*rap*1A into viral-K-*ras*-transformed NIH 3T3 cells resulted in the partial morphologic reversion of approximately 30% of the transfected cells, followed by the subsequent appearance of a near-complete reversion of a small percentage of the transfected cells. Apparently, high-level expression of Krev1/*rap*1A is required to achieve this suppression. The suppression activity of Krev1/*rap*1A may be achieving reversion of *ras* transformation by competing for a common target or regulatory protein, such as GAP. Alternatively, Krev1 may modulate a negative growth-regulatory pathway that indirectly counteracts the positive regulatory pathway modulated by *ras*.

ras and signal transduction

By virtue of the membrane localization of *ras*, and its structural and functional homologies with the regulatory G proteins, it has been proposed that *ras* proteins function as intermediaries between surface receptors to modulate intracellular processes [81–83]. While *ras* proteins share amino acid sequence homologies with G proteins, these shared sequences are principally restricted to the four regions that are shared among a wide variety of other guanine nucleotide-binding proteins [85,88]. Furthermore, no analogous beta and gamma subunits have been identified to interact with *ras* proteins. Thus, while it is likely that *ras* may be similarly modulated by the binding of guanine nucleotides, it remains to be determined whether *ras* proteins may function analogously to the G proteins in signal transduction pathways. Candidates for the membrane receptors that function through *ras* have been suggested [194–198], but no definitive evidence for any of these has been generated. Described below are the studies addressing the possible signal transduction systems *ras* has been proposed to modulate. Despite intensive research efforts, proof of a specific involvement of *ras* proteins in signal transduction remains elusive. Thus, while there is evidence for some influence of *ras* in several second messenger systems, a direct role of ras proteins in signal transduction remains to be established.

ras *and adenylate cyclase.* The extensive structural and biochemical homologies between the human and yeast ras proteins, coupled with the ease of genetic manipulations of yeast, suggested that the study of ras function in yeast would provide the best route to elucidate the function of ras in mammalian cells. Indeed, extensive genetic analysis of the function of the two yeast ras genes, *RAS1* and *RAS2*, in *S. cerevisiae* have identified an important role of yeast ras in regulating intracellular levels of cAMP via the regulation of the adenylate cyclase system [11].

The observation that mammalian ras proteins can stimulate yeast adenylate cyclase indicated a similar stimulatory role for ras in mammalian cells. However, attempts to extrapolate a role for mammalian ras in the regulation of the adenylate cyclase pathway have indicated that ras may function by a different mechanism in mammalian cells [199–206]. Studies addressing the relationship between ras transformation and adenylate cyclase activity have shown differing results. Mammalian fibroblast and epithelial cells transformed by ras have shown either a decrease [201,202,205], increase [199,200], or no change [203] in adenylate cyclase activities. Furthermore, Beckner et al. [205] have demonstrated that neither mammalian nor bacterially expressed ras proteins are able to stimulate or inhibit mammalian adenylate cyclase activity in vitro. Additionally, demonstrations that ras activities in either *Xenopus* oocyte maturation [204] or the fission yeast *S. pombe* [207] are unrelated to adenylate cyclase activities suggest that ras may function via different effector systems in different organisms. Consequently, it appears unlikely that ras proteins directly modulate adenylate cyclase activities in mammalian cells in a fashion analogous to the Gs and Gi proteins.

ras *and phospholipid metabolism.* Circumstantial evidence has suggested that the phospholipase C responsible for phosphatidylinositol (PI) breakdown is coupled to receptors via a putative G protein, designated as G_p. The involvement of ras proteins in the regulation of phosphatidylinositol metabolism has also been proposed [208,209]. Extensive studies in both yeast and mammalian cells have implicated the role of ras in regulating another second messenger system, via the regulation of phosphatidylinositol 4, 5-biphosphate (PIP2) levels. It is known that PIP2 hydrolysis is stimulated by hormones, neurotransmitters, serum, and growth factors. These ligands induce a rapid breakdown of PIP2 to generate two second messengers, diacylglycerol (DAG) and inositol 1, 4, 5-trisphosphate (IP3), which seem to act as intracellular regulators of growth. DAG activates protein kinase C, which is involved in functions relating to cellular growth and differentiation [210]. IP3 stimulates Ca^{+2} release from intracellular vesicles into the cytosol.

Earlier studies comparing ras-transformed cells with their untransformed counterparts indicated that PI turnover is altered in the transformed cells

[202,211–214]. Consistent with these observations, Wakelam et al. [194] demonstrated an increased coupling of growth factors such as bombesin to inositol phospholipid breakdown in NIH 3T3 cells overexpressing the normal N-*ras* protein. Additionally, it has been shown that NIH 3T3 cells overexpressing normal H-*ras* displayed an amplified response to platelet-derived growth factor, while cells expressing an oncogenic *ras* protein raised the basal rate of PI turnover in the absence of added growth factor [195]. Recently, it was shown that the microinjection of a monoclonal antibody to PIP2 into *ras*-transformed NIH 3T3 cells caused a decrease in proliferation and reversion to a normal cell morphology [215]. These results suggest a direct involvement of *ras* in the regulation of PI metabolism.

In contrast to the data from studies suggesting that *ras* proteins may be the G_p protein, results from a number of other studies do not find a direct association between *ras* transformation and an increased phospholipase C activity. Wolfman and Macara [216] and Lacal et al. [217] observed no significant alteration in inositol phosphates in H-*ras*-transformed NIH 3T3 cells, and phospholipase C activity in H-*ras* or K-*ras*-transformed hamster fibroblasts remained unchanged [218]. Microinjection of the Y13-259 *ras* neutralizing antibody into NIH 3T3 cells inhibited the proliferative response to agents that imitate the action of phospholipase C or phospholipase A2. These results suggest that *ras* is unlikely to function to control the action of these phospholipases [219]. Finally, while DAG levels are frequently elevated in *ras*-transformed cells, the absence of similar elevations of inositol phosphates suggest that *ras* is not likely to regulate PI metabolism directly [216,217,220,271]. However, the frequent elevation of DAG levels associated with *ras* transformation, coupled with evidence for functional relationships between *ras* proteins and protein kinase C, suggest some involvement of *ras* in the modulation of protein kinase C activity [198,216,219,221,222], which is involved in the relay of extracellular signals regulating cell growth and differentiation [210].

Involvement of other cellular oncogenes. Results from several lines of investigation have implicated *ras* proteins in signal transduction pathways involving other oncogenes. Smith et al. [223] demonstrated that microinjection of the anti-*ras* neutralizing antibody, Y13-259, into NIH3T3 cells transformed by membrane-associated, receptor–like proteins (*src*, *fms*, and *fes*) resulted in the reversion to a normal morphology. In contrast, the microinjection of cells transformed by two cytoplasmic viral oncogenes (*mos* and *raf*) did not reverse their transformed morphology. The dependence of receptor oncogenes on *ras*, and the independence of cytoplasmic oncogenes on *ras*, suggest a scheme wherein *ras* functions in a pathway that regulates cellular proliferation.

A similar signal transduction pathway involving oncogenes has also been suggested by a H-*ras* mutant that inhibits the proliferation of NIH 3T3 cells [224]. This mutant protein contains a substitution of asparagine for serine at position 17 of v-H-*ras*, which results in a 20–40-fold reduction in GTP-binding affinity, without significantly affecting the affinity for GDP. NIH 3T3 cells transfected with this mutant were inhibited in their proliferation. While NIH 3T3 cells transformed by v-*src* were sensitive to inhibition, cells transformed by v-*mos* and v-*raf* were resistant to inhibition by the 17-Asn mutant. Since the *mos* and *raf* oncogenes encode cytoplasmic protein kinases, these transforming proteins may act downstream of *ras* in a signal transduction pathway.

The interaction of *ras* with another oncogene has been demonstrated by the induction of *fos* expression in NIH 3T3 cells microinjected with oncogenic *ras* proteins [225]. Similarly, oncogenic *ras* induces a 20-fold induction of *fos* expression in rat PC12 pheochromocytoma cells. Analysis of various structural and biochemical mutants of H-*ras* demonstrated a direct correlation between the induction of PC12 differentiation and *fos* induction, suggesting that *ras* may induce differentiation via a signal transduction pathway mediated by *fos* [278].

Role of cellular *ras* genes in carcinogenesis

Transduction into oncogenic retroviruses

The first suggestion that cellular *ras* genes represent potential cellular oncogenes comes from studies on the viral oncogenes of the Harvey (v-H-*ras*) and Kirsten (v-K-*ras*) sarcoma viruses (table 3). These highly oncogenic RNA viruses represent rare isolates from tumors derived from rats following the passage of murine leukemia viruses [226,227]. These viruses can efficiently transform cells in culture and can induce tumors in infected animals at a high frequency within a short latency period of several weeks. Their oncogenicity can be ascribed to viral sequences that represent transduced cellular *ras* sequences [5,6]. The retroviral Harvey *ras* gene was derived from the rat H-*ras* gene. The Kirsten viral oncogene represents a transduced version of the rat K-*ras* gene sequences. Rasheed-MSV [228], BALB-MSV [229], AF-1 [230], and NS.C58 MSV-1 and NS.C58 MSV-2 [231] are additional isolates of oncogenic retroviruses containing oncogenic *ras* sequences as transduced versions of cellular H-*ras* genes (table 3). Of the three known cellular *ras* genes, only N-*ras* has not been identified as transduced into an oncogenic retrovirus genome.

Activation in human tumors

A second avenue of research that has resulted in the unveiling of cellular *ras* oncogenes comes from gene transfer studies utilizing the NIH 3T3 mouse fibroblast cell line [163,232]. These studies for the detection of biologically active transforming genes in cellular DNA are based on the experiments of Hill and Hillova [233], who demonstrated the transfection of chicken embryo fibroblasts with DNA from Rous sarcoma virus-transformed rat cells. Subsequent studies have utilized NIH 3T3 cells because of their capacity to stably integrate exogenously added DNA with relatively high efficiencies. Detection of transforming activity by transfection of NIH 3T3 cells has provided a very powerful biological assay for the identification and isolation of transforming genes that are activated in a large variety of animal and human tumor cells [4,10,163].

In the vast majority of transfection studies, the detected oncogene represents a member of the cellular *ras* gene family. The presence of activated *ras* genes in human tumors was first identified in a human bladder carcinoma (H-*ras*) cell line [7–9] and a human lung carcinoma (K-*ras*) cell line [7]. Subsequently, a third activated *ras* gene, N-*ras*, was detected in a human neuroblastoma cell line [234,235]. Extensive studies have now identified activated *ras* genes in a wide variety of human neoplasms, including carcinomas, sarcomas, leukemias, and lymphomas [236]. Data from an extensive body of transfection studies suggested that 10%–20% of human tumors contained activated *ras* sequences. However, with the application of more sensitive molecular detection techniques, the frequency of *ras* activation appears to be significantly higher. For example, activated K-*ras* sequences have been found in approximately 40% of human colorectal tumors [237,238] and in up to 95% of human pancreatic carcinomas [239].

Although the presence of a specific activated *ras* gene does not correlate absolutely with a specific tumor, several general tendencies can be observed. First, although H-*ras* activation has been routinely associated with experimentally induced rodent carcinomas [240–243], H-*ras* activation has only been observed infrequently in human tumors. Second, activated K-*ras* sequences have been identified in a variety of human tumors, with a frequent association observed with lung, colon, and pancreatic carcinomas. Finally, while N-*ras* activation has also been detected in a range of human tumors, a high frequency has been found in acute myelogenous [34,244–247] and acute lymphocytic [246,248] leukemias.

In a number of studies, where an activated *ras* gene was detected in a tumor isolate, normal cellular DNA from the same patient contained only the normal gene, suggesting that *ras* gene activation is a consequence of somatic mutations rather than germ-line mutations [249–251]. In a study characterizing the presence of activated K-*ras* and N-*ras* genes in human colorectal carcinomas, the activated genes were present in both benign and malignant regions of the tumor, suggesting that *ras* activation represented an early event in tumor progression [237]. Whether an activated *ras* induces the progression of benign adenomas to malignant carcinomas is not known. Similarly, the detection of activated *ras* in preleukemia patients is consistent with *ras* involvement in the early stages of human leukemia [252, 253]. The detection of activated H-*ras* in chemically induced benign papillomas in mice also supports the involvement of *ras* in the early stages of tumor progression [242,243]. Similarly, activated H-*ras* genes were identified in benign and self-regressing keratoacanthomas in both humans and rabbits, implying that the presence of an activated *ras* gene was not sufficient to maintain a neoplastic phenotype, although it may play a role in the early stages of tumorigenesis [254]. However, the persistence of the activated gene in metastatic tumors suggests the active involvement of the *ras* oncogene in tumor progression to the malignant state [239,255]. Consequently, whether *ras* activation is an initiating event, or contributes to tumor cell heterogeneity, remains to be determined. Long-term studies of large numbers of cases will be necessary to address this question.

In addition to the presence of structurally altered *ras* proteins in human tumors, a contribution of *ras* overexpression in tumor development has been suggested from several experimental observations. First, amplification of *ras* sequences in human tumors has been documented [75,264–266]. Second, elevated *ras* expression has been observed in some tumors when compared to the levels observed in normal tissue [21,238,266–268).

Activation in experimental carcinogenesis

Further implicating evidence for a role for *ras* activation in tumor development comes from a number of carcinogenesis studies performed on rodent systems. In a study by Barbacid and colleagues, female rats treated with methyl-nitrosomethylurea developed mammary carcinomas with 86% containing an activated H-*ras* gene [240,241]. Mice treated with the carcinogen dimethylbenz(a)anthracene, followed by promotion with the promoting agent 12-0-tetradecanoyl-phorbol-13-acetate, demonstrated a high frequency of H-*ras* activation in skin carcinomas [242,243]. Mice treated with either gamma radiation or the chemical carcinogen n-nitrosomethylurea resulted in the development of thymic lymphomas that displayed a frequent activation of K-*ras* or N-*ras* [256,257]. Thus, the treatment of animals with a specific physical agent resulted in the frequent induction of the same neoplasm and in the corresponding activation of a *ras* gene, supporting the involvement of these oncogenes in tumor development.

Acknowledgments

I would like to thank Charles Van Beveren, Adrienne Cox, and Marsha MacDonald for their critical comments on this chapter, and Tami Clevenger for excellent preparation of the text. CJD is supported by PHS grant CA42978.

References

1. Bishop JM: Cellular oncogenes and retroviruses. Annu Rev Biochem 52:301–354, 1983.
2. Varmus HE: The molecular genetics of cellular oncogenes. Annu Rev Genet 18:553–612, 1984.

3. Bishop JM: The molecular genetics of cancer. Science 235:305–311, 1987.
4. Der CJ: Cellular oncogenes and human carcinogenesis. Clin Chem 33:641–646, 1988.
5. DeFeo D, Gonda MA, Young HA, Chang EH, Lowy DR, Scolnick EM, Ellis RW: Analysis of two divergent rat genomic clones homologous to the transforming gene of Harvey murine sarcoma virus. Proc Natl Acad Sci USA 78:3328–3332, 1981.
6. Ellis RW, DeFeo D, Shih TY, Gonda MA, Young HA, Tsuchida H, Lowy DR, Scolnick EM: p21 src genes of Harvey and Kirsten sarcoma viruses originate from divergent members of a family of normal vertebrate genes. Nature 292:506–511, 1981.
7. Der CJ, Krontiris TG, Cooper GM: Transforming genes of human bladder and lung carcinoma cell lines are homologous to the *ras* genes of Harvey and Kirsten sarcoma viruses. Proc Natl Acad Sci USA 79:3637–3640, 1982.
8. Parada LF, Tabin CJ, Shih C, Weinberg RA: Human EJ bladder carcinoma oncogene is homologue of Harvey sarcoma virus *ras* gene. Nature 297:474–478, 1982.
9. Santos E, Tronick SR, Aaronson SA, Pulciani S, Barbacid M: T24 human bladder carcinoma oncogene is an activated form of the normal human homologue of Balb- and Harvey-MSV transforming genes. Nature 298:343–347, 1982.
10. Barbacid M: *ras* genes. Ann Rev Biochim 56:779–827, 1987.
11. Tamanoi F: Yeast *ras* genes. Biochim Biophys Acta 948:1–15, 1988.
12. Lacal JC, Tronick SR: The *ras* oncogene. In: Reddy EP, Skalka AM, Curran T (eds): Oncogenes. Amsterdam: Elsevier Science Publishers, 1988, pp 257–304.
13. Chang EH, Gonda MA, Ellis RW, Scolnick EM, Lowy DR: Human genome contains four genes homologous to transforming genes of Harvey and Kirsten murine sarcoma viruses. Proc Natl Acad Sci USA 79:4848–4852, 1982.
14. McGrath JP, Capon DJ, Smith DH, Chen EY, Seebury PH, Goeddel DV, Levinson AD: Structure and organization of the human Ki-*ras* proto-oncogene and a related processed pseudogene. Nature 304:501–506, 1983.
15. Shimizu K, Goldfarb M, Suard Y, Perucho M, Li Y, Kamata T, Feramisco J, Stavnezer E, Fogh J, Wigler MH: Three human transforming genes are related to the viral *ras* oncogenes. Proc Natl Acad Sci USA 80:2112–2116, 1983.
16. Hall A, Marshall CJ, Spurr NK, Weiss RA: Identification of transforming gene in two human sarcoma cell lines as a new member of the *ras* gene family located on chromosome 1. Nature 303:396–400, 1983.
17. Taparowsky E, Shimizu K, Goldfarb M, Wigler M: Structure and activation of the human N-*ras* gene. Cell 34:581–586, 1983.
18. Capon DJ, Chen EY, Levinson AD, Seeburg PH, Goeddel DV: Complete nucleotide sequences of the T24 human bladder carcinoma oncogene and its normal homologue. Nature 302:33–37, 1983.
19. Langbeheim H, Shih TY, Scolnick EM: Identification of a normal vertebrate cell protein related to the p21 src of Harvey murine sarcoma virus. Virology 106:292–300, 1980.
20. Furth ME, Davis LJ, Fleurdelys B, Scolnick EM: Monoclonal antibodies to the p21 products of the transforming gene of Harvey murine sarcoma virus and of the cellular *ras* gene family. J Virol 43:294–304, 1982.
21. Capon DJ, Seeburg PH, McGrath JP, Hayflick JS, Edman U, Levinson AD, Goeddel DV: Activation of Ki-*ras* 2 gene in human colon and lung carcinomas by two different point mutations. Nature 304:507–513, 1983.
22. Shimizu K, Birnbaum D, Ruley EA, Fasano O, Suard Y, Edlund L, Taparowsky E, Goldfarb M, Wigler M: Structure of the Ki-*ras* gene of the human lung carcinoma cell line Calu-1. Nature 304:497–500, 1983.
23. McCoy MS, Bargmann CI, and Weinberg RA: Human colon carcinoma Ki-*ras*2 oncogene and its corresponding proto-oncogene. Mol Cell Biol 4:1577–1582, 1984.
24. McBridge OW, Swan DC, Tronick SR, Gol R, Klimanis D, Moore DE, Aaronson SA: Regional chromosomal localization of N-*ras*, K-*ras* and *myb* oncogenes in human cells. Nucleic Acids Res 11:8221–8236, 1983.
25. O'Brien SJ, Nash WG, Goodwin JL, Lowy DR, Chang EH: Dispersion of the *ras* family of

transforming genes of four different chromosomes in man. Nature 302:839–842, 1983.
26. Jhanwar SC, Neel BG, Hayward WS, Ghaganti RSK: Localization of c-*ras* oncogene family on human germ-line chromosomes. Proc Natl Acad Sci USA 80:4794–4797, 1983.
27. Popescu NC, Amsbaugh SC, DiPaolo JA, Tronick SR, Aaronson SA, Swan DC: Chromosomal localization of three human *ras* genes by in situ molecular hybridization. Somatic Cell Mol Genet 11:149–155, 1985.
28. Ryan J, Barker PE, Shimizu K, Wigler M, Ruddle FH: Chromosomal assignment of a family of human oncogenes. Proc Natl Acad Sci USA 80:4460–4463, 1983.
29. Sakaguchi AY, Zabel BU, Grzeschik K–H, Law ML, Ellis RW, Scolnick EM, Naylor SL: Regional localization of two human cellular Kirsten *ras* genes on chromosomes 6 and 12. Mol Cell Biol 4:989–993, 1984.
30. Huerre C, Despoisse S, Gilgenkrantz S, Lenoir GM, Junien C: c-Ha-*ras*1 is not detected in aniridia-Wilms' tumour association. Nature 305:638–641, 1983.
31. Van Kessel AG, Nusse R, Slater R, Tetteroo P, Hagemeyer A: Localization of the oncogene c-Ha-*ras* 1 outside the Aniridia—Wilm's tumor-associated deletion of chromosome 11 (del 11p13) using somatic cell hybrids. Cancer Cytogenet 15:79–84, 1985.
32. Krontiris TG, DiMartino NA, Colb M, Parkinson DR: Unique allelic restriction fragments of the Ha-*ras* locus in leukocyte and tumour DNAs of cancer patients. Nature 313:369–374, 1985.
33. Theillet C, Lidereau R, Escot C, Hutzell P, Brunet M, Gest J, Schlom J, Callahan R: Loss of a c-H-*ras*-1 allele and aggressive human primary breast carcinomas. Cancer Res 46: 4776–4781, 1986.
34. Farr CJ, Saiki RK, Erlich HA, McCormick F, Marshall CJ: Analysis of *ras* gene mutations in acute myeloid leukemia by polymerase chain reaction and oligonucleotide probes. Proc Natl Acad Sci USA 85:1629–1633, 1988.
35. Gerhard DS, Dracopoli NC, Bale SJ, Houghton AN, Watkins P, Payne CE, Greene MH, Housman DE: Evidence against Ha-*ras*-1 involvement in sporadic and familial melanoma. Nature 325:73–75, 1987.
36. Olson EN, Spizz G, Tainsky MA : The oncogenic forms of N-*ras* or H-*ras* prevent skeletal myoblast differentiation. Mol Cell Biol 7:2104–2111, 1987.
37. Westaway D, Papkoff J, Moscovici C, Varmus HE: Identification of a provirally activated c-Ha-*ras* oncogene in an avian nephroblastoma via a novel procedure: cDNA cloning of a chimeric viral–host transcript. EMBO J 5:301–309, 1986.
38. Nemoto N, Kodama K–I, Tazawa A, Masahito P, Ishikawa T: Extensive sequence homology of the goldfish *ras* gene to mammalian *ras* genes. Differentiation 32:17–23, 1986.
39. Neuman-Silberberg FS, Schejter E, Hoffmann FM, Shilo BZ: The *Drosophila ras* oncogenes: structure and nucleotide sequence. Cell 37:1027–1033, 1984.
40. Mozer B, Marlor R, Parkhurst S, Corces V: Characterization and development expression of a *Drosophila ras* oncogene. Mol Cell Biol 5:885–889, 1985.
41. Schejter ED, Shilo B: Characterization of functional domains of p21 *ras* by use of chimeric genes. EMBO J 4:407–412, 1985.
42. Defeo-Jones D, Scolnick EM, Koller R, Dhar R: *ras*-related gene sequences identified and isolated from *Saccharomyces cerevisiae*. Nature 306:707–709, 1983.
43. Powers S, Kataoka T, Fasano O, Goldfarb M, Strathern J, Breach J, Wigler M: Genes in *S. cerevisiae* encoding proteins with domains homologous to the mammalian *ras* proteins. Cell 36:607–612, 1984.
44. Fukui Y, Kaziro Y: Molecular cloning and sequence analysis of a *ras* gene from *Schizosaccharomyces pombe*. EMBO J 4:687–691, 1985.
45. Reymond CD, Gomer RH, Mehdy MC, Firtel RA: Developmental regulation of a *Dictyostelium* gene encoding a protein homologous to a mammalian *ras* protein. Cell 39:141–149, 1984.
46. Swanson ME, Elste AM, Greenberg SM, Schwartz JH, Aldrich TH, Furth ME: Abundant expression of *ras* proteins in *Aplysia* neurons. J Cell Biol 103:485–492, 1986.
47. Gallwitz D, Donath C, Sander C: A yeast gene encoding a protein homologous to the

human c-*has/bas* proto-oncogene product. Nature 306:704–707, 1983.
48. Touchot N, Chardin P, Tavitian A: Four additional members of the *ras* gene superfamily isolated by an oligonucleotide strategy: Molecular cloning of YPT-related cDNAs from a rat brain library. Proc Natl Acad Sci USA 84:8210–8214, 1987.
49. Zahraoui A, Touchot N, Chardin P, Tavitian A: Complete coding sequences of the *ras* related *rab* 3 and 4 cDNAs. Nucleic Acids Res 16:1204, 1988.
50. Haubruck H, Disela C, Wagner P, Gallwitz D: The *ras*-related *ypt* protein is an ubiquitous eukaryotic protein: Isolation and sequence analysis of mouse cDNA clones highly homologous to the yeast *YPT1* gene. EMBO J 6:4049–4053, 1987.
51. Salminen A, Novick PJ: A *ras*-like protein is required for a post-Golgi event in yeast secretion. Cell 49:527–538, 1987.
52. Madaule P, Axel R: A novel *ras*-related gene family. Cell 41:31–40, 1985.
53. Madaule P, Axel R, Myers AM: Characterization of two members of the *rho* gene family from the yeast *Saccharomyces cerevisiae*. Proc Natl Acad Sci 84:779–783, 1987.
54. Chardin P, Madaule P, Tavitian A: Coding sequence of human *rho* cDNAs clone 6 and clone 9. Nucleic Acids Res 16:2717, 1988.
55. Yeramian P, Chardin P, Madaule P, Tavitian A: Nucleotide sequence of human *rho* cDNA clone 12. Nucleic Acid Res 15:1869, 1987.
56. Chardin P, Tavitian A: The *ral* gene: a new *ras* related gene isolated by the use of a synthetic probe. EMBO J 5:2203–2208, 1986.
57. Lowe DG, Capon DJ, Delwart E, Sakaguchi AY, Naylor SL, Goeddel DV: Structure of the human and murine R-*ras* genes, novel genes closely related to *ras* proto-oncogenes. Cell 48:137–146, 1987.
58. Pizon V, Chardin P, Lerosey I, Olfsson B, Tavitian A: Human cDNAs *rap*1 and *rap*2 homologous to the Drosophila gene D*ras*3 encode proteins closely related to *ras* in the 'effector' region. Oncogene 3:201–204, 1988.
59. Pizon V, Lerosey I, Chardin P, Tavitian A: Nucleotide sequence of a human cDNA encoding a *ras*-related protein (*rap*1B). Nucleic Acids Res 16:7719, 1988.
60. Noda M, Kitayama H, Matsuzaki, Sugimoto Y, Okayama H, Bassin RH, Ikawa Y: Detection of genes with a potential for suppressing the transformed phenotype associated with activated *ras* genes. Proc Natl Acad Sci USA, 86:162–166, 1989.
61. Kitayama H, Sugimoto Y, Matsuzaki T, Ikawa Y, Noda M: A *ras*-related gene with transformation suppressor activity. Cell, 56:77–84, 1989.
62. Tabin CJ, Bradley SM, Bargmann CI, Weinberg RA, Papageorge AG, Scolnick EM, Dhar R, Lowy DR, Change EH: Mechanism of activation of a human oncogene. Nature 300: 143–149, 1982.
63. Reddy EP, Reynolds RK, Santos E, Barbacid M: A point mutation is responsible for the acquisition of transforming properties by the T24 human bladder carcinoma oncogene. Nature 300:149–152, 1982.
64. Taparowsky E, Suard Y, Fasano O, Shimizu K, Goldfarb M, Wigler M: Activation of T24 bladder carcinoma transforming gene is linked to a single amino acid change. Nature 300:762–765, 1982.
65. Yuasa Y, Srivastava SK, Dunn CY, Rhim JS, Reddy EP, Aaronson SA: Acquisition of transforming properties by alternative point mutations within c-*bas/has* human proto-oncogene. Nature 303:775–779, 1983.
66. Bos JL, Toksoz D, Marshall CJ, Verlaan-deVries M, Veeneman GH, van der Eb AJ, van Boom J, Janssen JWG, Steenvoorden ACM: Amino-acid substitutions at codon 13 of the N-*ras* oncogene in human acute myeloid leukaemia. Nature 315:726–730, 1985.
67. Fasano O, Aldrich T, Tamanoi F, Taparowsky E, Furth M, Wigler M: Analysis of the transforming potential of the human H-*ras* gene by random mutagenesis. Proc Natl Acad Sci USA 71:4008–4012, 1984.
68. Walter M, Clark SG, Levinson AD: The oncogenic activation of human p21*ras* by a novel mechanism. Science 233:649–652, 1986.
69. Sigal IS, Gibbs JB, D'Alonzo JS, Temeles GL, Wolanski BS, Socher SH, Scolnick EM:

Mutant *ras*-encoded proteins with altered nucleotide binding exert dominant biological effects. Proc Natl Acad Sci USA 83:952–956, 1986.
70. Der CJ, Weissman B, MacDonald MJ: Altered guanine nucleotide binding and H-*ras* transforming and differentiating activities. Oncogene 3:105–112, 1988.
71. Seeburg PH, Colby WW, Hayflick JS, Capon DJ, Goeddel DV, Levinson AD: Biological properties of human c-Ha-*ras*1 genes mutated at codon 12. Nature 312:71–75, 1984.
72. Chipperfield RG, Jones SS, Lo K–M, Weinberg RA: Activation of Ha-*ras* p21 by substitution, deletion and insertion mutations. Mol Cell Biol 5:1809–1813, 1985.
73. Der CJ, Finkel T, Cooper GM: Biological and biochemical properties of human *ras*H genes mutated at codon 61. Cell 44:167–176, 1986.
74. Chang EH, Furth ME, Scolnick EM, Lowy DR: Tumorigenic transformation of mammalian cells induced by a normal human gene homologous to the oncogene of Harvey murine sarcoma virus. Nature 297:479–483, 1982.
75. McCoy MS, Toole JJ, Cunningham JM, Chang EH, Lowy DR, Weinberg RA: Characterization of a human colon/lung carcinoma oncogene. Nature 302:79–81, 1983.
76. Stacey DW, Kung H-F: Transformation of NIH/3T3 cells by microinjection of Ha-*ras* p21 protein. Nature 310:508–511, 1984.
77. Winter E, Perucho M: Oncogene amplification during tumorigenesis of established rat fibroblasts reversibly transformed by activated human *ras* oncogenes. Mol Cell Biol 6: 2562–2570, 1986.
78. Spandidos DA, Wilkie NM: Malignant transformation of early passage rodent cells by a single mutated human encogene. Nature 310:469–475, 1984.
79. Cohen JB, Levinson AD: A point mutation in the last intron responsible for increased expression and transforming activity of the c-Ha-*ras* oncogene. Nature 334:119–124, 1988.
80. Ricketts MH, Levinson AD: High-level expression of c-H-*ras*1 fails to fully transform Rat-1 cells. Mol Cell Biol 8:1460–1468, 1988.
81. Gilman AG: G proteins and dual control of adenylate cyclase. Cell 36:577–579, 1984.
82. Hurley JB, Simon MI, Teplow DB, Robishaw JD, Gilman AG: Homologies between signal transducing G proteins and *ras* gene products. Science 226:860–862, 1984.
83. Lochrie MA, Hurley JB, Simon MI: Sequence of the alpha subunit of photoreceptor G protein: homologies between transducin, *ras*, and elongation factors. Science 228:96–99, 1984.
84. Gilman AG: G proteins: Transducers of receptor-generated signals. Annu Rev Biochem 56:615–649, 1987.
85. Masters SB, Stroud RM, Bourne HR: Family of G protein alpha chains: amphipathic analysis and predicted structure of functional domains. Pro Eng 1:47–54, 1986.
86. Halliday K: Regional homology in GTP-binding proto-oncogene products and elongation factors. J Cyclic Nucl Res 9:431–448.
87. Leberman R, Egner U: Homologies in the primary structure of GTP-binding proteins: the nucleotide-binding site of EF-Tu and p21. EMBO J 3:339–341, 1984.
88. Dever TE, Glynias MJ, Merrick WC: GTP-binding domain: Three consensus sequence elements with distinct spacing. Proc Natl Acad Sci USA 84:1814–1818, 1987.
89. Finkel T, Der CJ, Cooper GM: Activation of *ras* genes in human tumors does not affect subcellular localization, post-translational modification or guanine nucleotide binding properties of p21. Cell 37:151–158, 1984.
90. McGrath JP, Capon DJ, Goeddel DV, Levinson AD: Comparative biochemical properties of normal and activated human *ras* p21 protein. Nature 310:644–649, 1984.
91. Sweet RW, Yokoyama S, Kamata T, Feramisco JR, Rosenberg M, Gross M: The product of *ras* is a GTPase and the T24 oncogenic mutant is deficient in this activity. Nature 311:273–275, 1984.
92. Gibbs JB, Ellis RW, Scolnick EM: Intrinsic GTPase activity distinguishes normal and oncogenic *ras* p21 molecules. Proc Natl Acad Sci USA 81:5704–5708, 1984.
93. Manne V, Yamazaki S, Kung H: Guanosine nucleotide binding by highly purified Ha-*ras*-encoded p21 protein produced in *Escherichia coli*. Proc Natl Acad Sci USA 81:6953–6957, 1984.

94. Temeles GL, Gibbs JB, D'Alonzo JS, Sigal IS, Scolnick EM: Yeast and mammalian *ras* proteins have conserved biochemical properties. Nature 313:700–703, 1985.
95. Trahey M, Milley RJ, Cole GE, Innis M, Paterson H, Marshall CJ, Hall A, McCormick F: Biochemical and biological properties of the human N-*ras* p21 protein. Mol Cell Biol 7: 541–544, 1987.
96. Lacal JC, Srivastava SK, Anderson PS, Aaronson SA: *ras* p21 proteins with high or low GTPase activity can efficiently transform NIH/3T3 cells. Cell 44:609–617, 1986.
97. Trahey M, McCormick F: A cytoplasmic protein stimulates normal N-*ras* p21 GTPase, but does not affect oncogenic mutants. Science 238:542–545, 1987.
98. Vogel US, Dixon RAF, Schaber MD, Diehl RE, Marshall MS, Scolnick EM, Sigal IS, Gibbs JB: Cloning of bovine GAP and its interaction with oncogenic *ras* p21. Nature 335:90–93, 1988.
99. Calés C, Hancock JF, Marshall CJ, Hall A: The cytoplasmic protein GAP is implicated as the target for regulation by the *ras* gene product. Nature 332:548–551, 1988.
100. Gibbs JB, Schaber MD, Allard WJ, Sigal IS, Scolnick EM: Purification of *ras* GTPase activating protein from bovine brain. Proc Natl Acad Sci USA 85:5026–5030, 1988.
101. Hoshino M, Kawakita M, Hattori S: Characterization of a factor that stimulates hydrolysis of GTP bound to *ras* gene product p21 (GTPase-activating protein) and correlation of its activity to cell density. Mol Cell Biol 8:4169–4173, 1988.
102. Lacal PM, Pennington CY, Lacal JC: Transforming activity of *ras* proteins translocated to the plasma membrane by a myristoylation sequence from the *src* gene product. Oncogene 2:533–538, 1988.
103. Adari H, Lowy DR, Willumsen BM, Der CJ, McCormick F: Guanosine triphosphatase activating protein (GAP) interacts with the p21 *ras* effector binding domain. Science 240:518–521, 1988.
104. Der CJ, Pan B–T, Cooper GM: *ras*H mutants deficient in GTP binding. Mol Cell Biol 6:3291–3294, 1986.
105. Clanton DJ, Lu Y, Blair DG, Shih TY: Structural significance of the GTP-binding domain of *ras* p21 studied by site-directed mutagenesis. Mol Cell Biol 7:3092–3097, 1987.
106. Feig LA, Corbley M, Pan B–T, Roberts TM, Cooper GM: Structure/function analysis of *ras* using random mutagenesis coupled with functional screening assays. Mol Cell Endocrinol 1:127–136, 1987.
107. Feig LA, Cooper GM: Relationship among guanine nucleotide exchange, GTP hydrolysis, and transforming potential of mutated *ras* proteins. Mol Cell Biol 8:2472–2478, 1988.
108. McCormick F, Clark BF, laCour TFM, Kjeldgoard M, Norskov-Lauritsen L, Nyborg J: A model for the tertiary structure of p21, the product of the *ras* oncogene. Science 230:78–82, 1985.
109. de Vos AM, Tong L, Milburn MV, Matias PM, Jancarik J, Noguchi S, Nishimura S, Miura K, Ohtsuka ES, Kim S–H: Three-dimensional structure of an oncogene protein: Catalytic domain of human c-H-*ras* p21. Science 239:888–893, 1988.
110. Clark R, Wong G, Arnheim N, Nitecki D, McCormick F: Antibodies specific for amino acid 12 of the *ras* oncogene product inhibit GTP binding. Proc Natl Acad Sci USA 82:5280–5284, 1985.
111. Feramisco JR, Clark R, Wong G, Arnheim N, Milley R, McCormick F: Transient reversion of *ras* oncogene-induced cell transformation by antibodies specific for amino acid 12 of *ras* protein. Nature 314:639–642, 1985.
112. Hattori S, Ulsh LS, Halliday K, Shih TY: Biochemical properties of a highly purified v-*ras*H p21 protein overproduced in *Escherichia coli* and inhibition of its activities by a monoclonal antibody. Mol Cell Biol 5:1449–1455, 1985.
113. Mulcahy LS, Smith MR, Stacey DW: Requirement for *ras* proto-oncogene function during serum-stimulated growth of NIH 3T3 cells. Nature 313:241–243, 1985.
114. Kung H–F, Smith MR, Bekesi E, Manne V, Stacey DW: Reversal of transformed phenotype by monoclonal antibodies against Ha-*ras* p21 proteins. Exp Cell Res 162:363–371, 1986.
115. Lacal JC, Aaronson SA: Monoclonal antibody Y13–259 recognizes an epitope of the p21 *ras* molecule not directly involved in the GTP-binding activity of the protein. Mol Cell Biol

6:1002–1009, 1986.
116. Willumsen BM, Papageorge AG, Kung H-F, Bekesi E, Robins T, Johnsen M, Vass WC, Lowy DR: Mutational analysis of a ras catalytic domain. Mol Cell Biol 6:2646–2654, 1986.
117. Lacal JC, Aaronson SA: ras p21 deletion mutants and monoclonal antibodies as tools for localization of regions relevant to p21 function. Proc Natl Acad Sci USA 83:5400–5404, 1986.
118. Goodrich GA, Burrell HR: Micromeasurement of nucleotide 5'-triphosphates using coupled bioluminescence. Anal Biochem 127:395–401, 1982.
119. Proud CG: Guanine nucleotides, protein phosphorylation and the control of translation. TIBS 11:73–77, 1986.
120. Reynolds SH, Stowers SJ, Patterson RM, Maronpot RR, Aaronson SA, Anderson MW: Activated oncogenes in B6C3F1 mouse liver tumors: Implications for risk assessment. Science 237:1309–1316, 1987.
121. Willingham MC, Pastan I, Shih TY, Scolnick EM : Localization of the src gene product of the Harvey strain of MSV to the plasma membrane of transformed cells by electron microscopic immunocytochemistry. Cell 19:1005–1014, 1980.
122. Shih TY, Weeks MO, Gruss P, Dhar R, Oroszlan S, Scolnick EM: Identification of a precursor in the biosynthesis of the p21 transforming protein of Harvey murine sarcoma virus. J Virol 42:253–261, 1982.
123. Sefton BM, Trowbridge IS, Cooper JA, Scolnick EM: The transforming proteins of Rous sarcoma virus, Harvey sarcoma virus and Abelson virus contain tightly bound lipid. Cell 31:465–474, 1982.
124. Willumsen BM, Christensen A, Hubbert NL, Papageorge AG, Lowry DR: The p21 ras C-terminus is required for transformation and membrane association. Nature 310:583–586, 1984.
125. Buss JE, Sefton BM: Direct identification of palmitic acid as the lipid attached to p21 ras. Mol Cell Biol 6:116–122, 1986.
126. Chen Z–Q, Ulsh LS, DuBois G, Shih T: Post-translational processing of p21 ras proteins involves palmitylation of the C-terminal tetrapeptide containing cysteine-186. J Virol 56: 607–612, 1985.
127. Tamanoi F, Hsueh EC, Goodman LE, Cobitz AR, Detrick RJ, Brown WR, Fujiyama A: Posttranslational modification of ras proteins: detection of a modification prior to fatty acid acylation and cloning of a gene responsible for the modification. J Cell Biochem 36: 261–273, 1988.
128. Magee AI, Gutierrez L, McKay IA, Marshall CJ, Hall A: Dynamic fatty acylation of p21N-ras. EMBO J 6:3353–3357, 1987.
129. Backlund PS, Aksamit RR: Guanine nucleotide-dependent carboxyl methylation of mammalian membrane proteins. J Biol Chem 263:15864–15867, 1988.
130. Willumsen BM, Norris K, Papageorge AG, Hubbert NL, Lowy DR: Harvey murine sarcoma virus p21 ras protein: Biological and biochemical significance of the cysteine nearest the carboxy terminus. EMBO J 3:2581–2585, 1984.
131. Sefton BM, Buss JE: The covalent modification of eukaryotic proteins with lipid. J Cell Biol, 1987.
132. Buss JE, Solski PA, Schaeffer JP, MacDonald MJ, Der CJ: Activation of the cellular proto-oncogene product p21c-ras by addition of a myristylation signal. Science 243:1600–1603, 1989
133. Signal IS, Gibbs JB, D'Alonzo JS, Scolnick EM : (1986). Identification of effector residues and a neutralizing epitope of Ha-ras-encoded p21. Proc Natl Acad Sci USA 83:4725–4729.
134. Stone JC, Vass, WC, Willumsen BM, Lowy DR: p21-ras effector domain mutants constructed by "cassette" mutagenesis. Mol Cell Biol 8:3565–3569, 1988.
135. Trahey M, Wong G, Halenbeck R, Rubinfeld B, Martin GA, Ladner M, Long CM, Crosier WJ, Watt K, Koths K, McCormick F: Molecular cloning of two types of GAP complementary DNA from human placenta. Science 242:1697–1700, 1988.
136. Furth ME, Aldrich TH, Cordon-Cardo C: Expression of ras proto-oncogene proteins in

normal human tissues. Oncogene 1:47–58, 1987.
137. Papageorge AG, Defeo-Jones D, Robinson P, Temeles G, Scolnick EM: *Saccharomyces cerevisiae* synthesizes proteins related to the p21 gene product of *ras* genes found in mammals. Mol Cell Biol 4:23–29, 1984.
138. Pawson T, Amiel T, Hinze E, Auersperg N, Neave N, Sobolewski A, Weeks G: Regulation of a *ras*-related protein during development of *Dictyostelium discoideum*. Mol Cell Biol 5:33–39, 1985.
139. Hattori S, Clanton DJ, Satoh T, Nakamura S, Kaziro Y, Kawakita M, Shih TY: Neutralizing monoclonal antibody against *ras* oncogene product p21 which impairs guanine nucleotide exchange. Mol Cell Biol 7:1999–2002, 1987.
140. Rasheed S, Norman GL, Heidecker G: Nucleotide sequence of the Rasheed rat sarcoma virus oncogene: New mutations. Science 221:155–157, 1983.
141. Lautenberger JA, Ulsh L, Shih TY, Papas TS: High-level expression in *Escherichia coli* of enzymatically active Harvey murine sarcoma virus p21*ras* protein. Science 221:858–860, 1983.
142. Lacal JC, Santos E, Notario V, Barbacid M, Yamazaki S, Kung H, Seamans C, McAndrew S, Crowl R: Expression of normal and transforming H-*ras* genes in *Escherichia coli* and purification of their encoded p21 proteins. Proc Natl Acad Sci USA 81:5305–5309, 1984.
143. Nakano ET, Rao MM, Perucho M, Inouye M: Expression of the Kirsten *ras* viral and human proteins in *Escherichia coli*. J Virol 61:302–307, 1987.
144. Buss JE, Der CJ, Solski PA: The six amino-terminal amino acids of p60*src* are sufficient to cause myristylation of p21v-*ras*. Mol Cell Biol 8:3960–3963, 1988.
145. Jurnak F: Structure of the GDP domain of EF-Tu and location of the amino acids homologous to *ras* oncogene proteins. Science 230:32–36, 1985.
146. Jurnak F: The three-dimensional structure of c-H-*ras* p21: Implications for oncogene and G protein studies. TIBS 13:195–198, 1988.
147. Gibbs JB, Schaber MD, Marshall MS, Scolnick EM, Sigal IS: Identification of guanine nucleotides bound to *ras*-encoded proteins in growing yeast cells. J Biol Chem 262: 10426–10429, 1987.
148. Satoh T, Nakamura S, Nakafuku M, Kaziro Y: Studies on *ras* proteins. Catalytic properties of normal and activated *ras* proteins purified in the absence of protein denaturants. Biochim Biophys Acta 25(949):97–109, 1988.
149. Field J, Broek D, Kataoka T, Wigler M: Guanine nucleotide activation of, and competition between, *ras* proteins from *Saccharomyces cerevisiae*. Mol Cell Biol 7:2128–2133, 1987.
150. Satoh T, Nakamura S, Kaziro Y: Induction of neurite formation in PC12 cells by microinjection of proto-oncogenic Ha-*ras* protein incubated with guanosine-5 -0-(3-thiotriphosphate). Mol Cell Biol 7:4553–4556, 1987.
151. Segev N, Mulholland J, Botstein D: The yeast GTP-binding YPT1 protein and a mammalian counterpart are associated with the secretion machinery. Cell 52:915–924, 1988.
152. Bourne HR: Do GTPases direct membrane traffic in secretion? Cell 53:669–671, 1988.
153. Goud B, Salminen A, Walworth NC, Novick PJ: A GTP-binding protein required for secretion rapidly associates with secretory vesicles and the plasma membrane in yeast. Cell 53:753–768, 1988.
154. Anderson PS, Lacal JC: Expression of the *Aplysia californica rho* gene in *Escherichia coli*: Purification and characterization of its encoded p21 product. Mol Cell Biol 7:3620–3628, 1987.
155. Kikuchi A, Yamamoto K, Fujita T, Takai Y: ADP-ribosylation of the bovine brain *rho* protein by botulinum toxin type C1. J Biol Chem 263:16303–16308, 1988.
156. Narumiya S, Sekine A, Fujiwara M: Substrate for botulinum ADP-ribosyltransferase, Gb, has an amino acid sequence homologous to a putative *rho* gene product. J Biol Chem 263:17255–17257, 1988.
157. Knight DE, Tonge DA, Baker PF: Inhibition of exocytosis in bovine adrenal medullary cells by botulinum toxin type D. Nature 317:719–721, 1985.
158. Bar-Sagi D, Feramisco JR: Induction of membrane ruffling and fluid-phase pinocytosis in

quiescent fibroblasts by *ras* proteins. Science 233:1061–1068, 1986.
159. Burgoyne RD: G proteins. Control of exocytosis. Nature 328:112–113, 1987.
160. Adam-Vizi V, Knight D: The *ras* protein is not associated with exocytosis. Nature 328: 581, 1987.
161. Lowe DG, Goeddel DV: Heterologous expression and characterization of the human R-*ras* gene product. Mol Cell Biol 7:2845–2856, 1987.
162. Lowe DG, Ricketts M, Levinson AD, Goeddel DV: Chimeric proteins define variable and essential regions of Ha-*ras*-encoded protein. Proc Natl Acad Sci USA 85:1015–1019, 1988.
163. Cooper GM: Cellular transforming genes. Science 217:801–806, 1982.
164. Taparowsky EJ, Heaney ML, Parsons JT: Oncogene-mediated multistep transformation of C3H10T1/2 cells. Cancer Res 47:4125–4129, 1987.
165. Land H, Parada LF, Weinberg RA: Tumorigenic conversion of primary embryo fibroblasts requires at least two cooperating oncogenes. Nature 304:596–606, 1983.
166. Yancopoulos GD, Nisen PD, Tesfaye A, Kohl NE, Goldfarb MP, Alt FW: N-*myc* co-operates with *ras* to transform normal cells in culture. Proc Natl Acad Sci USA 82: 5455–5459, 1985.
167. Land H, Chen AC, Morgenstern JP, Parada LF, Weinberg RA: Behavior of *myc* and *ras* oncogenes in transformation of rat embryo fibroblasts. Mol Cell Biol 6:1917–1925, 1986.
168. Ruley HE: Adenovirus early region 1A enables viral and cellular transforming genes to transform primary cells in culture. Nature 304:602–606, 1983.
169. Schwartz RC, Stanton LW, Riley SC, Marcu KB, Witte ON: Synergism of v-*myc* and v-Ha-*ras* in the *in vitro* neoplastic progression of murine lymphoid cells. Mol Cell Biol 6:3221–3231, 1986.
170. Fusco A, Berlingieri MT, Di Fiore PP, Portella G, Grieco M, Vecchio G: One- and two-step transformations of rat thyroid epithelial cells by retroviral oncogenes. Mol Cell Biol 7:3365–3370, 1987.
171. Weissman BE, Aaronson SA: BALB and Kirsten murine sarcoma viruses alter growth and differentiation of EGF-dependent BALB/c mouse epidermal keratinocyte lines. Cell 32: 599–606, 1983.
172. Weissman BE, Aaronson SA: Members of the *src* and *ras* oncogene families supplant the epidermal growth factor requirement of BALB/MK-2 keratinocytes and induce distinct alterations in their terminal differentiation program. Mol Cell Biol 5:3386–3396, 1985.
173. Jenkins JR, Rudge K, Currie GA: Cellular immortalization by a cDNA clone encoding the transformation-associated phosphoprotein p53. Nature 312:651–654, 1984.
174. Ridley AJ, Paterson HF, Noble M, Land H: *ras*-mediated cell cycle arrest is altered by nuclear oncogenes to induce Schwann cell transformation. EMBO J 7:1635–1645, 1988.
175. Schwab M, Varmus HE, Bishop JM: Human N-*myc* gene contributes to neoplastic transformation of mammalian cells in culture. Nature 316:160–162, 1985.
176. Eliyahu D, Raz A, Gruss P, Givol D, Oren M: Participation of p53 cellular tumour antigen in transformation of normal embryonic cells. Nature 312:646–649, 1984.
177. Parada LF, Land H, Weinberg RA, Wolf D, Rotter V: Cooperation between genes encoding p53 tumour antigen and *ras* in cellular transformation. Nature 312:649–651, 1984.
178. Namba M, Nishitani K, Fukushima F, Kimoto T, Nose K: Multistep process of neoplastic transformation of normal human fibroblasts by 60Co gamma rays and Harvey sarcoma viruses. Int J Cancer 37:419–423, 1986.
179. Sager R, Tanaka K, Lau CC, Ebina Y, Anisowicz A: Resistance of human cells to tumorigenesis induced by cloned transforming genes. Proc Natl Acad Sci USA 80:7601–7605, 1983.
180. Yoakum GH, Lechner JF, Gabrielson EW, Korba BE, Malan-Shibley L, Willey JC, Valerio MG, Shamsuddin AM, Trump BF, Harris CC: Transformation of human bronchial epithelial cells transfected by Harvey *ras* oncogene. Science 227:1174–1179, 1985.
181. Rhim JS, Jay G, Arnstein P, Price FM, Sanford KK, Aaronson SA: Neoplastic transformation of human epidermal keratinocytes by AD12-SV40 and Kirsten sarcoma virus. Science 227:1250–1252, 1985.

182. Spandidos DA, Wilkie NM: Malignant transformation of early passage rodent cell's by a single mutated human oncogene. Nature 310:469–475, 1984.
183. Noda M, Ko M, Ogura A, Liu D-G, Amano T, Takano T, Ikawa Y: Sarcoma viruses carrying *ras* oncogenes induce differentiation-associated properties in a neuronal cell line. Nature 318:73–75, 1985.
184. Bell JC, Jardine K, McBurney MW: Lineage-specific transformation after differentiation of multi-potential murine stem cells containing a human oncogene. Mol Cell Biol 6:617–725, 1986.
185. Schubert D, Heinemann S, Kodokoro Y: Cholinergic metabolism and synapse formation by a rat nerve cell line. Proc Natl Acad Sci USA 74:2579–2583, 1977.
186. Greene LA, Tischler AS: Establishment of noradrenergic clonal line of rat adrenal pheochromocytoma cells which respond to nerve growth factor. Proc Natl Acad Sci USA 73:2424–2428, 1976.
187. Hagag N, Halegoua S, Viola M: Inhibition of growth factor-induced differentiation of PC12 cells by microinjection of antibody to *ras* p21. Nature 319:680–682, 1986.
188. Nakagawa T, Mabry M, De Bustros A, Ihle JN, Nelkin BD, Baylin SB: Introduction of v-Ha-*ras* oncogene induces differentiation of cultured human medullary thyroid carcinoma cells. Proc Natl Acad Sci USA 84:5923–5927, 1987.
189. Craig RW, Sager R: Suppression of tumorigenicity in hybrids of normal and oncogene-transformed CHEF cells. Proc Natl Acad Sci USA 82:2062–2066, 1985.
190. Geiser AG, Der CJ, Marshall CJ, Stanbridge EJ: Suppression of tumorigenicity with continued expression of the c-Ha-*ras* oncogene in EJ bladder carcinoma-human fibroblast hybrid cells. Proc Natl Acad Sci USA 83:5209–5213, 1986.
191. Benedict WF, Weissman BE, Mark C, Stanbridge EJ: Tumorigenicity of human HT1080 fibrosarcoma X normal fibroblast hybrids: Chromosome dosage dependency. Cancer Res 44:3471–3479, 1984.
192. Schaefer R, Iyer J, Iten E, Nirkko AC: Partial reversion of the transformed phenotype in H*ras*-transfected tumorigenic cells by transfer of a human gene. Proc Natl Acad Sci USA 85:1590–1594, 1988.
193. Noda M, Selinger Z, Scolnick EM, Bassin RH: Flat revertants isolated from Kirsten sarcoma virus-transformed cells are resistant to the action of specific oncogenes. Proc Natl Acad Sci USA 80:5602–5606, 1983.
194. Wakelam MJO, Davies SA, Houslay MD, McKay I, Marshall CJ, Hall A: Normal p21N-*ras* couples bombesin and other growth factor receptors to inositol phosphate production. Nature 323:173–176, 1986.
195. Marshall CJ: Oncogenes and growth control. Cell 49:723–725, 1987.
196. Korn LJ, Siebel CW, McCormick F, Roth RA: *ras* p21 as a potential mediator of insulin action in Xenopus oocytes. Science 236:840–843, 1987.
197. Kamata T, Feramisco JR: Epidermal growth factor stimulates guanine nucleotide binding acitivity and phosphorylation of *ras* oncogene proteins. Nature 310:147–150, 1987.
198. Jeng AY, Srivastava SK, Lacal JC, Blumberg PM: Phosphorylation of *ras* oncogene product by protein kinase C. Biochem Biophys Res Commun 145:782–788, 1987.
199. Spina A, Di Donato A, Colella G, Illiano G, Berlingieri MT, Fusco A, Grieco M: Increased adenylate cyclase activity in rat thyroid epithelial cells expressing viral *ras* genes. Biochem Biophys Res Commun 142:527–535, 1987.
200. Franks DJ, Whitfield JF, Durkin JP: A viral K-*ras* protein increases the stimulability of adenylate cyclase by cholera toxin in NRK cells. Biochem Biophys Res Commun 147: 596–601, 1987.
201. Salterelli Biochem Biophys Res Commun 127:318–325, 1985.
202. Chiarugi V, Porciatti F, Pasquali F, Bruni P: Transformation of BALB/3T3 cells with EJ/T24/H-*ras* oncogene inhibits adenylate cyclase response to beta-adrenergic agonist while increases muscarinic receptor dependent hydrolysis of inositol lipids. Biochem Biophys Res Commun 132:900–907, 1985.
203. Levitzki A, Rudick J, Pastan I, Vass WC, Lowy DR: Adenylate cyclase activity of NIH/3T3

cells morphologically transformed by *ras* genes. FEBS Lett 197:134–138, 1986.
204. Birchemeier C, Broek D, Wigler M: *ras* proteins can induce meiosis in Xenopus oocytes. Cell 43:615–621, 1985.
205. Beckner SK, Hatton S, Shih TY: The *ras* oncogene product is not a regulatory component of adenylate cyclase. Nature 317:71–72, 1985.
206. Tarpley WG, Hopkins NK, Gorman RR: Reduced hormone-stimulated adenylate cyclase activity in NIH-3T3 cells expressing the EJ human bladder *ras* oncogene. Proc Natl Acad Sci USA 83:3703–3707, 1986.
207. Fukui Y, Kozasa T, Kaziro Y, Takeda T, Yamamoto M: Role of a *ras* homolog in the life cycle of *Schizosaccaromyces pombe*. Cell 44:329–336, 1986.
208. Mitchell B: Oncogenes and inositol lipids. Nature 308:770–770, 1984.
209. Berridge MJ, Irvine RF: Inositol trisphosphate, a novel second messenger in cellular signal transduction. Nature 312:315–321, 1984.
210. Nishizuka Y: Studies and perspectives of protein kinase C. Science 233:305–312, 1986.
211. Fleishman LF, Chahwala SB, Cantley L: *ras*-transformed cells: Altered levels of phosphatidylinositol-4,5-bisphosphate and catabolites. Science 231:407–410, 1986.
212. Parries G, Hoebel R, Racker E: Opposing effects of a *ras* oncogene on growth factor-stimulated phosphoinositide hydrolysis: Desensitization to platelet-derived growth factor and enhanced sensitivity to bradykinin. Proc Natl Acad Sci 84:2648–2652, 1987.
213. Benjamin CW, Connor JA, Tarpley WG, Gorman RR: NIH-3T3 cells transformed by the EJ-*ras* oncogene exhibit reduced platelet-derived growth factor-mediated Ca2+ mobilization. Proc Natl Acad Sci USA 85:4345–4349, 1988.
214. Preiss J, Loomis CR, Bishop WR, Stein R, Niedel JE, Bell RM: Quantitative measurement of sn-1,2-diacylglycerols present in platelets, hepatocytes and *ras*- and *sis*-transformed normal rat kidney cells. J Biol Chem 261:8597–8600, 1986.
215. Fukami K, Matsuoka K, Nakanishi O, Yamakawa A, Kawai S, Takenawa T: Antibody to phosphatidylinositol 4,5-bisphosphate inhibits oncogene-induced mitogenesis. Proc Natl Acad Sci USA 85:9057–9061, 1988.
216. Wolfman A, Macara IG: Elevated levels of diacylglycerol and decreased phorbol ester sensitivity in *ras*-transformed fibroblasts. Nature 325:359–361, 1987.
217. Lacal JC, Moscat J, Aaronson SA: Novel source of 1,2-diacylglycerol elevated in cells transformed by Ha-*ras* oncogene. Nature 330:269–272, 1987.
218. Seuwen K, Lagarde A, Pouyssegur J: Deregulation of hamster fibroblast proliferation by mutated *ras* oncogenes is not mediated by constitutive activation of phosphoinositide-specific phospholipase C. EMBO J 7:161–168, 1988.
219. Yu C–L, Tsai M–H, Stacey DW: Cellular *ras* activity and phospholipid metabolism. Cell 52:63–71, 1988.
220. Lacal JC, de la Pena P, Moscat J, Garcia-Barreno P, Anderson PS, Aaronson SA: Rapid stimulation of diacylglycerol production in Xenopus oocytes by microinjection of H-*ras* p21. Science 238:533–536, 1987.
221. Ballester R, Furth ME, Rosen OM: Phorbol ester- and protein kinase C-mediated phosphorylation of the cellular Kirsten *ras* gene product. J Biol Chem 262:2688–2695, 1987.
222. Lacal JC, Fleming TP, Warren HS, Blumberg PM, Aaronson SA: Involvement of functional protein kinase C in the mitogenic response to the H-*ras* oncogene product. Mol Cell Biol 7:4146–4149, 1987.
223. Smith MR, DeGudicibus SJ, Stacey DW: Requirement for c-*ras* proteins during viral oncogene transformation. Nature 320:540–543, 1986.
224. Feig LA, Cooper GM: Inhibition of NIH 3T3 cells proliferation by a mutant *ras* protein with preferential affinity for GDP. Mol Cell Biol 8:3235–3243, 1988.
225. Stacey DW, Watson T, Kung H–F, Curran T: Microinjection of transforming *ras* protein induces c-*fos* expression. Mol Cell Biol 7:523–527, 1987.
226. Harvey JJ: An unidentified virus which causes the rapid production of tumors in mice. Nature 204:1104–1105, 1964.
227. Kirsten WH, Mayer LA: Morphologic responses to a murine erythroblastosis virus. J Natl

Cancer Inst 39:311–334, 1967.
228. Rasheed S, Gardner MB, Huebner RJ: *In vitro* isolation of stable rat sarcoma viruses. Proc Natl Acad Sci USA 75:2972–2976, 1978.
229. Peters RL, Rabstein LS, Van Vleck R, Kelloff GJ, Huebner RJ: Naturally occurring sarcoma virus of the BALB/cCr mouse. J Natl Cancer Inst 53:1725–1729, 1984.
230. Franz T, Lohler J, Fusco A, Pragnell I, Nobis P, Padua R, and Ostertag W: Transformation of mononuclear phagocytes *in vivo* and malignant histiocytosis caused by a novel murine spleen focus-forming virus. Nature 315:149–151, 1985.
231. Frederickson TN, O'Neill RR, Rutledge TS, Theodore TS, Martin MA, Ruscetti SK, Austin JB, Hartley JW: Biologic and molecular characterization of two newly isolated *ras*-containing murine leukemia viruses. J Virol 61:2109–2119, 1987.
232. Weinberg RA: The action of oncogenes in the cytoplasm and nucleus. Science 230:770–776, 1985.
233. Hill M, Hillova J: Virus recovery in chicken cells tested with Rous sarcoma cell DNA. Nature 237:35–39, 1972.
234. Shimizu K, Goldfarb M, Perucho M, Wigler M: Isolation and preliminary characterization of the transforming gene of a human neuroblastoma cell line. Proc Natl Acad Sci USA 80:383–387, 1983.
235. Hall A, Marshall CJ, Spurr NK, Weiss RA: Identification of transforming gene in two human sarcania cell lines as a new member of the *ras* gene family located on chromosome 1, Nature 303: 396–400, 1983.
236. Bos JL: The *ras* gene family and human carcinogenesis: Mutation Res 195:255–271, 1987.
237. Bos JL, Fearon ER, Hamilton SR, Verlaan-de Vries M, van Boom JH, van der Eb, AJ Vogelstein R: Prevalence of *ras* gene mutations in human colorectal cancers. Nature 327: 293–297, 1987.
238. Forrester K, Almoguera C, Han K, Grizzle WE, Perucho M: Detection of high incidence of K-*ras* oncogenes during human colon tumorigenesis. Nature 327:298–303, 1987.
239. Almoguera C, Shibata D, Forrester K, Martin J, Arnheim N, Perucho M: Most human carcinoma of the exocrine pancreas contain mutant c-K-*ras* genes. Cell 53:549–554, 1988.
240. Sukumar S, Notario V, Martin-Zanca D, Barbacid M: Induction of mammary carcinomas in rats by nitroso-methylurea involves malignant activation of H-*ras*-1 locus by single point mutations. Nature 306:658–662, 1983.
241. Zarbl H, Sukumar S, Arthur AV, Martin-Zanca D, Barbacid M: Direct mutagenesis of Ha-*ras*-1 oncogenes by N-nitroso-N-methylurea during initiation of mammary carcinogenesis in rats. Nature 315:382–385, 1985.
242. Balmain A, Pragnell IB: Mouse skin carcinomas induced *in vivo* by chemical carcinogens have a transforming Harvey-*ras* oncogene. Nature 303:72–74, 1983.
243. Balmain A, Ramsden M, Bowden GT, Smith J: Activation of the mouse cellular Harvey-*ras* gene in chemically induced benign skin papillomas. Nature 307:658–660, 1984.
244. Gambke C, Signer E, Moroni C: Activation of N-*ras* gene in bone marrow cells from a patient with acute myeloblastic leukemia. Nature 307:476–478, 1984.
245. Bos JL, Toksoz D, Marshall CJ, Verlaan-deVries M, Veeneman GH, van der Eb AJ, van Boom J, Janssen JWG, Steenvoorden ACM: Amino-acid substitutions at codon 13 of the N-*ras* oncogene in human acute myeloid leukaemia. Nature 315:726–730, 1985.
246. Neri A, Knowles DM, Greco A, McCormick F, Dalla-Favera R: Analysis of *ras* oncogene mutations in human lymphoid malignancies. Proc Natl Acad Sci USA 85:9268–9272, 1988.
247. Bos JL, Verlaan-de Vries M, van der Eb AJ, Janssen JWG, Delwel R, Lowenberg B, Colly LP: Mutations in N-*ras* predominate in acute myeloid leukemia. Blood 69:1237–1241, 1987.
248. Rodenhuis S, Bos JL, Slater RM, Behrendt H, van 't Veer M, Smets LA: Absence of oncogene amplifications and occasional activation of N-*ras* in lymphoblastic leukemia of childhood. Blood 67:1698–1704, 1986.
249. Santos E, Martin-Zanca D, Reddy EP, Pierotti MA, Della-Porta G, Barbacid M: Malignant activation of a K-*ras* oncogene in lung carcinoma but not in normal tissue of the same

patient. Science 223:661–664, 1984.
250. Feig LA, Bast RC Jr, Knapp RC, Cooper GM: Somatic activation of *ras*K gene in a human ovarian carcinoma. Science 223:698–701, 1984.
251. O'Hara BM, Oskarsson M, Tainsky MA, Blair DG: Mechanism of activation of human *ras* genes cloned from a gastric adenocarcinoma and a pancreatic carcinoma cell line. Cancer Res 46:4695–4700, 1986.
252. Liu E, Hjelle B, Morgan R, Hecht F, Bishop JM: Mutations of the Kirsten-*ras* proto-oncogene in human preleukemia. Nature 330:186–188, 1987.
253. Hirai H, Kobayashi Y, Mano H, Hagiwara K, Maru Y, Omine M, Mizoguchi H, Nishida J, Takaku F: A point mutation at codon 13 of the N-*ras* oncogene in myelodysplastic syndrome. Nature 327:430–432, 1987.
254. Leon J, Kamino H, Steinberg JJ, Pellicer A: H-*ras* activation in benign and self-regressing skin tumors (keratoacanthomas) in both humans and an animal model system. Mol Cell Biol 8:786–793, 1988.
255. Albino AP, Le Strange R, Oliff AI, Furth ME, Old LJ: Transforming *ras* genes from human melanoma: A manifestation of tumor heterogeneity. Nature 308:68–72, 1984.
256. Guerrero I, Calzada P, Mayer A, Pellicer A: A molecular approach to leukemogenesis: Mouse lymphomas contain an activated c-*ras* oncogene. Proc Natl Acad Sci USA 81:202–205, 1984.
257. Diamond LE, Guerrero I, Pellicer A: Concomitant K- and N-*ras* gene point mutations in clonal murine lymphoma. Mol Cell Biol 8:2233–2236, 1988.
258. Kataoka T, Powers S, McGill C, Fasaro O, Strathern J, Broach J, Wigler M: Genetic analysis of yeast *RAS* 1 and *RAS* 2 genes. Cell 37:437–445, 1984.
259. Tatchell K, Chaleff DT, Defeo-Jones D, Scolnick EM: Requirement of either of a pair of *ras* related genes of *Saccharomyces cerevisiae* for spore viability, Nature 309:523–527, 1984.
260. Schmitt HD, Wagner P, Pfaff E, Gallwitz D: The *ras*-related *YPT1* gene product in yeast: A GTP-binding protein that might be involved in microtubule organization. Cell 47:401–412, 1986.
261. Segev N, Botstein D: The *ras*-like yeast *YPT1* gene is itself essential for growth, sporulation, and starvation response. Mol Cell Biol 7:2367–2377, 1987.
262. Schmitt HD, Puzicha M, Gallwitz D: Study of a temperature-sensitive mutant of the *ras*-related *YPT1* gene product in yeast suggests a role in the regulation of intracellular calcium. Cell 53:635–647, 1988.
263. Madaule P, Axel R, Myers AM: Characterization of two members of the *rho* gene family from the yeast Saccharomyces cerevisiae. Proc Natl Acad Sci USA 84:779–783, 1987.
264. Bos JL, Verlaan-de Vries M, Marshall CJ, Veeneman GH, van Boom JH, van der Eb AJ: A human gastric carcinoma contains a single mutated and an amplified normal allele of the Ki-*ras* oncogene. Nucleic Acids Res 14:1209–1217, 1986.
265. Filmus JE, Buick RN: Stability of c-K-*ras* amplification during progression in a patient with adenocarcinoma of the ovary. Cancer Res 45:4468–4472, 1985.
266. Winter E, Yamamoto F, Almoguera C, Perucho M: A method to detect and characterize point mutations in transcribed genes: amplification and overexpression of the mutant c-Ki-*ras* allele in human tumor cells. Proc Natl Acad Sci USA 82:7575–7579, 1985.
267. Slamon DJ, deKernion JB, Verma IM, Cline MJ: Expression of cellular oncogenes in human malignancies. Science 224:256–262, 1984.
268. Spandidos DA, Kerr IB: Elevated expression of the human *ras* oncogene family in premalignant and malignant tumours of the colorectum. Br J Cancer 49:681–688, 1984.
269. Clanton DJ, Hattori S, Shih TY: Mutations of the *ras* gene product p21 that abolish guanine nucleotide binding. Proc Natl Acad Sci USA 83:5076–5080, 1986.
270. Lacal JC, Aaronson SA: Activation of *ras* p21 transforming properties associated with an increase in the release rate of bound guanine nucleotide. Mol Cell Biol 6;4214–4220, 1986.
271. Alonso T, Morgan RO, Marvizon JC, Zarbl H, Santos E: Malignant transformation by *ras* and other oncogenes produce common alterations in inositol phospholipid signaling pathways. Proc Natl Acad Sci USA 85:4271–4275, 1988.

272. Santos E, Reddy EP, Pulciani S, Feldmann RJ, Barbacid M: Spontaneous activation of a human proto-oncogene. Proc Natl Acad Sci USA 80:4679–4682, 1983.
273. Thein SL, Oscier DG, Flint J, Wainscoat JS: Ha-*ras* hypervariable alleles in myelodysplasia. Nature 321:84–85, 1986.
274. McCormick F: *ras* GTPase activating protein: Signal transmitter and signal terminator. Cell 56:5–8, 1989.
275. Feig LA, Pan BT, Roberts TM, Cooper GM: Isolation of *ras* GTP binding mutants using an *in situ* colony–binding assay. Proc Natl Acad Sci USA 83:4607–4611, 1986.
276. Clarke S, Vogel JP, Deschenes RJ, Stock J: Posttranslational modification of the Ha-*ras* oncogene protein: Evidence for a third class of protein carboxyl methyltransferases. Proc Natl Acad Sci USA 85:4643–4647, 1988.
277. Kamps MP, Buss JE, Sefton BM: Mutation of N-terminal glycine of p60*src* prevents both myristoylation and morphological transformation. Proc Natl Acad Sci USA 82:4625–4628, 1985.
278. Sassone-Corsi P, Der CJ, Verma IM: *Ras*-induced differentiation of PC12 cells: Possible involvement of *fos* and *jun*. Mol Cell Biol, in press.
279. Molenaar CMT, Prange R, Gallwitz D: A carboxyl-terminal cysteine residue is required for palmitic acid binding and biological activity of the *ras*-related yeast YPT1 protein. EMBO J 7:971–976, 1988.
280. Oshimura M, Gilmer TM, Barrett JC. Nonrandom loss of chromosome 15 in Syrian hamster tumours induced by v-Ha-*ras* plus v-*myc* oncogenes. Nature 316:636–639, 1985.
281. Katan M, Parker PJ: Oncogenes and cell control. Nature 332:203, 1988.

5. *src*-related protein tyrosine kinases

André Veillette and Joseph B. Bolen

Tyrosine protein kinases (TPKs) catalyze the transfer of phosphate groups from nucleotide triphosphates to tyrosine residues on proteins and peptides. While phosphorylation of proteins on tyrosine residues is a well-known post-translational event detected in different regulatory systems, only a small number of cellular proteins are known substrates for TPKs [1]. Coupled with the likelihood that many of these modifications are rapidly turned over, it is not surprising that the abundance of phosphotyrosine in most cells is less than 0.05% of the steady-state phosphoamino-acids [2]. There are about 30 mammalian TPKs that have been identified to date (table 1); however, this number is expected to increase as strategies for cloning new genes belonging to this group become more refined. Most TPKs can be divided into two major groups (table 1): those corresponding to growth factor receptors (such as the epidermal growth factor receptor) and those associated with the internal portion of the plasma membrane (such as the c-*src* protein). The growth factor receptors are covered elsewhere (see chapters 8 and 9).

Three different groups of tyrosine kinase genes known or predicted to encode products associated with the inner aspect of the cytoplasmic membrane have been described: the *src* family, the *fes/fps* family, and the *abl* family. The members of a given family are likely to be derived from a single ancestor gene since their exon–intron structures appear to be highly conserved and since they encode closely related products. However, as will be discussed later, the different members of these gene families can vary significantly in their tissue distribution and have notable structural differences. These observations have led to the speculation that the different families and even different members within a single family provide unique functions in normal cellular physiological processes. It is also clear from a variety of experimental systems that gene products belonging to each of these families possess the ability to participate in oncogenic transformation.

This review will focus on the *src*-related family of gene products, since this group provides several of the best examples of our current understanding of the regulation and function of non-growth-factor-receptor protein tyrosine kinases. The *src* family is currently comprised of seven members: c-*src* [3–5], c-*yes* [6], c-*fgr* [7–9], *fyn* [10,11], *lck* [12,13], *hck* [14–16], and *lyn* [17]. A

Table 1. Mammalian protein tyrosine kinase genes

Growth-factor-receptor tyrosine kinase genes
1. Epidermal growth factor receptor family
   - EGFR: epidermal growth factor receptor gene (homologue of the v-*erb*B oncogene from avian erythroblastosis virus)
   - *neu*: cellular oncogene found in rat neuroblastomas
2. Insulin receptor gene family
   - INS.R: insulin receptor gene
   - IGF1R: insulinlike growth factor 1 receptor gene
   - c-*ros*: homologue of the UR2 avian sarcoma virus oncogene
   - *trk*: cellular oncogene from colon carcinoma activated through genetic recombination
   - *met*: N-methyl-N-nitro-N-nitrosoguanidine – induced cellular oncogene
   - *ltk*: leukocyte tryosine kinase gene
   - *eph*: tyrosine kinase gene related to growth factor receptor genes
3. Platelet-derived growth factor receptor gene family
   - PDGFR: platelet-derived growth factor receptor gene
   - CSF1R: colony stimulating factor-1 receptor gene (homologue of the v-*fms* McDonough feline sarcoma virus oncogene)
   - c-*kit*: homologue of the Hardy-Zuckerman 4 feline sarcoma virus oncogene
   - *ret*: cellular oncogene from T-cell lymphoma activated through genetic recombination

Non-growth-factor-receptor tyrosine kinase genes
1. *src* family
   - c-*src*: homologue of the v-*src* Rous sarcoma virus oncogene
   - c-*yes*: homologue of the v-*yes* Yamaguchi 73 sarcoma virus oncogene
   - c-*fgr*: homologue of the v-*fgr* Gardner–Rasheed sarcoma virus oncogene
   - *fyn*: tyrosine protein kinase gene related to *src* and *yes*
   - *lck*: lymphoid cell tyrosine protein kinase gene
   - *lyn*: lymphoid cell tyrosine protein kinase gene
   - *hck*: hematopoietic cell tyrosine protein kinase gene
   - *tkl*: *lck*-like tyrosine protein kinase gene
2. *abl* family
   - c-*abl*: homologue of the v-*abl* Abelson leukemia virus oncogene
   - *arg*: tyrosine protein kinase gene related to c-*abl*
3. *fes/fps* family
   - c-*fes*/c-*fps*: homologues of Gardner–Arnstein, Snyder–Theilen, Fujinami, and PRCII sarcoma virus oncogenes

potential additional member (*tkl*) has recently been described [18], and it is possible that other closely related genes will be discovered in the future. The members of the *src* family are all predicted or known to be membrane-associated phosphoproteins that lack amino acid sequences required for transmembrane insertion. This lack of transmembrane and cell surface domains structurally distinguishes this gene family from the tyrosine kinases which function as peptide hormone receptors.

General properties

The genomic organization of the various members of the *src* family of genes is thought to be highly conserved, although the genomic sequences of most family members have not been rigorously evaluated. For avian c-*src*, the genomic sequence contains 11 coding exons [5] with the initiating methionine codon in exon 2 and the amber codon located in exon 12. While the structure of the avian and human c-*src* genes is similar, the introns of the human c-*src* gene are significantly larger than their avian counterparts [19,20]. The overall size of the c-*src* gene in either species is not precisely known since additional 5' and 3' noncoding exons are continuing to be delineated.

The DNA sequences required for the transcriptional control of the members of the c-*src* gene family have not been determined, although analysis of upstream elements of c-*src* and *lck* are currently underway by several groups. Transcriptional control is an important issue to be addressed for at least some of the members of this gene family for which expression levels in different cell types appear to be controlled primarily at the RNA level. This has been clearly documented for *lck* [12,21] in a variety of normal cell and tissue types. Current studies from this laboratory indicate that the abundance of the *c-yes* and *fyn* gene products in a variety of human cells also correlates very closely with the relative levels of *c-yes* and *fyn* RNAs (A. Veillette, I.D. Horak, and J.B. Bolen, unpublished). It has not yet been established whether the abundance of RNA is regulated primarily at the transcriptional or posttranscriptional level.

Evaluation of the murine LSTRA cells has provided evidence suggesting that the expression of the *lck* gene product ($p56^{lck}$) may also be regulated at the translational level [22]. The marked overexpression of $p56^{lck}$ in this Moloney Murine Leukemia Virus (M-MuLV) induced thymoma cell line results at least partially from increased levels of *lck* transcripts as a consequence of an insertion of the retroviral Long Terminal Repeat (LTR) upstream of the *lck* gene [12,13,23]. The LTR insertion also removes several AUGs located upstream of the initiating codon on the mature *lck* mRNA molecule, allowing for more efficient translation of the RNA and further increase in the levels of $p56^{lck}$ [22]. While similar AUGs are present in other *src*-related tyrosine kinase mRNAs [7,10,11,14–16], it remains to be determined if translational regulation plays an important role in physiologically relevant expression control mechanisms.

The tissue distribution of the different *src*-related tyrosine kinases is varied (table 2). Some have been found to be expressed in virtually all cell types (c-*src*, *c-yes* and *fyn*), with others having a more restricted pattern of tissue expression (*lck*, *c-fgr*, *lyn*, and *hck*). While it is believed that the *src*-related kinases all aid in the mediation of various cellular signaling pathways, organization of the *src*-related genes into 'ubiquitous' and 'tissue-specific' expression subgroups reflects the potential for two functional classes of gene products within this family. The first group, represented by c-*src*, might be important for basic cellular signal transduction processes such as those mediating proliferation and differentiation pathways [24–30], while the second group, represented by *lck*, might be involved in more specialized functions such as signal transduction events during the activation of lymphoid cells by antigen [31,32].

Table 2. src-related tyrosine kinase genes

Gene	Chromosome	mRNA (kb)	Protein[a] (kDa)	Tissue
c-src	20q13.3	5.0	60	High in brain and platelets;
c-yes	18q21.3	4.8	62	High in kidney and liver
fyn	6q21	3.0	60	High in brain and T-cells
c-fgr	1p36.1	3.0	59	Granulocytes; macrophages
lck	1p32-p35	2.2	56	T-cells
hck	20q11-q12	2.2	(55)	Granulocytes; macrophages
lyn	8q13-qter.	3.2	(56)	B-cells
tkl	?	?	?	?

[a] Number in parentheses indicates predicted molecular weight.

Primary translation product

Carboxy-terminal region

The primary translation products of the src-related genes vary between 505 and 543 amino acids in length, with predicted molecular weights of 55 to 62 kilodaltons (kDa) (figure 1). The sequences of the src-related proteins are most highly conserved over their carboxy-terminal halves, which grossly encompass the catalytic region responsible for the protein kinase functions (figures 1 and 2). In avian pp60^{c-src}, this region extends approximately from residue 260 to residue 516. This domain contains the ATP binding site centered around lysine 295 (K295) [33] and the major autophosphorylation site at tyrosine residue 416 (Y416) [34,35]. There are other conserved sequence motifs in this domain that are found in other protein kinases (including the growth factor receptors and cAMP-dependent protein kinase) that are thought to be important for nucleotide triphosphate and divalent cation binding and/or for the actual catalytic process. These sequences include the Gly-X-Gly-X-X-Gly (actual sequence Gly-Gln-Gly-Cys-Phe-Gly) motif, which extends from residue 274 to 279, and the Asp-X-X-X-X-Asn (actual sequence Asp-Leu-Arg-Ala-Ala-Asn) motif, located between amino acids 386 and 391 in the avian c-src gene product. The first of these motifs is found in a wide variety of nucleotide-binding proteins and is believed to form part of the nucleotide-binding fold [36]. The second motif, along with another region between amino acids 425 and 432 (Pro-Ile-Lys-Trp-Thr-Ala-Pro-Glu) [37], may be involved in identifying the appropriate hydroxyamino acid target (i.e., tyrosine versus serine/threonine) on substrate peptides and proteins. Site-specific mutational analysis of these and other sequences in this group of enzymes will undoubtedly provide an interesting area for future research.

A highly conserved 'regulatory' domain of the src family of protein kinases is located at the carboxy terminus of the molecules adjacent to the catalytic domain [5] (figure 2). In avian c-src, the regulatory domain consists of 17 amino acids representing residues 517 to 533 (Glu-Asp-Tyr-Phe-Thr-Ser-Thr-

```
C-SRC  MGSSKSKP-KDP----SQRRRSLEPPDSTHHGGFPASQTPNKTAAPDTHRTPS-RSF--------GTVATEPKLFGFNTS
C-YES  MGCIKSKENKSPAIKRPENTPEPVST-SVS--HYGAEPTT-VSPCPSSSAKGTAVNFSSLSMTPFGGSSGVTPFGGASSS
FYN    MGCVQCKD-KEATKLTEERDGSL---NQSSGYRYGTDPTPQHYPSFGVTSIPNYVNNF---HAA--GGQGLTV-FGGVNSS
C-FGR  MGCVFCKKLEPVATAKEDAGLEGDFRSYGAADHYGPDPTKARPASSFAH-IPNYSNFSSQAINP-GFLDSGTI-RGVSG-
LCK    MGCVCSS-NPE----------------------DDWMENIDVCENCHYPIVPL-DSKISLPIRNGSEVRDPL
HCK    MGCMKSK---------------------FLQVGGNTFSKTETSASPHCPVYVP-DPTSTIKPGPNSHNSNTP
LYN    MGCIKSK------------------GKDSLSDDGVDLKTQPVRNTERT-------IYVR-DPTSNKQQRPVPESLLPG
tkl    *****************************************************************PL


C-SRC  DTVTSPQRAGALAGGVTTFVALVDYESRTETDLSFKKGERFQIVNNT-EGDWWLARSLTTGQTGYIPSNYVAPSDSIQAE
C-YES  FSVVPSSYPAGLTGGVTIFVALYDYEARTTEDLSFKKGERFQIINNT-EGDWWEARSIATGKNGYIPSNYVAPADSIQAE
FYN    SHTGTLRTRGG-T-GVTLFVALYDYEARTEDDLSFHKGEKFQILNSS-EGDWWEARSLTTGETGYIPSNYVAPVDSOQAE
C-FGR  -------------IGVTLFIALYDYEARTEDDLTFTKGEKFHILNNT-EGDWWEARSLSSGKTGCIPSNYVAPVDSIQAE
LCK    VTYEGSLPPASPL-QDNLVIALHSYEPSHDGDLGFEFKEQLRILEQS--GEWWKAQSLTTGQEGFIPFNFVAKANSLEPE
HCK    ----GIREAGSEDI---IVVALYDVEAIHHEDLSFQKGDQMVVLEES--GEWWKARSLATRKEGYIPSNYVARVDSLETE
LYN    ----QRFQTKDPEEQGDIVVALVPYDGIHPDDLSFKKGEKMKVLEER--GEWWKAKSLLTKKEGFIPSNYVAKLNTLETE
tkl    VS-EAMSPPCSPL-QDKLVVALYDYEPTHDGDLGLKQGEQLRVLEES--GEWWRAQSLTTGQEGLIPHNFVAMVNSLEPE


C-SRC  EWYFGKITRRESERLLLNPENPRGTFLVRESETTKGAYCLSVSDFDNAKGLNVKHYKIRKLDSGGFYITSRTQFSSLQQL
C-YES  EWYFGKMGRKDAERLLLNPGNQRGIFLVRESETTKGAYSLSIRDWDEIRGDNVKHYKIRKLDNGGYYITTRAQFDTLQKL
FYN    EWYFGKLGRKDAERQLLSFGNPRGTFLIRESETTKGAYSLSIRDWDDMKGDHVKHYKIRKLDNGGYYITTRAQFETLQQL
C-FGR  EWYFGKIGRKDAERQLLSPGNPQGAFLIRESETTKGAYSLSIRDWDQTRGDHVKHYKIRKLDMGGYYITTRVQFNSVQEL
LCK    FWFFKNLSRKDAERQLLAPGNTHGSFLIRESESTAGSFSLSVRDFDQNQGEVVKHYKIRNLDNGGFYISPRITFPGLHDL
HCK    EWFFFKGISRKDAERQLLAPGNMEDLGSFMIRDSETTKGSYSLSVRDYDPRQGDTVKHYKIRTLDNGGFYISPRSTFSTLQEL
LYN    EWFFKDITRKDAERQLLAPGNSAGAFLIRESETLKGSFSLSVRDFDPYHGDVIKHYKIRSLDNGGYYISPRITFPCISDM
tkl    PWPPLNLSRKNAEARLLASGNTHGSFLIRESETSKGSYSLSVRDFDQNQGETVKHYKIRNMDNGGYYISPRVTFSSLHEL


                                                                            1
C-SRC  VAYYSKHADGLCHRLTNVCPTSKPQTQGL---AKDAWEIPRESLRLEVKLGQGCFGEVWMGTWNGTTRVAIKTLKPGNMSP
C-YES  VKHYTEHADGLCHKLTTVCPTVKPQTQGL---AKDAWEIPRESLRLEVKLGQGCFGEVWMGTWNGTTKVAIKTLKPGTMMP
FYN    VQRYSERAAGLCCRLVVPCHKGMPRLTDLSVKTKDVWEIPRESLQLIKRLGNGQFGEVWMGTWNGNTKVAIKTLKPGTMSP
C-FGR  VQHYMEVNDGLCNLLIAPCTIMKPQTLGL---AKDAWEISRSSITLERRLGTGCFGDVWLGTWNGSTKVAVKTLKPGTMSP
LCK    VRHYTNASDGLCTKLSRPCQTQKPQKP----WWEDEWEVPRETLKLVERLGAGQFGEVWMGYVNGHTKVAVKSLKQGSMSP
HCK    VDHYKKGNDGLCQKLSVPCMSSKPQKP----WEKDAWEIPRESLKLVERLGAGQFGEVWMGVYNGHTKVAVKSLKQGSMSP
LYN    IKHYQKQADGLCRRLEKACISPKPQKP----WDKDAWEIPRESIKLVKRLGAGQFGEVWMGVYNNSTKVAVKTLKPGTMSV
tkl    VEYYSSSSDGLCTRLGKPCRTQKPQKP----WWJQDEWEVPRESLKLVEKLGAGQFGEVWMGFYNGHTKVAIKNLKQGSMSP


C-SRC  EAFLQEAQVMKKLRHEKLVQLYAVVS-EEPIYIVTEYMSKGSLLDFLKGEMGKYLRLPQLVDMAAQIASGMAYVERMNYVH
C-YES  EAFLQEAQIMKKLRHDKLVPLYAVVS-EEPIYIVTEFMSKGSLLDFLKEGDGKYVLKLPQLVDMAAQIADGMAYIERMNIH
FYN    ESFLEEAQIMKKLKHDKLVQLYAVVS-EEPIYIVTEYMNKGSLLDFLKDGEGRALKLPNLVDMAAQVAAGMAYIERMNYIH
C-FGR  KAFLEEAQVMKLLRHDKLVQLYAVVS-EEPIYIVTEFMCHGSLLDFLKNPEGQDLRLPQLVDMAAQVAEGMAYMERMNYIH
LCK    DAFLAEANLMKQLQHPRLVRLYAVVT-QEPIYIITEYMENGSLVDFLKTPSGIKLNVNKLLDMAAQIAEGMAFIEEQNYIH
HCK    EAFLAEANVMKTLQHDKLVKLHAVVT-KEPIYIITEFMAKGSLLDFLKSDEGSKQPLPKLIDFSAQIAEGMAFIEQRNYIH
LYN    QAFLEEANLMKTLQHDKLVRLYAVVTREEPIYIITEYMAKGSLLDFLKSDEGGKVLLPKLIDFSAQIAEGMAYIERKNYIH
tkl    SAFLAEANLMKNLQHPRLVR-YAVVT-KEPIYIITEYMEKGSLVDFLKTSEGIKLSINKLLDMAAQIAEGMAFIEAKNYIH


                                     2
C-SRC  RDLRAANILVGENLVCKVADFGLARLIEDNEYTARQGAKFPIKWTAPEAALYGRFTIKSDVWSFGILLTELTTKGRVPYPG
C-YES  RDLRAANILVGENLVCKIADFGLARLIEDNEYTARQGAKFPIKWTAPEAALYGRFTIKSDVWSFGILQTELVTKGRVPYPG
FYN    RDLRAANILVGNGLICKIADFGLARLIEDNEYTARQGAKFPIKWTAPEAALYGRFTIKSDVWSFGILLTELVTKGRVPYPG
C-FGR  RDLRAANILVGERLACKIADFGLARLIKDDEYNPCQGSKFPIKWTAPEAALFGRFTIKSDVWSFGILLTELITKGRIPYPG
LCK    RDLRAANILVSDTLSCKIADFGLARLIEDNEYTAREGAKFPIKWTAPEAINYGTFTIKSDVWSFGILLTEIVTHGRIPYPG
HCK    RDLRAANILVSASLVCKIADFGLARVIEDNEYTAREGAKFPIKWTAPEAINFGSFTIKSDVWSFGILLMEIVTYGRIPYPG
LYN    RDLRAANVLVSESLMCKIADFGLARVIEDNEYTAREGAKFPIKWTAPEAINFGCFTIKSDVWSFGILLYEIVTYGKIPYPG
tkl    RDLRAANILVSEALCCKIADFGLARLIEDNEYTAREGAKFPIKWTAPEAINYGTFTIKSDVWSFGILLTEIVTYGRIPYPG


                                                                 3
C-SRC  MVNREVLDQVERGYRMPCPPECPESLHDLMCQCWRKDPEERPTFEYLQAFLEDYFTSTEPQYQPGENL
C-YES  MVNREVLEQVERGYRMPCPQGCPESLHELMNLCWKKDPERPTFEYIQSFLEDYFTATEPQYQPGENL
FYN    MNNREVLEQVERGVRMPCPQDCPISLHELMIHCWKKDPEERPTFEYLQSFLEDYFTATEPQYQPGENL
C-FGR  MNKREVLEQVEQGVHMPCPPGCPASLYEAMEQTWRLDPEERPTFEYLQSFLEDYFTSAEPQYQPGDQT
LCK    MTNPEVIQNLERGYRVMRPDNCPEELYHLMMLCWKERPEDRPTFDYLRSVLDDFFTATEGQYQPQP
HCK    RTNADVMTALSQGYRMPRVENCPDELYDIMKMCWKEKAEERPTFDYLQSVLDDFYTATEGQYQQQP
LYN    RTNADVMTALSQGYRMPRVENCPDELYDIMKMCWKEKAEERPTFDYLQSVLDDFYTATEGQYQQQP
tkl    MTNPEVIQNLERGYRMPQPDNCPQELTELMNQCWKEQPEERPTFEYMKSVLEDFFTATEGQYQQQP
```

(1) Lysine at ATP binding site (2) Tyrosine autophosphorylation site (3) Major in vivo tyrosine phosphorylation site

Figure 1. Predicted amino acid sequences of the *src* family of protein tyrosine kinases.

Glu-Pro-Gln-*Tyr*-Gln-Pro-Gly-Glu-Asn-Leu). The consensus sequence for the *src* gene family is X-Asp-Tyr-Phe-Thr-X-X-Glu-X-Gln-Tyr-Gln-X-X-X-X-X. This region includes the major site of in vivo tyrosine phosphorylation (Y527) [38,39]. The relevance of these carboxy-terminal sequences in the regulation of the enzymatic activity of *src*-related kinases will be addressed in a later section.

AVIAN pp60[c-src]

```
 M                P¹      P²
 ▼                ▼       ▼
MGSSKSKPKD  PSQRRRSLEP  PDSTHHGGFP  ASQTPNKTAA  PDTHRTPSRS  FGIVATEPKL   60
  2           12   17
                                                            ┌RKVDVR┐
FGGFNTSDTV  TSPQRAGALA  GGVTTFVALY  DYESRTETDL  SFKKGERLQI  VNNTEGDWWL  120
                                ┌→SHR
ARSLTTGQTG  YIPSNYVAPS  DSIQAEEWYF  GKITRRESER  LLLNPENPRG  TFLVRESETT  180
 SHR←┐
KGAYCLSVSD  FDNAKGLNVK  HYKIRKLDSG  GFYITSRTQF  SSLQQLVAYY  SKHADGLCHR  240
                      ┌→K                                   ATP
                                                             ▼
LTNVCPTSKP  QTQGLAKDAW  EIPRESLRLE  VKLGQGCFGE  VWMGTWNGTT  RVAIKTLKPG  300
                                                              295
NMSPEAFLQE  AQVMKKLRHE  KLVQLYAVVS  EEPIYIVTEY  MSKGSLLDFL  KGEMGKYLRL  360
                                                                  P³
                                                                   ▼
PQLVDMAAQI  ASGMAYVERM  NYVHRDLRAA  NILVGENLVC  KVADFGLARL  IEDNEYTARQ  420
                                                              416
GAKFPIKWTA  PEAALYGRFT  IKSDVWSFGI  LLTELTTKGR  VPYPGMVNRE  VLDQVERGYR  480
                                    K←┬→R       P⁴          R←┐
                                                ▼
MPCPPECPES  LHDLMCQCWR  KDPEERPTFE  YLQAFLEDYF  TSTEPQYQPG  ENL        533
                                                  527
```

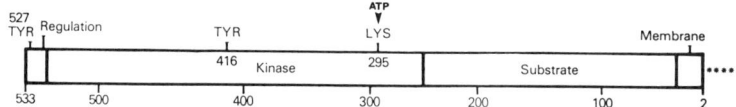

Figure 2. Structural organization and posttranslational modifications of avian pp60[c-src]. M: site of glycine 2 myristylation; P^1: site of serine 12 phosphorylation; P^2: site of serine 17 phosphorylation; RKVDVR: neuronal-specific amino acid insertion; SHR: short homology region; K: beginning of kinase domain; ATP: ATP binding site at lysine 295; P^3: autophosphorylation site at tyrosine 416; R: beginning of regulatory domain; P^4: site of phosphorylation at tyrosine 527. The lower panel shows a schematic representation of several of the features indicated along the amino acid sequence with the designation of the substrate interactive domain, as well as the myristylation and membrane-association domain.

Amino-terminal region

The amino-terminal half of the *src*-related protein kinases contains sequences essential for myristylation, membrane transport, stable membrane association, and, most likely, substrate interaction [40–42]. Additionally, there is accumulating evidence suggesting that this region interacts with the carboxy-terminal domain to modulate the enzymatic activity of these molecules. As might be expected from the list of functions assigned to the amino-terminal portions of the *src*-related proteins, the overall sequence homology between family members varies significantly, although selected motifs retain conserved distribution and sequence identity (figure 1).

Despite the fact that pp60[c-src] is translated on free ribosomes [43], this protein and all the other *src* family gene products tested thus far have proven to be predominantly membrane-associated. Work with the *src* protein has established that this cellular localization results from the cotranslational addition of a fatty acid (myristate) to the penultimate amino-terminal amino acid glycine (G2) (the initiating methionine is also cleaved during translation) [44,45]. Myristate addition is also dependent upon the sequence of the first several distal amino acids of the protein, which are also likely to be critical for transport and targeting to the cytoplasmic face of the plasma membrane [40]. Mutation of the G2 residue results in the localization of pp60^{c-src} to the cytoplasm and renders pp60^{v-src} incapable of transforming NIH3T3 fibroblasts [46,47]. It has recently been shown that stable association of pp60^{v-src} with the membrane phospholipid bilayer is also dependent upon the presence of other cell membrane-associated components [41,42]. While the nature of these membrane factors is not known, it has been suggested that these components may represent internal membrane receptors [41,42]. Since G2 is conserved in all members of the *src*-family, it is probable that all are myristylated and membrane-associated. Thus, the subcellular locale of this group of enzymes suggests that they are ideally positioned to communicate with cell surface components and with other membrane-associated molecules.

The region between avian c-*src* residues 8 and 80 is notable both for the lack of sequence homology with other members of the *src* family and for the fact that this region possesses multiple sites of serine/threonine phosphorylation [24,25,48–51]. It has also been proposed that this domain is the site of specific regulatory alterations and may help regulate the interaction of this group of enzymes with specific cellular substrates. With regard to phosphorylation, serine residue 17 of the c-*src* protein has been shown to be phosphorylated by the cAMP-dependent protein kinase [52], while serine 12 is modified by protein kinase C [50]. There are additional sites of amino-terminal serine and threonine phosphorylation in pp60^{c-src} that have not been precisely mapped or associated with the action of a specific protein kinase [24,25]. The avian pp60^{c-src} serines 12 and 17 are not conserved in the other members of the *src* family, and it has been suggested that modifications of these amino acids by phosphorylation represent important pp60^{c-src}-specific regulatory changes. While site specific mutagenesis of these serine residues has not yielded c-*src* molecules with detectable alterations in function ([53]; D. Shalloway, personal communication), phosphorylation at these sites may nevertheless be important for yet undefined pp60^{c-src} functions. It remains to be established if other members of the *src* family are also subject to similar phosphorylation events within this non-conserved domain.

The amino acid sequences between residues 144 and 190 in avian c-*src* are conserved in all *src*-related tyrosine kinases as well as in the c-*abl* and c-*fes/fps* proteins. This region has been designated as SH2 (for Short Homology Region 2) [54]. Various mutations in this region have been shown to modify the transforming properties of the v-*fps* protein [55], apparently due to alterations in the interaction of this domain with cellular substrates or cellular regulators. Interestingly, a similar domain has recently been described in a phospholipase C isoenzyme [56] and in the retroviral oncogenic protein p47$^{gag-crk}$ [57]. Although these two gene products do not possess tyrosine kinase activity, the conservation of the SH2 region raises the possibility that these different proteins may be under the control of common regulatory processes or may be able to interact with a common set of cellular substrates. Support for this idea is provided by the observation that transformation by the viral *crk* oncogene is associated with a marked increase in the phosphorylation of cellular proteins on tyrosine residues [57].

Post translational regulation: Phosphorylation

Carboxy-terminal region

There is a high degree of phosphate occupancy of tyrosine residue 527 (Y527) on pp60^{c-src} molecules expressed in fibroblasts [39]. Mutation of this residue by substituting Y527 with a phenylalanine [58–60] or truncation of the carboxy-terminal portion of pp60^{c-src} distal to leucine 516 [61] results in a marked (5 to 10-fold) increase in tyrosine phosphotransferase activity of the protein as measured by immune-complex kinase assays. These changes in pp60^{c-src} protein kinase-specific activity are associated with the acquisition of the ability of these mutant proteins to transform cells of fibroblastic lineage (see below). The importance of the occupancy state of Y527 in the regulation of the enzymatic activity of pp60^{c-src} is further supported by experiments in which dephosphorylation of pp60^{c-src} by potato acid phosphatase was shown to result in an elevation of the specific activity of the enzyme [62]. The notion that conformational changes play an important role in this process is strongly suggested by other experiments showing that binding of peptide antibodies to this c-*src* regulatory region increases the protein kinase activity of pp60^{c-src} even in the presence of fully phosphorylated tyrosine 527 [62]. Therefore, the conformation induced by occupancy of this tyrosine residue seems to be critical for decreasing c-*src* tyrosine kinase activity. Since, as indicated above, the phosphate occupancy of the Y527 in vivo is thought to be high (at least in fibroblasts), the protein kinase activity of pp60^{c-src} is considered to be normally repressed. Thus, the tyrosine kinase(s) and phosphatase(s) controlling the dynamics of the phosphorylation state of this residue represent potentially potent regulators of enzyme activity. While there is no experimental evidence that transient hypophosphorylation of Y527 on pp60^{c-src} occurs in physiologic responses where c-*src* has been implicated, this may simply reflect our inability to detect this potentially short-lived intermediate.

Conservation of the c-*src* carboxy-terminal tyrosine 527 residue and surrounding sequences in all the *src*-related tyrosine kinases suggests that this tyrosine residue is a common site of in vivo phosphorylation, which regulates tyrosine kinase enzymatic activity. Consistent with this view are experiments demonstrating that Y505 is the major site of in vivo tyrosine phosphorylation of p56^{lck} molecules expressed in cloned normal T-lymphocytes [31]. Replacement of Y505 by phenylalanine results in p56^{lck} molecules capable of transforming NIH3T3 fibroblasts [63,64]. However, the relevance of this observation to the role of Y505 phosphorylation in the regulation of *lck* in T-cells remains unclear.

Currently, it is not clear what cellular TPK is responsible for maintaining phosphorylation of Y527. The majority of the evidence suggests that this TPK is not pp60^{c-src} itself. The experiments supporting this view include those which demonstrate the low capacity for pp60^{c-src} to autophosphorylate Y527 in vitro, the low degree of Y527 occupancy following c-src expression in yeast [65,66] (yeast have no detectable endogenous c-src and have very low levels of other TPKs), and the capacity of c-src mutants that lack the ability to bind ATP (K295 mutants) and/or associate with the plasma membrane (myristylation mutants) to nevertheless possess Y527 phosphorylation in mammalian, but not yeast cells [65]. However, some recent evidence suggests that c-src molecules may posses the capacity to more efficiently phosphorylate Y527 residues on other c-src molecules through intermolecular mechanisms [67], thereby providing an autoregulatory function. Since multiple *src* family members are usually expressed in the same cell, one possibility arising from this observation is that some family members may play a role in regulating the activity of others within the family.

In common with many other protein kinases, the *src*-related protein kinases are capable of carrying out intramolecular and intermolecular autophosphorylation reactions in vitro [34,35]. The major site of avian pp60^{c-src} autophosphorylation is at tyrosine residue 416 (Y416), which is located in the catalytic domain of the enzyme [34, 35]. In the absence of Y527 phosphorylation in vivo, increased specific activity of pp60^{c-src} in fibroblasts is usually associated with a significant degree of Y416 phosphorylation. This has been documented for pp60^{v-src} [52], c-src Y527 mutants [58–60], a variety of transforming c-src proteins carrying mutations in the amino-terminal region or within the catalytic domain [68,69], and the pp60^{c-src} molecules complexed by the polyomavirus transforming protein middle T-antigen [70]. Additional studies have shown that the presence of an intact Y416 residue is important for the phenotypic changes (increased kinase activity, oncogenic transformation, and decreased cell-to-cell communication) resulting from the expression of c-src point mutants lacking Y527 [58,71]. In contrast, the absence of phosphorylatable Y416 was not found to inhibit the protein kinase activity of the transforming v-*src* gene product (which carries more extensive mutations than the Y527 mutant) nor did site-specific mutagenesis of Y416 suppress the ability of pp60^{v-src} to transform avian fibroblasts [72,73]. However, tumor formation in chickens by avian retroviruses carrying the v-*src* Y416 to F416 mutant was diminished [72–74]. Taken together, these data suggest that the presence of an intact Y416 residue (and presumably its phosphorylation) appear to be important for the altered properties of c-*src* molecules carrying relatively weak oncogenic mutations (such as Y527 point mutants). Recent data [75] have demonstrated that treatment of NIH3T3 fibroblasts overexpressing avian pp60^{c-src} with the tyrosine phosphatase inhibitor vanadate results in c-*src* molecules with increased in vivo phosphorylation of Y416 and elevated specific kinase activity. Such data further support the view that the Y416 residue can participate in the modulation of the c-*src*-associated tyrosine kinase activity.

Amino-terminal region

An increasing number of cellular responses initiated by cell surface interactions with external factors have been found to be associated with alterations of the phosphorylation state in the amino-terminal portion of the *src*-related tyrosine kinases. For example, exposure of normal murine T-lymphocytes to activating signals such as mitogenic lectins or antibodies to the T-cell receptor complex leads to rapid modifications of the *lck* protein characterized by reduced *lck* electrophoretic mobility and the appearance of several novel sites of amino-terminal serine phosphorylation [31]. Similarly, rapid amino-terminal serine and tyrosine phosphorylations of pp60^{c-src} have been observed following treatment of fibroblasts with platelet-derived growth factor (PDGF) [25,76]. Furthermore, during mitosis, a large fraction of the c-*src* molecules expressed in fibroblasts acquire numerous novel sites of amino-terminal phosphorylation both on serine and threonine residues [24]. The alterations in pp60^{c-src} amino-terminal phosphorylation detected during mitosis and following PDGF treatment were found to be associated with a 3- to 7-fold increase in specific activity [25,76]. Interestingly, neither the PDGF nor the mitosis-related alterations in enzymatic activity of pp60^{c-src} were found to be associated with detectable changes in the ratio of Y527 to Y416 phosphorylation [24,25].

These results raise the possibility that a potentially important mechanism of physiologic regulation of the *src*-related tyrosine kinases may be through phosphorylation of specific residues within their unique amino-terminal sequences. Such modifications would not only allow for 'cross-talk' between the serine/threonine and tyrosine kinases but would also permit changes in *src* family members' substrate specificity and/or enzymatic activity by a mechanism independent of any change in the phosphate occupancy of the regulatory carboxy-terminal tyrosine residues.

Oncogenic potential

src was the first genetically and functionally defined oncogene [77,78]. It was identified as the transforming gene of a replication-competent avian sarcoma retrovirus (Rous Sarcoma Virus). This viral gene, denoted as v-*src* (its 60-kDa product being named pp60^{v-src}), was ultimately found to be a mutated form of a cellular gene appropriately termed c-*src* (its product being pp60^{c-src}) [5]. Two other *src*-related tyrosine kinase genes, c-*yes* and c-*fgr*, were also originally identified as the oncogenes of the Y73 sarcoma virus [79] (c-*yes*) and Gardner-Rasheed Feline sarcoma virus [80] (c-*fgr*). All the other members of this gene family were identified as a result of their nucleic acid homology with known *src*-related tyrosine kinase genes, although the identification of the *lck* gene postdated the description of its protein product in membranes of normal and transformed murine lymphocytes [81–83]. Despite the fact that naturally occurring oncogenic versions of the remaining members of the *src*-related tyrosine kinase genes have not been found, the conserved ability to mutate these normal cellular genes into genes possessing oncogenic potential justifies their classification as proto-oncogenes [63,64,84].

Even when expressed 10 to 20 times the endogenous level, pp60^{c-src} is unable to transform NIH3T3 fibroblasts and chicken embryo fibroblasts [85,86] although some alterations in anchorage-independent growth capacity and increased focus formation have been noted when pp60^{c-src} is highly (50-fold) overexpressed [87]. Interestingly, cotransfection of NIH3T3 fibroblasts with c-*src* and a variety of nuclear oncogenes (c-*myc*, v-*myc*, adenovirus E1A, and the 5' half of polyoma large T) induces anchorage-independent growth and increased focus formation [88]. Cotransfection with polyoma large T results in an increased pp60^{c-src}-specific activity, lack of Y527 phosphorylation with increased occupancy of Y416 in vivo, and confers tumorigenicity in immunocompetent mice [88]. The significance and the biochemical basis of the ability of nuclear oncogenes to complement c-*src* in the transformation of NIH3T3 fibroblasts remains unclear. It is not known what the effect of overexpression of other *src* family members might have on parameters of cell transformation.

The requirements for converting the nontransforming cellular *src* gene into an oncogene have been intensively studied over the past decade. The general functional requirements for the transformation competence of *src*-derived oncogene products are possession of enzymatic activity (which is usually activated several-fold) and the ability to associate with plasma membrane components. Thus, *src*-related oncogene products such as pp60^{v-src} that have either been site-specifically mutated to prevent ATP binding [88,90] or have mutations affecting myristylation [46,47] are incapable of transformation. These results predict that the *src* substrates important for transformation contain phosphorylatable tyrosine residues and are in or around the cell membrane. Unfortunately, the rather large number of cellular proteins phosphorylated on tyrosine residues in *src*-related oncogene-transformed cells has created problems in identifying which are the critical targets. An emerging concept in this area is that the restriction of *src*-related gene products to interact with important substrates might be dependent upon the capacity of a tyrosine kinase to associate with the cytoskeletal components in the region near the plasma membrane. Indeed, analysis of a variety of transforming and nontransforming *src*-related proteins revealed a close correlation between their transforming potential and their association with the detergent-insoluble (cytoskeleton) fraction of cells [91].

There are numerous sequence differences betwen c-*src* and v-*src*. These changes consist of several point mutations scattered throughout the coding region and a carboxy-terminal deletion/substitution in v-*src* that ablates the regulatory domain (including Y527) [5]. As mentioned above, it has been established that a single amino acid alteration (Y527 to F527) is sufficient for the conversion of the nononcogenic c-*src* gene to a gene with oncogenic potential [58–60]. These results are all consistent with the idea that constitutive deregulation of normal cellular phosphorylation of tyrosine residues within the carboxy-terminal domain of the c-*src* protein is a major factor in determining the oncogenic potential. However, it should be noted that some of the amino-terminal mutations found in the v-*src* gene product are sufficient for converting c-*src* into an oncogene [68,69]. These oncogenic mutations of c-*src* also add to the concept that the amino terminus of this group of enzymes can communicate with and affect the function of the catalytic domain.

Since most of the experiments concerning transformation have to date been performed with fibroblasts or fibroblast-derived cell lines, the impact of the *src*-related genes on the phenotype of other cell types is not well defined. For example, overexpression of the normal *lck* gene product in NIH3T3 cells does not result in transformation [63,64]. However, overexpression of p56^{lck} and elevated levels of phosphotyrosine have been detected in the murine thymoma cell line LSTRA [80,81,91]. Analysis of complementary DNA clones corresponding to the *lck* gene demonstrated that the primary structure of the p56^{lck} expressed in LSTRA cells is identical to that expressed in normal lymphocytes [12,13]. Currently available data suggest that p56^{lck} is neither mutated nor 'activated' in LSTRA cells and that its overexpression alone is responsible for the elevation in cellular phosphotyrosine. Although it remains to be established that the *lck* gene product participates in the transformed phenotype of these cells, it is possible that the overexpression of wild-type *lck* protein in lymphocytes might have transforming potential.

While it appears that the normal products of the *src* family of genes do not generally participate in the initiation of cellular transformation, analysis of polyomavirus has revealed that normal pp60^{c-src} and potentially other family members are involved in the mechanism through which this virus transforms cells. The ability of polyomavirus to transform rodent cells is dependent upon the ability of the virus to encode the membrane-associated middle T-antigen (for a recent review see [93]). Middle T-antigen possesses an associated tyrosine kinase activity that was originally detected by the in vitro phosphorylation of middle T-antigen on tyrosine residues [94]. Subsequent analysis revealed that middle T-antigen forms a complex with pp60^{c-src} [95,96] and that the c-*src* molecules residing in this complex have elevated protein kinase activity [96]. The pp60^{c-src} molecules associated with middle T represent only 5%–10% of all the *src* molecules present in a fibroblast [97] and lack Y527 phosphorylation while possessing a significant degree of occupancy of Y416 [70]. These observations support the concept that these c-*src* molecules are enzymatically activated. Evaluation of a variety of middle T mutants [96,98–100] and c-*src* antisense experiments [101] confirmed that the interaction of middle T with pp60^{c-src} is essential for transformation. By engineering a large number of c-*src* mutants, it was established that residues aspartic acid 518 to proline 525 of pp60^{c-src} are required for the stable association with middle T [102]. Since the important residues are in close proximity with Y527, these observations suggest that middle T-antigen might activate pp60^{c-src} by altering the dynamics of phosphorylation/dephosphorylation of this regulatory tyrosine residue. Alternatively, middle T-antigen could associate more avidly with c-*src* molecules with unoccupied Y527, thereby maintaining these molecules in an 'activated' state. Since antibodies directed against the regulatory domain also are capable of stimulating pp60^{c-src} kinase activity [62], binding of middle T-antigen to this region of pp60^{c-src} might also act in the process of activation independently of changes in tyrosine phosphorylation.

The middle T-antigen of polyomavirus is also capable of forming complexes with both the c-*yes* [103] and *fyn* [104–106] gene products. While it appears that p62^{c-yes} is activated to a small degree in the middle T-antigen complexes [103], p60^{fyn} has not been found to be detectably activated [104–106]. Since all three of these *src* family members are expressed in most cells capable of being transformed by middle T-antigen (I.D. Horak, and J.B. Bolen, unpublished), it is not clear what role the individual *src*-related kinases play in the transformation process. Additional genetic analysis of these proteins will hopefully aid in these determinations. It is noteworthy that increases in pp60^{c-src} kinase activity have been observed in adenovirus, Simian virus 40 (SV40), and bovine papilloma virus type I transformed hamster fibroblasts [107], and in chemically transformed Syrian hamster fibroblasts [108]. Interestingly, the changes in pp60^{c-src} enzyme activity were found to be independent of alterations in Y527/Y416 phosphorylation [108] and independent of complex formation with other cellular proteins or viral encoded oncogenes [107]. These observations suggest that activation of pp60^{c-src} enzyme activity in these types of transformed cells might involve novel mechanisms of posttranslational activation. Since the SV40 large T-Antigen and adenovirus E1A proteins (which are responsible for the oncogenic potential of these viruses) have recently been shown to bind the 105-kDa product of the tumor-suppressor retinoblastoma gene [109,110], a pathway involving changes in the function of nuclear regulatory proteins might therefore promote alterations in the activity of the TPKs.

Despite the strong evidence that *src*-related tyrosine kinases are implicated in the oncogenic potential of certain RNA viruses and DNA viruses (polyoma and potentially others), there is no unambiguous evidence to implicate these gene products in the genesis of human tumors. While the activity of pp60^{c-src} has been found to be elevated in certain types of human solid tumors including colon [111–114] and breast ([113]; J. O'Shaughnessy, N. Rosen and J.B. Bolen, unpublished observations) carcinomas, the molecular basis and the importance of the $pp60^{c-src}$ activation observed in these tumors remain undefined. In the absence of detectable activating mutations of the *src*-related genes in human tumor tissues, the determination of the role of this gene family in human oncogenesis must await a more thorough understanding of the biology of each of the family members.

Functions of normal cellular products

Little is known about the normal physiologic functions of the different members of the *src* family of tyrosine kinases. Their cellular localization and the several known examples of alterations of *src*-related tyrosine kinases during programmed cellular responses suggest that they have the potential to play a role in some aspects of cellular proliferation and differentiation. It is also clear that our understanding of the normal functions of this group of enzymes has been complicated by the lack of reagents required to simultaneously study multiple family members in different types of cells. Since the largest battery of reagents available have been those detecting $pp60^{c-src}$, the majority of what is known about the *src* family in normal cells results from the analysis of the *c-src* gene product. The isolated study of $pp60^{c-src}$ may not be adequate to evaluate the role of *src*-related tyrosine kinases in cellular physiology since $pp60^{c-src}$ is usually expressed with $pp62^{c-yes}$, $p60^{fyn}$, and potentially other family members in almost all cells and tissues.

The abundance and even the primary structure of the *c-src* gene product is known to be altered in certain cell types. This fact may be indicative of situations where $pp60^{c-src}$ is providing a specialized function more amenable to study. Elevated levels of $pp60^{c-src}$ were first noted in embryonic chicken brain [114]. The expression of the *c-src* gene was subsequently found to be modulated during embryogenesis in various mammalian and avian neural tissues [26,117]. Furthermore, the expression of $pp60^{c-src}$ is also maintained at relatively high levels in adult neural tissues and neuronal-derived cells in culture [28,116–119]. The *c-src* gene product has also been shown to be abundant in membrane fractions derived from platelets [120]. The high levels of $pp60^{c-src}$ expressed in these postmitotic cells (platelets and neurons) indicate that this tyrosine kinase is not only a potential signal transducer of proliferating cells but also can be implicated in differentiated cell functions such as degranulation or release of neurotransmitters. High levels of $pp62^{c-yes}$ [121,122] and $p60^{fyn}$ (I.D. Horak, and J.B. Bolen, unpublished) have also been found in neural cells and tissues. Potential functions of the other *src* family members expressed in these cells need to be evaluated.

Neural cells of avian and mammalian origin express an altered form of pp60^{c-src} which was initially noticed because of its slower migration on sodium dodecyl sulfate-polyacrylamide gels [27–29,118,123]. This 'isoenzyme' of pp60^{c-src} has since been shown to be exclusively expressed in neural cells and arises as the result of alternative splicing events generating an additional 18-base-pair exon derived from sequences located in the third intron [124, 125]. Interestingly, the six amino acids encoded by this 'neural-specific' exon (Arg-Lys-Val-Asp-Val-Arg) (figure 2) are inserted in the amino-terminal portion of the molecule and have been shown to be identical in the neuronal forms of chicken and mouse pp60^{c-src} [124,125]. Preliminary data suggest that the p60^{fyn} detected in neural cells does not have a gel migration different from that of the fibroblast *fyn* protein (P. Thompson, I.D. Horak, and J.B. Bolen, unpublished).

The restricted expression of some *src*-related tyrosine kinases to certain cellular lineages (e.g., p56^{lck} in T-cells, *hck* protein in granulocytes/macrophages, *lyn* protein in B-cells, and c-*fgr* protein in granulocytes/macrophages) is consistent with the theory that these gene products are involved in some aspects of specialized cellular physiology. Currently, the best-characterized member of this group is the *lck* gene product, which is expressed in cells of lymphoid origin and is the most abundant *src* family member to be expressed in T-lymphocytes [31]. From the tissue distribution and abundance of l*ck* expression, we and others have suggested that p56^{lck} may be important for some normal functions of T-cells [12,21]. This concept is supported by the finding that p56^{lck} is abundantly expressed in both helper-inducer (CD4$^+$) and cytotoxic-suppressor (CD8$^+$) T-cell subsets [32,126]. During the process of T-cell activation, the p56^{lck} expressed in normal T-lymphocytes is rapidly modified into a protein migrating at approximately 59 kDa on sodium dodecyl sulfate – polyacrylamide gels. Additional experiments revealed that this physical alteration in the *lck* gene product is likely to be dependent upon phosphorylation of multiple serine residues within the amino-terminal portion of the protein [30]. More recently, it has been found that p56^{lck} forms a noncovalent complex with the CD4 and CD8 T-cell surface glycoproteins [31,127]. Since the CD4/CD8 cell surface proteins have been shown to be important both for the major histocompatibility complex restriction of T-cell responses and for signal transduction during T-cell activation (for a review, see [128]), these data strongly support the idea that p56^{lck} plays a central role in T-cell activation through the mediation of CD4 and CD8 signaling events. These results also raise the possibility that the other members of the *src* family that demonstrate restricted tissue expression may be similarly participating in differentiated functions related to cell-to-cell communication.

Important concepts concerning cellular signal transduction and oncogenic transformation mechanisms are emerging from the study of the *src* family of tyrosine kinase genes. The major focus to date has been the molecular analysis of these genes, which has uncovered their structural and regulatory complexities as well as their uniform oncogenic potential. Recent analysis of some family members with restricted tissue expression (such as *lck*) is now allowing for the design of experiments that will potentially define the physiological functions of at least some of the members of the src family of proteins. However, as these gene products continue to be studied individually, additional efforts will be needed to evaluate the respective participation of multiple members of the src family in physiological processes.

Acknowledgments

We thank the other members of the Laboratory of Tumor Virus Biology for helpful suggestions. A.V. is supported by a fellowship grant from the National Cancer Institute of Canada.

References

1. Hunter T Cooper JA: Protein tyrosine kinases. Annu Rev Biochem 54:897–930, 1985.
2. Hunter T, Sefton BM: Transforming gene product of Rous sarcoma virus phosphorylates tyrosine. Proc Natl Acad Sci USA 77:1311–1315, 1980.
3. Parker RC, Varmus HE, Bishop Jm: Cellular homologue (c-src) of the transforming gene of Rous Sarcoma Virus: isolation, mapping, and transcriptional analysis of c-src and flanking regions. Proc Natl Acad Sci USA 78:5842–5846, 1981.
4. Shalloway D, Zelentz A, Cooper GM: Molecular cloning and characterization of the chicken gene homologous to the transforming gene of Rous Sarcoma Virus. Cell 24:531–541, 1981.
5. Takeya T, Hanafusa H: Structure and sequence of the cellular gene homologous to the RSV src gene and the mechanism for generating the transforming virus. Cell 32:881–890, 1983.
6. Sukegawa J, Semba K, Yamanashi Y, Nishizawa M, Miyajima N, Yamamoto T, Toyoshima K: Characterization of cDNA clones for the human c-yes gene. Mol Cell Biol 7:41–47, 1989.
7. Katamine S, Notario V, Rao CD, Miki T, Cheah MSC, Tronick SR, Robbins KC: Primary structure of the human fgr proto-oncogene product pp55^{c-fgr}. Mol Cell Biol 8:259–266, 1988.
8. Nishizawa M, Semba K, Yoshida MC, Yamamoto T, Toyoshima K: Structure, expression, and chromosomal location of the human c-fgr gene. Mol Cell Biol 6:511–517, 1986.
9. Inoue K, Ikawa S, Semba K, Sukegawa T, Yamamoto T, Toyoshima T: Isolation and sequencing of cDNA clones homologous to the v-fgr oncogene from a human B-lymphocyte cell line, IM-9. Oncogene 1:301–304, 1987.
10. Semba K, Nishizawa M, Miyajima N, Yoshida MC, Sukegawa J, Yamanashi Y, Sasaki M, Yamamoto T, Toyoshima K: yes-related protooncogene, syn, belongs to the protein tyrosine kinase family. Proc Natl Acad Sci USA 83:5459–5463, 1986.
11. Kawakami T, Pennington CY, Robbins KC: Isolation and oncogenic potential of a novel human src-like gene. Mol Cell Biol 6:4195–4201, 1986.
12. Marth JD, Peet R, Krebs EG, Perlmutter RM: A lymphocyte-specific protein tyrosine kinase is rearranged and overexpressed in the murine T cell lymphoma LSTRA. Cell 43:393–404, 1985.
13. Voronova AF, Sefton BM: Expression of a new tyrosine protein kinase is stimulated by retrovirus promoter insertion. Nature 319:682–685, 1986.
14. Quintrell N, Lebo R, Varmus H, Bishop JM, Pettenati MJ, LeBeau MM, Diaz MO, Rowley JD: Identification of a human gene (HCK) that encodes a protein-tyrosine kinase and is expressed in hemopoeitic cells. Mol Cell Biol 7:2267–2275, 1987.

15. Ziegler SF, Marth JD, Lewis DB, Perlmutter RM: Novel protein-tyrosine kinase gene (*hck*) preferentially expressed in cells of hematopoietic origin. Mol Cell Biol 7:2276–2285, 1987.
16. Holtzman DA, Cook WD, Dunn AR: Isolation and sequence of a cDNA corresponding to a *src*-related gene expressed in murine hemopoeitic cells. Proc Natl Acad Sci USA 84:8325–8329, 1987.
17. Yamanashi Y, Fukushige SI, Semba K, Sukegawa J, Miyajima N, Matsubara KI, Yamamoto T, Toyoshima K: The *yes*-related cellular gene *lyn* encodes a possible tyrosine kinase similar to p56^{lck}. Mol Cell Biol 7:237–243, 1987.
18. Strebhardt K, Mullins JI, Bruck C, Rubsamen-Waigmann H: Additional member of the protein-tyrosine kinase family: the *src*- and *lck*-related protooncogene c-*tkl*. Proc Natl Acad Sci USA 84:8778–8782, 1987.
19. Anderson SK, Gibbs CP, Tanaka A, Kung H-J, Fujita DJ: Human cellular *src* gene: nucleotide sequence and derived amino-acid sequence of the region coding for the carboxy-terminal two-thirds of pp60^{c-src} Mol Cell Biol 5:1122–1129, 1985.
20. Tanaka A, Gibbs CP, Arthur RR, Anderson SK, Kung H-J, Fujita DJ: DNA sequence encoding the amino-terminal region of the human c-*src* protein: implications of sequence divergence among *src*-type kinase oncogenes. Mol Cell Biol 7:1978–1983, 1987.
21. Veillette A, Foss FM, Sausville EA, Bolen JB, Rosen N: Expression of the *lck* tyrosine kinase gene in human colon carcinoma and other non-lymphoid human tumor cell lines. Oncogene Res 1:357–374, 1987.
22. Marth JD, Overell RW, Meier KE, Krebs EG, Perlmutter RM: Translational activation of the *lck* proto-oncogene. Nature 332:171–173, 1988.
23. Garvin AM, Pawar S, Marth JD, Perlmutter RM: Structure of the murine *lck* gene and its rearrangement in a murine lymphoma cell line. Mol Cell Biol 8:3058–3064, 1988.
24. Chackalaparampil I, Shalloway D: Altered phosphorylation and activation of pp60^{c-src} during fibroblast mitosis. Cell 52:801–810, 1988.
25. Gould KL, Hunter, T: Platelet-derived growth factor induces multisite phosphorylation of pp60^{c-src} and increases its protein-tyrosine kinase activity. Mol Cell Biol 8:3345–3356, 1988.
26. Sorge LK, Levy BT, Maness PF: pp60^{c-src} is developmentally regulated in the neural retina. Cell 36:249–257, 1984.
27. Lynch SA, Brugge JS, Levine JM: Induction of altered c-*src* product during neural differentiation of embryonal carcinoma cells. Science 234:873–876, 1986.
28. Cartwright CA, Simantov R, Kaplan PL, Hunter T, Eckhart W: Alterations in pp60^{c-src} accompany differentiation of neurons from rat embryo striatum. Mol Cell Biol 7:1830–1840, 1987.
29. Wiestler OD, Walter G: Developmental expression of two forms of pp60^{c-src} in mouse brain. Mol Cell Biol 8:502–504, 1988.
30. Barnekow A, Gessler M: Activation of the pp60^{c-src} kinase during differentiation of monomyelocytic cells *in vitro*. EMBO J 5:701–705, 1986.
31. Veillette A, Horak ID, Horak EM, Bookman MA Bolen JB: Alterations of the lymphocyte-specific protein tyrosine kinase (p56^{lck}) during T-cell activation. Mol Cell Biol 8:4353–4361, 1988.
32. Veillette A, Bookman MA, Horak EM, Bolen JB: The CD4 and CD8 T-cell surface antigens are associated with the internal membrane tyrosine kinase p56^{lck}. Cell 55:301–308, 1988.
33. Kamps MP, Taylor SS, Sefton BM: Direct evidence that oncogenic typrosine kinases and cyclic AMP-dependent protein kinase have homologous ATP-binding sites. Nature 310:589–592, 1984.
34. Patschinski T, Hunter T, Esch FS, Cooper JA, Sefton BM: Analysis of the sequence of amino acids surrounding sites of tyrosine phosphorylation. Proc Natl Acad Sci USA 79:973–977, 1982.
35. Smart JE, Oppermann H, Czernilofski AP, Purchio Af, Erikson RL, Bishop JM: Characterization of sites for tyrosine phosphorylation in the transforming protein of Rous

Sarcoma Virus (pp60^{src}) and its normal cellular homologue (pp60^{c-src}). Proc Natl Acad Sci USA 78:6013–6017, 1981.
36. Toner-Webb J, Taylor SS: Inhibition of the catalytic subunit of cAMP-dependent protein kinase by dicyclohexylcarbodiimide. Biochemistry 26:7371–7378, 1987.
37. Hanks SK, Quinn AM, Hunter T: The protein kinase family: conserved features and deduced phylogeny of the catalytic domains. Science 241:42–52, 1988.
38. Laudano AP, Buchanan JM: Phosphorylation of tyrosine in the carboxy-terminal tryptic peptide of pp60^{c-src}. Proc Natl Acad Sci USA 83:892–896, 1986.
39. Cooper JA, Gould KL, Cartwright CA, Hunter T: Tyr^{527} is phosphorylated in pp60^{c-src}: implications for regulation. Science 231:1431–1434, 1986.
40. Garber EA, Cross FR, Hanafusa H: Processing of p60^{v-src} to its myristylated membrane-bound form. Mol Cell Biol 5:2781–2788, 1985.
41. Resh MD: Reconstitution of the Rous Sarcoma Virus transforming protein pp60^{v-src} into phospholipid vesicles. Mol Cell Biol 8:1896–1905, 1988.
42. Deichaite I, Casson LP, Ling H-P, Resh MD: In vitro synthesis of pp60^{v-src}: myristylation in cell-free system. Mol Cell Biol 8:4295–4301, 1988.
43. Lee JS, Varmus HE, Bishop JM: Virus-specific messenger RNAs in permissive cells infected by avian sarcoma virus. J Biol Chem 254:8015–8022, 1979.
44. Buss JE, Sefton BM: Myristic acid, a rare fatty acid, is attached to the transforming protein in Rous sarcoma virus and its cellular homologue. J Virol 53:7–12, 1985.
45. Schultz AM, Henderson LE, Orozlan S, Garber EA, Hanafusa H: Amino terminal myristylation of the protein kinase p60^{src}, a retroviral transforming protein. Science 227:427–429, 1985.
46. Cross FR, Garber EA, Pellman D, Hanafusa H: A short sequence in the pp60^{src} N-terminus is required for pp60^{src} myristylation and membrane association, and for cell transformation. Mol Cell Biol 4: 1834–1842, 1984.
47. Kamps MR, Buss JE, Sefton BM: Rous Sarcoma Virus transforming protein lacking myristic acid phosphorylates known polypeptide substrates without inducing transformation. Cell 45:105–112, 1986.
48. Cross FR, Hanafusa H: Local mutagenesis of Rous Sarcoma Virus: the major sites of tyrosine and serine phosphorylation of pp60^{src} are dispensable for transformation. Cell 34:597–607, 1983.
49. Purchio AF, Shoyab M, Gentry LE: Treatment of RSV-transformed cells with a tumor promoter. Science 229:1393–1395, 1985.
50. Gould KL, Woodgett JR, Cooper JA, Buss JE, Shalloway D, Hunter T: Protein kinase C phosphorylates pp60^{src} at a novel site. Cell 42:849–857, 1985.
51. Gentry LE, Chaffin KE, Shoyab M, Purchio AF: Novel serine phosphorylation of pp60^{c-src} in intact cells after tumor promoter treatment. Mol Cell Biol 6:735–738, 1986.
52. Collett MS, Erikson E, Erikson RL: Structural analysis of the avian sarcoma virus transforming protein: sites of phosphorylation. J Virol 29:770–781, 1979.
53. Hirota Y, Kato J-Y, Takeya T: Substitution of ser-17 of pp60^{c-src}: biological and biochemical characterization in chicken embryo fibroblasts. Mol Cell Biol 8:1826–1830, 1988.
54. Sadowski I, Stone JC, Pawson T: A noncatalytic domain conserved among cytoplasmic protein-tyrosine kinases modifies the kinase function and transforming activity of Fujinami Sarcoma Virus p130$^{gag-fps}$. Mol Cell Biol 6:4396–4408, 1986.
55. DeClue JE, Sadowski I, Martin GS, Pawson T: A conserved domain regulates interactions of the v-fps protein-tyrosine kinase with the host cell. Proc Natl Acad Sci USA 84:9064–9068, 1987.
56. Stahl ML, Ferenz CR, Kelleher KL, Kriz RW, Knopf JL: Sequence similarity of phospholipase C with the non-catalytic region of src. Nature 332:269–272, 1988.
57. Mayer BJ Hamaguchi M, Hanafusa H: A novel viral oncogene with a structural similarity to phospholipase C. Nature 332:272–275, 1988.
58. Kmiecik TE, Shalloway D: Activation and suppression of pp60^{c-src} transforming ability by

mutation of its primary sites of tyrosine phosphorylation. Cell 49:65–73, 1987.
59. Piwnica-Worms H, Saunders KB, Roberts TM, Smith AE, Cheng SH: Tyrosine phosphorylation regulates the biological and biochemical properties of pp60^{c-src}. Cell 49:75–82, 1987.
60. Cartwright CA, Eckhart WE, Simon S, Kaplan PL: Cell transformation by pp60^{c-src} mutated in carboxy-terminus regulatory domain. Cell 49:83–91, 1987.
61. Yaciuk P, Shalloway D: Features of pp60^{v-src} carboxyl terminus that are required for transformation. Mol Cell Biol 6:2807–2819, 1986.
62. Cooper JA, King CS: Dephosphorylation or antibody binding to the carboxy terminus stimulates pp60^{c-src}. Mol Cell Biol 6:4467–4477, 1986.
63. Marth JD, Cooper JA, King CS, Ziegler SF, Tinker DA, Overell RW, Krebs EG, Perlmutter RM: Neoplastic transformation induced by an activated lymphocyte-specific protein tyrosine kinase (pp56^{lck}). Mol Cell Biol 8:540–550, 1988.
64. Amrein KE, Sefton BM: Mutation at a site of tyrosine phosphorylation in the lymphocyte-specific tyrosine protein kinase, p56^{lck}, reveals its oncogenic potential in fibroblasts. Proc Natl Acad Sci USA 85:4247–4251, 1988.
65. Jove R, Kornbluth S, Hanafusa H: Enzymatically inactive p60^{c-src} mutant with altered ATP-binding site is fully phosphorylated in its carboxy-terminal regulatory region. Cell 50:937–943, 1987.
66. Shuh SM, Brugge JS: Investigation of factors that influence phosphorylation of pp60^{c-src} on tyrosine 527. Mol Cell Biol 8:2465–2471, 1988.
67. Cooper JA, MacAuley A: Potential positive and negative autoregulation of p60^{c-src} by intermolecular phosphorylation. Proc Natl Acad Sci USA 85:4232–4236, 1988.
68. Levy JB, Iba H, Hanafusa H: Activation of the transforming potential of p60^{c-src} by a single amino-acid change. Proc Natl Acad Sci USA 83:4228–4232, 1986.
69. Kato J-Y, Takeya T, Grandori C, Iba H, Levy JB, Hanafusa H: Amino acid substitutions sufficient to convert the nontransforming p60^{c-src} protein to a transforming protein. Mol Cell Biol 6:4155–4160, 1986.
70. Cartwright CA, Kaplan PL, Cooper JA, Hunter T, Eckhart W: Altered sites of tyrosine phosphorylation in pp60^{c-src} associated with polyoma virus middle tumor antigen. Mol Cell Biol 6:1562–1570, 1986.
71. Azarnia R, Reddy S, Kmiecik TE, Shalloway D, Loewenstein WR: The cellular *src* gene product regulates junctional cell-to-cell communication. Science 239:398–401, 1988.
72. Snyder MA, Bishop JM, Colby WW, Levinson AD: Phosphorylation of tyrosine-416 is not required for the transforming properties and kinase activity of pp60^{v-src}. Cell 32:891–901, 1983.
73. Cross FR, Hanafusa H: Local mutagenesis of Rous sarcoma virus: the major sites of tyrosine and serine phosphorylation of p60^{src} are dispensable for transformation. Cell 34:597–607, 1983.
74. Snyder MA Bishop JM: A mutation of the major phosphotyrosine in pp60^{src} alters oncogenic potential. Virology 136:375–386, 1984.
75. Kmiecik TE, Johnson PJ, Shalloway D: Regulation by the autophosphorylation site in overexpressed pp60^{c-src}. Mol Cell Biol 8:4541–4546, 1988.
76. Ralston R, Bishop JM: The product of the protooncogene c-*src* is modified during the cellular response to platelet-derived growth factor. Proc Natl Acad Sci USA 82:7845–7849, 1985.
77. Brugge JS, Erikson RL: Identification of a transforming specific antigen induced by an avian sarcoma virus. Nature 269:346–348, 1977.
78. Collett MS, Purchio AF, Erikson RL: Avian sarcoma virus transforming protein, p60^{src} shows protein kinase activity specific for tyrosine. Nature 285:167–169, 1980.
79. Kitamura N, Kitamura K, Toyoshima K, Hirayama Y, Yoshida M: Avian sarcoma virus Y73 genome sequence and structural similarity of its transforming gene product to that of Rous sarcoma virus. Nature 297:205–208, 1982.
80. Naharro G, Robbins KC, Reddy EP: Gene product of v-*fqr* onc: hybrid protein containing

a portion of actin and a tyrosine-specific protein kinase. Science 223:63–66, 1984.
81. Casnellie JE, Harrison ML, Pike LJ, Hellstrom KE, Krebs EG: Phosphorylation of synthetic peptides by a tyrosine protein kinase from the particulate fraction of a lymphoma cell line. Proc Natl Acad Sci USA 79:282–286, 1982.
82. Gacon G, Gisselbrecht S, Piau JP, Boissel JP, Tolle J, Fischer S: High level of tyrosine protein kinase in a murine lymphoma cell line induced by Moloney leukemia virus. EMBO J 1:1579–1582, 1982.
83. Earp HS, Austin KS, Buessow SC, Dy R, Gillespie GY: Membranes from T and B lymphocytes have different patterns of tyrosine phosphorylation. Proc Natl Acad Sci USA 81:2347–2351, 1984.
84. Kawakami T, Kawakami Y, Aaronson SA, Robbins KC: Acquisition of transforming properties by FYN, a normal SRC-related human gene. Proc Natl Acad Sci USA 85:3870–3874, 1988.
85. Shalloway D, Coussens PM, Yaciuk P: Overexpression of the c-*src* protein does not induce transformation of NIH3T3 cells. Proc Natl Acad Sci USA 81:7071–7075, 1984.
86. Parker RC, Varmus HE, Bishop JM: Expression of v-*src* and chicken c-*src* in rat cells demonstrates qualitative differences between $pp60^{v-src}$ and $pp60^{c-src}$. Cell 37:131–139, 1984.
87. Johnson PJ, Coussens PM, Danko AV Shalloway D: Overexpressed $pp60^{c-src}$ can induce focus formation without complete transformation of NIH3T3 cells. Mol Cell Biol 5:1073–1083, 1985.
88. Shalloway D, Johnson PJ, Freed EO, Coulter D, Flood WA Jr: Transformation of NIH3T3 cells by cotransfection with c-*src* and nuclear oncogenes. Mol Cell Biol 7:3582–3590, 1987.
89. Snyder MA, Bishop JM, MacGrath JP, Levinson AD: A mutation at the ATP-binding site of $pp60^{v-src}$ abolishes kinase activity, transformation, and tumorigenicity. Mol Cell Biol 5:1772–1779, 1985.
90. Kamps MP, Sefton BM: Neither arginine nor histidine can carry out the function of Lys 295 at the ATP-binding site of $p60^{src}$. Mol Cell Biol 6:751–757.
91. Hamaguchi M, Hanafusa H: Association of $p60^{src}$ with Triton X-100-resistant cellular structure correlates with morphological transformation. Proc Natl Acad Sci USA 84:2312–2316. 1987.
92. Casnellie JE, Harrison ML, Hellstrom KE, Krebs EG: A lymphoma cell line expressing elevated levels of tyrosine protein kinase activity J Biol Chem 258:10738–10742, 1983.
93. Markland W, Smith AE: Mutants of polyomavirus middle-T antigen. Biochem Biophys Acta 907:299–321, 1987.
94. Eckhardt W, Hutchinson MA, Hunter T: An activity phosphorylating tyrosine in polyoma T antigen immunoprecipitates. Cell 18:925–934, 1979.
95. Courtneidge SA, Smith AE: Polyoma virus transforming protein associates with the product of the c-*src* cellular gene. Nature 303:435–439, 1984.
96. Bolen JB, Thiele CJ, Israel MA, Yonemoto W, Lipsich LA, Brugge JS: Enhancement of cellular *src* gene product associated tyrosyl kinase activity following polyoma virus infection and transformation. Cell 38:767–777, 1985.
97. Bolen JB, DeSeau V, O'Shaughnessy J, Amini S: Analysis of middle tumor antigen and $pp60^{c-src}$ interactions in polyomavirus-transformed rat cells. J Virol 61:3299–3305, 1987.
98. Courtneidge SA, Smith AE: The complex of polyoma virus middle-T antigen and $pp60^{c-src}$. EMBO J 3: 585–591, 1984.
99. Bolen JB, Israel MA: Middle tumor antigen of polyomavirus transformation-defective mutant NG59 is associated with $pp60^{c-src}$. J Virol 53:114–119, 1985.
100. Cartwright CA, Hutchinson MA, Eckhardt W: Structural and functional modification of $pp60^{c-src}$ associated with polyoma middle tumor antigen from infected or transformed cells. Mol Cel Biol 5:2647–2652, 1985.
101. Amini S, DeSeau V, Reddy S, Shalloway D, Bolen JB: Regulation of $pp60^{c-src}$ synthesis by inducible RNA complementary to c-*src* mRNA in polyomavirus-transformed rat cells. Mol Cell Biol 6:2305–2316, 1986.

102. Cheng SH, Piwnica-Worms H, Harvey RW, Roberts TM, Smith AE: The carboxy terminus of pp60^{c-src} is a regulatory domain and is involved in complex formation with the middle-T antigen of polyomavirus. Mol Cell Biol 8:1936–1747, 1988.
103. Kornbluth S, Sudol M, Hanafusa H: Association of the polyomavirus middle-T antigen with c-*yes* protein. Nature 325: 171–173, 1987.
104. Kypta RM, Hemming A, Courtneidge SA: Identification and characterization of p59^{fyn} (a src-like protein tyrosine kinase) in normal and polyoma virus transformed cells. EMBO J 7:3837–3844, 1988.
105. Cheng SH, Harvey R, Estino PC, Semba K, Yamamoto T, Toyoshima K, Smith AE: Peptide antibodies to the human c-*fyn* gene product demonstrate that pp59^{c-fyn} is capable of complex formation with the middle T antigen of polyomavirus. EMBO J 7:3845–3856, 1988.
106. Horak ID, Kawakami T, Gregory F, Robbins KC, Bolen JB: Association of p60^{fyn} with middle tumor antigen in murine polyomavirus transformed rat cells. J Virol 63:2343–2347, 1989.
107. Amini S, Lewis AM, Israel MA, Butel JS, Bolen JB: Analysis of pp60^{c-src} protein kinase activity in hamster embryo cells transformed by simian virus 40, human adenoviruses, and bovine papillomavirus-1. J Virol 57:357–361, 1986.
108. Kanner SB, Parsons SJ, Parsons JT, Gilmer TM: Activation of pp60^{c-src} tyrosine kinase specific activity in tumor-derived Syrian hamster embryo cells. Oncogene 2:327–335, 1988.
109. Whyte P, Buchkovich KJ, Horowitz JM, Friend SH, Raybuck M, Weinberg RA, Harlow E: Association between an oncogene and an anti-oncogene: the adenovirus E1A proteins bind to the retinoblastoma gene product. Nature 334:124–129, 1988.
110. DeCaprio JA, Ludlow JW, Figge J, Shew J-Y, Huang C-M, Lee W-H, Marsilio E, Paucha E, Livingston DM: SV40 large tumor antigen forms a specific complex with the product of the retinoblastoma susceptibility gene. Cell 54:275–283, 1988.
111. Bolen JB, Veillette A, Schwartz AM, DeSeau V, Rosen N: Activation of pp60^{c-src} protein kinase in human colon carcinoma. Proc Natl Acad Sci USA 84:2251–2255, 1987.
112. Bolen JB, Veillette A, Schwartz AM, DeSeau V, Rosen N: Analysis of pp60^{c-src} in human colon carcinoma and normal human colon mucosal cells. Oncogene Res 1: 149–168, 1987.
113. Rosen N, Bolen JB, Schwartz AM, Cohen P, DeSeau V, Israel MA: Analysis of pp60^{c-src} protein kinase activity in human tumor cell lines and tissues. J Biol Chem 261:13754–13759, 1986.
114. DeSeau V, Rosen N, Bolen JB: Analysis of pp60^{c-src} tyrosine kinase activity and phosphotyrosyl phosphatase activity in human colon carcinoma and normal human colon mucosal cells. J Cell Biochem 35:113–128, 1987.
115. Jacobs C, Rubsamen H: Expression of pp60^{c-src} protein kinase in adult and fetal tissue: high activities in some sarcomas and mammary carcinomas. Cancer Res 43:1696–1702, 1983.
116. Cotton PC, Brugge JS: Neuronal tissues express high levels of the cellular *src* gene product pp60^{c-src}. Mol Cell Biol 3:1157–1162, 1983.
117. Sorge JP, Sorge LK, Maness PF: pp60^{c-src} is expressed in human fetal and adult brain. Am J Pathol 119, 151–157.
118. Brugge JS, Cotton PC, Queral AE, Barrett JN, Nonner D, Keane RW: Neurones express high levels of a structurally modified, activated form of pp60^{c-src}. Nature 316:554–557, 1985.
119. O'Shaughnessy J, DeSeau V, Amini S, Rosen N, Bolen JB: Analysis of the c-*src* gene product structure, abundance, and activity in human neuroblastoma and glioblastoma cells. Oncogene Res 2:1–18, 1987.
120. Golden A, Nemeth SP, Brugge JS: Blood platelets express high levels of the pp60^{c-src}-specific tyrosine kinase activity. Proc Natl Acad Sci USA 83:852–856, 1986.
121. Sudol M, Hanafusa H: Cellular proteins homologous to the viral *yes* gene product. Mol Cell Biol 6:2839–2846, 1986.
122. Sudol M, Alvarez-Buylla A, Hanafusa H: Differential developmental expression of cellular

yes and cellular *src* proteins in cerebellum. Oncogene Res 2:345–355, 1988.
123. Bolen JB, Rosen N, Israel MA: Increased pp60^{c-src} tyrosyl kinase activity in human neuroblastomas is associated with amino-terminal tyrosine phosphorylation of the *src* gene product. Proc Natl Acad Sci USA 82:7275–7279, 1985.
124. Martinez R, Mathey-Prevot B, Bernards A, Baltimore D: Neuronal pp60^{c-src} contains a six-amino acid insertion relative to its non-neuronal counterpart. Science 237:411–415, 1987.
125. Levy JB, Dorai T Wang L-H, Brugge JS: The structurally distinct form of pp60^{c-src} detected in neuronal cells is encoded by a unique c-*src* mRNA. Mol Cell Biol 7:4142–4145, 1987.
126. Perlmutter RM, Marth JD, Lewis DB, Peet R, Ziegler SF, Wilson CB: Structure and expression of *lck* transcripts in human lymphoid cells. J Cell Biochem in press.
127. Rudd CE, Trevillyan JM, Dasgupta JD, Wong LL, Schlossman SF: The CD4 receptor is complexed in detergent lysates to a protein-tyrosine kinase (pp 58) From human T lymphocytes. Proc Natl Acad Sci USA 85:5190–5194, 1988.
128. Swain SL: T-cell subsets and the recognition of MHC class. Immunol Rev 74:129–142, 1983.

6. The epidermal growth factor receptor and its ligands

Alan Wells

The stage

Appropriate response to growth and differentiation signals distinguishes normal development from neoplastic processes. A number of systems assure a regulated interaction with the surrounding environment. Polypeptide growth factors and their receptors constitute one such pathway by which cells interpret the external milieu. Acting via specific membrane-spanning moieties, these messengers initiate a cascade of enzymatic activities which lead to replication and/or differentiation. One class of receptors (figure 1) possesses an intrinsic tyrosine-specific kinase—an activity initially found in the viral oncogene v-*src*. While the nature of the secondary signal was similar in regulated and neoplastic growth, it was postulated that either the specificity or regulation of the signaling was altered. This view of oncogenesis by mutated growth factor receptors was cemented by the discovery of the Avian Erythroblastosis Virus (AEV) v-*erb*B gene as being a trucated version of the Epidermal Growth Factor Receptor (EGFR) [1–5]. Thus, the EGFR, a gene which in its normal configuration regulates growth in response to specific signals, can be mutated to induce uncontrolled proliferation.

It has long been known that certain tumors produce factors that induce the transformed phenotype in indicator cell lines. One such product is Transforming Growth Factor α(TGFα), an EGFR-specific mitogen. As the relationship between tyrosine-kinase oncogenes and growth factor receptors was being delineated, many investigators began to seek a role for receptors in the induction of naturally occurring human tumors. Both the EGFR and its ligand are aberrantly expressed in certain neoplastic states (see below). The weight of evidence suggests a causative role for this system in a number of tumors. However, the mechanism of action remains to be elucidated for both normal and aberrant signaling. Nevertheless, the EGFR system presents a model with which to decipher the subtleties and consequences of altered signaling.

Polypeptide growth factors interact with specific receptors that mediate most, if not all, of the effects [6,7]. The active member of this particular system, the EGF receptor, binds a number of ligands equally at its one ligand-

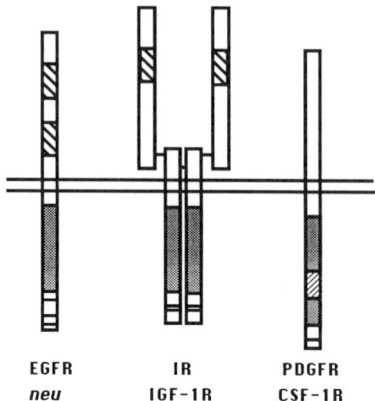

Figure 1. The tyrosine-kinase receptor families. A schematic representing the three families of growth factor receptors possessing intrinsic tyrosine kinase activity. Above the horizontal lines denotes the cell's exterior, below the cytoplasmic domain. Diagonal stripes demarcate the cysteine-rich regions, the heavy stipple the kinase domains, and the dark lines the autophosphorylation sites. Archetypical members include EGFR and c-*neu* for the first family, the insulin receptor (IR) and the insulin like growth factor I receptor (IGF-1R) for the second, and in the third group the receptors for the platelet-derived growth factor (PDGFR) and colony stimulating factor-I (CSF-1R).

binding site [8–10]. The initiators include EGF, TGFα, and a virally–encoded factor in poxviruses. Any discussion of this system needs to describe the various ligands along with the receptor and its derivative, the v-*erb*B oncogene [5,11–13]. The *neu* gene, a closely related putative growth factor receptor, also will be described. Finally, a mechanism for signaling will be proposed and its role in cellular proliferation and neoplastic change will be considered.

The players

The epidermal growth factor receptor

High-affinity receptors for EGF have been detected on a wide variety of cell types (for review, see [14]). Normal human cells bind on the order of 10,000 to 100,000 ligand [15,16]. A number of tumor cell lines present over a million sites per cell [17–19]. With the greater number of binding sites it has been possible to dissect two populations of high-affinity receptors. On A431 cells, the higher-affinity population (K_d = 0.3nM) represents 10% of the sites, whereas a larger, lower-affinity population exhibits a dissociation constant of 4nM [20–22]. While it is possible to distinguish these two populations immunologically, biochemical and molecular investigations have failed to detect differences in the receptors. Conformation differences are suggested as accounting for this difference [23–27], microaggregation state being the

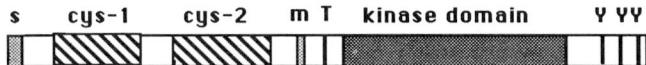

Figure 2. The topography of the EGFR is shown. The initial amino-terminus signal sequence (s) is cleaved from the mature polypeptide. There are two cysteine-rich domains (cys-1 and cys-2), a transmembrane domain (m), and a conserved kinase domain. Four phosphorylation sites are designated; a threonine (T) and three tyrosines (Y).

primary suspect. Contradictory evidence for dimerization accounting for the increased affinity has yet to be resolved.

The receptor is formed by posttranslational modification of a 1186-aminoacid, 130kDa polypeptide backbone [28,29]. Eleven to thirteen N-linked, but no O-linked, carbohydrate moieties bring the receptor to a functionally active, high mannose form [30–32]. Glycosylation is necessary for binding activity. This 160-kDa form is processed further to a mature receptor with a molecular weight of 170 kDa. Phosphorylation of the receptor occurs preferentially at four sites. Threonine at amino acid 654, just internal to the plasma membrane (figure 2), serves as the acceptor site for protein kinase C action [33–35]. Three tyrosine residues in the carboxy-terminal domain (amino acids 1173, 1148, and 1068) are the targets of intra- and intermolecular kinase activity [2,36,37].

The mature protein comprises four functional domains (figure 2). External to the cell lie two cysteine-rich regions, a feature conserved among this subfamily of receptors and the insulin receptor, but not the PDGF receptor group (figure 1) [38–43]. This is thought to be the site of ligand recognition. A short hydrophobic stretch of 23 amino acids forms the transmembrane span. A tyrosine kinase region is closely conserved with all of the other members of the superfamily. Lysine^{721} attaches ATP during the phosphorylation reaction [44]. The kinase domain is continuous, not interrupted as with PDGF and CSF-1 receptors [38, 45–47]. A specific carboxy terminus is thought to regulate the accessibility of the kinase domain [48–50]. Within this region lie the three autophosphorylation sites.

The gene covers over 110 kb on chromosome 7p11, constituting at least 26 exons [51,52]. Transcription initiation is controlled by a GC-rich element [53], similar to *ras* and the adenovirus gene E1a [54,55]. This control is distinct from that for c-*neu* (see below). The gene gives rise to two transcripts of 5.8 kb and 10.5 kb [2,4], though the rat gene produces only a single mRNA species [56]. The cause of this difference is unknown, though it is thought to represent elongation of the 3' untranslated region. In A431 cells a third transcript of 2.9 kb arises from a truncated gene. This leads to a secreted 115-kDa protein that consists of the external, lignad-binding domain [3,4,57]. This form might have arisen during amplicon formation. Similar occurrences have not been noted in other tissues or tumors. At the 5' end, the mRNA contain a signal sequence that directs the amino terminus to the exterior of the cell. These amino acids are cleaved from the maturing protein.

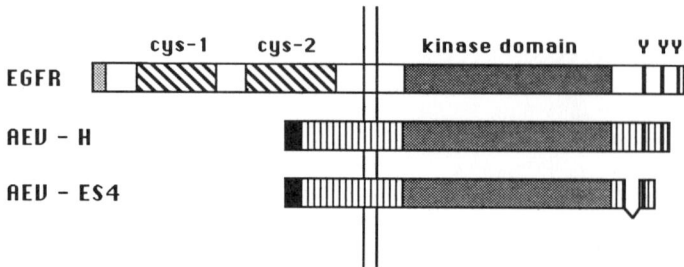

Figure 3. Comparison of the products of the EGFR and two AEV *erb*B genes. The various domains are as in figure 2. Both AEV genes are derived from the chicken homologue of the EGFR. The amino-terminus shaded region represents six amino acids from the viral *gag* gene.

The v-erbB oncogene

In 1936, Engelbreth-Holm and Meyer [58] isolated a virus that caused erythroblastosis in susceptible chickens. Various isolates of this virus, the avian erythroblastosis virus, have been analyzed. Common to all the viruses is the v-*erb*B gene, a membrane-spanning member of the tyrosine kinase family [59,60]. Molecular investigations of viral isolates have shown that while all are 5'-truncated versions of the chicken EGFR, differences exist in the integrity of the 3' coding sequences (figure 3) [13, 59–62]. Kung and others [11] studied a series of viral insertions in which all 5' integrations occurred within the same intron as that seen in the case of AEV-H and AEV-ES4. Carboxy-terminal truncations seem to dictate the disease spectrum of the resultant neoplasia. Virions with complete termini give rise to erythroblastosis, while those missing at least one phosphotyrosine acceptor site cause sarcomas [11,61,62]. However, this limitation has not been substantiated in mammalian tissue culture systems [63]. Point mutations seen amongst the various isolates and the parental gene seem not to play a role in transformation as the differences noted amount to conservative changes in neutral coding regions [5].

The AEV retroviral message consists of a spliced *gag-erb*B transcript (A. Bruskin, unpublished data). The splice acceptor represents a cellular intron–exon boundary in the second cystein-rich region [5,64]. The derived protein includes the amino-terminus six amino acids form *gag* and random amino acids at the carboxy terminus derived from the 3' *env* sequences of the retrovirus [59,60]. Thus, the polypeptide lacks an initial signal sequence, but still orients itself correctly in the plasma membrane [65]. This may be due to random integration [66] with specific degradation of the carboxy-external forms.

The protein product first appears as a 65-kDa polypeptide in the case of ES-4 [67] (the AEV-H protein is a few kilodaltons more massive [59]). Initial processing leads to a membrane-associated 68-kDa, high mannose form. Only a small percentage of label in pulse-chase experiments attain the final, cell surface form, which presents a broad band centered at 72 kDa [67,68]. Steady-state data suggest, however, that this may be the predominant species [63] though only a small fraction of translation products attain complete maturity. Use of inhibitors of glycosylation maturation [68] and temperature-sensitive mutants [69] provide evidence that transport to the cell surface is necessary for oncogenic potential.

Removal of the extracellular ligand-binding domain is postulated to lead to constitutive activation of the tyrosine kinase. Nevertheless, the absolute level of phosphotyrosine is elevated only marginally in infected cells [70]. This stands in contrast to other tyrosine kinase oncogenes and normal EGFR activation. Purified protein does not exhibit this kinase activity, since activating antibodies are necessary to demonstrate tyrosine phosphorylation in vitro [71,72]. It is likely that oncogenesis proceeds from compartmentalization of the protein or altered specificity as opposed to generalized increased enzymatic activity.

The neu *gene*

Two approaches led to the discovery of the *neu* gene, alternatively designated ERBB2 [73] or HER2 [41]. Treatment of pregnant rats with ethylnitrosourea induced neuro-/glio-blastomas in the newborn animals [74]. An oncogene was identified in the NIH3T3 focus-forming assay. Cloning and sequencing suggested a transmembrane growth factor receptor with intrinsic tyrosine kinase activity [40]. Sequence analysis foretold close homology with the EGFR. Independently, other groups were searching for genes with homology to EGFR/*erb*B. The human conterpart to the rat *neu* gene and these EGFR homologues were identical and mapped to chromosome 17q21 [41,75,76]. This second member of the EGFR family presents 44% homology in the extracellular cysteine-rich region, 82% in the conserved kinase region, and 32% in the specific tail segment [40,41,77]. In addition, *neu* contains both the internal phosphothreonine and the three phosphotyrosine sites. The topography of the product is identical to that of the EGFR (figure 1).

The c-*neu* gene regulation differs from EGFR in being under the control of TATA and CAAT boxes [78,79]. A single transcript of 4.6-kb is seen [80,81]. A truncated transcript of 2.3 kb, similar to the short EGFR message in A431 cells, has been detected in the gastric carcinoma cell line MKN-7 [75,80]. As this observation also is unique, the significance of such secreted receptor fragments remains speculative.

The *neu* gene product is a 185-kDa integral membrane glycoprotein with two external cysteine-rich regions and a cytoplasmic tyrosine kinase domain [82,83]. In spite of extensive searches the specific ligand has yet to be determined. The activated oncogene isolated from rat neuro-/glio-blastomas presents a tyrosine kinase activity that can be elicited from the cellular counterpart by activating antibodies [82,84]. The oncogenic version of the gene differs from the cellular homologue by presenting a charged amino acid in the middle of the transmembrane span [84]. It is speculated that this mutation affects the conformation or aggregation state of the receptor in the plasma membrane.

Both message and product are expressed in a tissue- and stage-specific manner [85]. In mid-gestational rat embryos, the gene is on in connective tissue, the nervous system, and secretory epithelium; in adult animals the gene is on only in secretory epithelium [85,86]. This pattern of the protein appearing predominantly in post mitotic cells is distinct from that of the EGFR.

The epidermal growth factor

The epidermal growth factor (EGF) was discovered by serendipity while investigating the effects of nerve growth factor (for review see [14]). This factor, extracted from the submaxillary gland, stimulated tooth eruption and eyelid opening in newborn animals. It subsequently was shown that urogastrone is the human homologue. The factor is a heat-stable, 6.2-kDa, 53-amino-acid polypeptide. There are three intramolecular disulphide bonds that are conserved among the EGF-like family (figure 4). The protein forms antiparallel sheets in solution with the carboxy terminus folding back upon this scaffolding [87–89]. Processing of the factor yields a form consisting of only the first 48 residues, which elicits only 10% of the mitogenic acitivity and lacks other functions [90]. Interestingly EGF proteins of high molecular weights have been isolated from a number of body fluids [91,92] and from the urine of patients with astrocytomas [93]. These hormones can replace EGF in biological assay systems and thus represent incomplete, aberrant processing of a larger precursor.

EGF is produced as a prohormone of 1207 amino acids [94–96]. This

```
hEGF               N S D S E C P L    S H D G Y C L H D G    V C M Y I E A L D
TGFα       V V S H F N K C P D        S H T Q Y C F H   G    T C R F L V Q E E
VGF        D I P A I R L C G P        E G D G Y C L H   G    D C I H A R D I D
SFGF       I V K H V K V C N H        D Y E N Y C L N N G    T C F T I   A L D N
MGF        I I K R I K L C N D        D Y K N Y C L N N G    T C F T V   A L N N

hEGF               K Y A C N C V      V G Y I G E R C Q Y    R D L K W W E L R
TGFα               K P A C V C H      S G Y V G V R C E H    A D L L A
VGF                G M Y C R C S      H G Y T G I R C Q H    V V L V D Y Q R S
SFGF       V S I T P F C V C R        I N Y E G S R C Q F    I N L V T Y
MGF        V S L N P F C A C H        I N Y V G S R C Q F    I N L I T I K
```

Figure 4. Comparison of the various EGFR ligands. The primary amino acid sequences of human EGF [95], rat TGF α [112], vaccinia virus growth factor (VGF) [120], Shope fibroma virus growth factor (SFGF) [1975], and myxoma virus growth factor (MGF) [196] are aligned to demonstrate homologies. Bold face denotes amino acids in common. The entire mature forms of EGF and TGF α are shown. The VGF sequence represents amino acids 38 to 92 of the prohormonal form. The other poxvirus sequences are deduced from codons 26 to 79 (SFGF) and 30 to 84 (MGF).

polypeptide takes the form of a membrane-anchored glycoprotein with a short cytoplasmic tail. The molecule contains eight EGF-like repeats exposed on the external surface, the innermost being the mature EGF. These repeats share homology with LDL receptor regions that have been implicated in acid-dissociable binding and receptor recycling [97,98]. Additional homologies with these repeats have been detected in Drosophila neurogenic genes [99,100] and nematode homeotic genes [101]. Lastly, there is distant relationship between the short cytoplasmic domain of pro-EGF and the serine/threonine kinase oncogene *mos* [102]. The significance of these relations remains a mystery, though the prohormonal form may subsume the role of a membrane receptor.

The prepro-EGF gene consists of at least 24 exons covering 110 kb at chromosome 4q24–26 [94]. This gene is actively transcribed in a number of epithelial tissues [103]. The highest level of synthesis is seen in salivary glands, where testosterone treatment greatly augments hormone production. While EGFR expression is seen to be differentiation-stage-related in embryos [104], ligand message appears only after weaning [105]. The physiologic relevant EGF in the pre- and perinatal periods is maternally derived [106,107].

Transforming growth factor α

Transforming growth factor α(TGF-α) was isolated as one component of the sarcoma growth factor (the other being TGF-β), a potent mitogen produced by various tumor lines. This 5.6-kDa, 50-amino-acid protein shares homology with EGF, including the three disulphide bridges (figure 4). The biological effects of EGF, including precocious eyelid opening, can be duplicated by this mitogen [108–111]. TGF-α has been shown to compete with EGF binding; antagonistic EGFR antibodies block TGF-α-associated responses [112]. This hormone binds to the EGFR with comparable affinity to EGF and activates the tyrosine kinase [113–115]. Thus EGFR serves as the target for both hormones, EGF and TGF. The only biologic difference between the two ligands concerns a small quantitative difference in vascular epithelial responsiveness [113].

The gene, on chromosome 2p11-13 [116], encodes a prohormone from [94]. The membrane-anchored 160-amino-acid polypeptide is glycosylated as well as conjoined with palmitate [115]. There is only one EGF-like sequence. Higher-molecular-weight forms of TGF-α have been noted. The role of this membrane form, like that of pro-EGF, remains speculative. Various workers have postulated that TGF-α represents an embryonal form of EGF. It is absent from most adult tissues but is expressed by a number of solid tumors and transformed cells [117]. Reports of TGF-α expression in rat embryos are misleading since the material is concentrated in the maternal decidua and is induced by implantation [118]. The embryonal form of the EGFR ligand remains maternally derived hormone.

Poxvirus growth factors

Poxviruses encode sequences that bear striking homology to the EGF family (figure 4). The best-characterized of these, the vaccinia growth factor or 19K early protein, is a 140-amino-acid protein [119]. This membrane-associated form is reminiscent of pre-TGF-α. One of the characteristics of poxvirus infection is a benign hyperproliferative response of the infected epithelium [120]. Definitive elucidation of the role of the viral growth factors (VGFs) awaits viral deletion mutants. However, VGF stimulates EGFR kinase activity directly [119]. Recognizing the same site as EGF, it effectively competes with ligand [121]. The viral factors may induce an autocrine loop in infected cells that present receptor.

The action

The ligands of the EGF family exert their effects either through or in conjunction with the EGFR. Thus, in discussing actions and mechanisms, the EGF ligand/receptor system will be considered as a functional unit.

The signaling pathway

EGFR presents two populations of receptors with dissociation constants on the order of 0.3nM and 4nM. Phorbol ester treatment of cells induces phosphorylation of threonine^{654} by protein kinase C, resulting in a shift of the high-affinity receptor to the lower-affinity form [48,122–125]. This treatment abrogates most EGF responses, arguing for the high-affinity group being the active receptors. The fact that submaximal binding of EGF initiates some effects also would support this contention [14]. Binding of ligand alters the aggregation state of the EGFR. While there is evidence pointing to a monomerization of receptor coincident with increased affinity, the weight of the data currently favors the opposite situation—that interaction with ligand shifts the EGFR to a dimerized form that binds ligand more tenaciously [22,24,25,126].

Aggregated receptors are recruited into coated pits, internalized, sequestered in endosomes, and degraded in an acidic environment [27, 127–129]. During aggregation, the tyrosine kinase is activated. The initial reaction kinetics suggests a bi–bi reaction leading to autophosphorylation of the carboxy-terminal tyrosines [130]. Kinase activity is sensitive to levels of ATP stores [131] and receptor concentration. Sufficient EGFR concentration triggers phosphorylation independently of ligand binding status [9,23,26,132]. Ligand increases the activity of monomers four-fold, but only marginally affects aggregated receptors [26]. Agonistic antibodies may exert their effects by cross-linking receptors and achieving this critical concentration [133]. One scenario presents kinase activation as secondary to receptor accumulation in coated pits, the role of ligand being a passive one that facilitates this EGFR movement.

Receptor hybrids have demonstrated the independence of the ligand-binding and kinase domains [134–137]. Insulin and IL-2 (TCGF) can activate the heterologous kinase in insulin receptor/EGFR and IL-2 receptor/EGFR hybrids, respectively. The role of ligand is nonspecific, a fact that supports conformation alterations or aggregation as being the initial mechanism of activation. The nature of the activating mutation in *neu* provides suggestive support for this concept. The kinase domains do impart some specificity [136]. *erb/src* hybrids share phenotypes of both oncogenes [138]. The external domain offers the ligand specificity while the cytoplasmic portion imparts the commands. The role of the most divergent region of the growth factor receptors, the tails, awaits the results of further structural studies. However, data from studies on *erb*B suggest that these short regions play major roles in determining cellular specificity of activation.

The threonine phosphorylation site constitutes a controlling element in EGFR functioning. Protein kinase C will phosphorylate this amino acid either after phorbol ester exposure or in a feedback mechanism secondary to EGF binding [122]. A second mechanism, independent of protein kinase C, results in phosphorylation of threonine^{654} subsequent to PDGF receptor activation [122,139,140]. Labeling of this residue causes receptor internalization and recycling instead of the lysozyme-directed specific degradation sequence (see below). Site-specific replacement of this amino acid also abrogates the natural sequence of internalization and degradation subsequent to ligand binding, leading to the nonmitogenic cycling motif [35,141].

Once internalized, the receptor is cleaved just proximal to the three phosphotyrosine sites ([142], author's unpublished observations). A calcium-dependent, neutral protease releases a protein of 150 kDa. Such removal of the terminal tyrosine autophosphorylation sites is a hallmark of viral transduction of tyrosine kinase proto-oncogenes [143]. Further proteolytic cleavages leave a 42-kDa core kinase domain that retains activity [144]. Interestingly, in vivo systems have traced labeled EGF and even intact receptor to peri- and intranuclear sites [145–150]. That the EGFR is closely associated with a DNA nicking molecule [151,152] is an intriguing coincidence.

Intramolecular tyrosine phosphorylation precedes exogenous substrate labeling [9,153]. The most carboxy-terminal tyrosine (tyr^{1173}) is rapidly phosphorylated, with the other two sites being labeled more slowly [36]. The tail is pictured as lying in the kinase active site, masking it. Upon activation, phosphorylation of these tyrosines unhinges this domain, opening the active cleft to other substrates [126]. A number of target proteins have been identified [143,153–155], but none have been shown to be of physiologic relevance.

Of the multitude of measureable responses to ligand binding (table 1), only aggregation proceeds independently of kinase activity. Aggregation has been demonstrated in mutants lacking the entire cytoplasmic region [156]. As

Table 1. Action of epidermal growth factor

Immediate	Early	Late
Aggregation	Internalization	Morphologic changes
Dimerization	Down-regulation	Nuclear accumulation
Monomerization	Degradation	DNA synthesis
Auto- & exo-kinase	S6 phosphorylation	Anchorage-independence
PI turnover	mRNA synthesis	
Ca^{++} flux	*myc, fos, jun*, EGFR	

stated above, internalization and down regulation of binding sites can be effected by heterologous regulation and nonactivating antibodies [157], and by ligand in kinase-negative mutants [158]. However, these reactions follow a different pathway than the normally witnessed one, failing to elicit the secondary responses.

Immediately upon ligand activation, phosphotidyl inositol (PI) is broken down to IP_3 and diacylgycerol (see chapter) [159,160]. There is a concommittant calcium flux, consisting mainly of mobilization of internal stores [161]. Shortly thereafter, the S6 ribosomal protein is phosphorylated on serine [162]. Increased transcription of various messages leads to higher levels of *fos, myc*, and the EGFR itself [163–166]. All of the above responses can be effected with activation of EGFR frozen on the cell surface, a situation in which mitogenesis is not accomplished [167]. In addition, evidence suggests that EGFR mitogenesis is not contingent upon PI turnover [168]. Thus, the roles of these initial responses in the mitogenic cascade remains unproven.

Internalization is thought to be necessary for morphological changes to occur. However, it is possible that internalization and subsequent degradation serve only to negatively regulate EGFR activation. Upon ligand stimulation, the cells assume a transformed phenotype [169,170]. At least six hours of constant exposure to EGF is needed to induce de novo DNA synthesis [14]. This is consistent with the view of EGF as a progression factor [171]. In the presence of EGF tissue culture fibroblasts and epithelial cells grow with a transformed phenotype; these cell are fully capable of proliferation in soft agar [172]. In this aspect a ligand/receptor exocrine loop recaptures the oncogenic phenotype.

The EGFR system is not activated in a vacuum. Other mitogens and proto-oncogenes are involved in the cascade. The oncogene *abl* cannot transform EGFR-negative lines [173]. Biochemical data link EGFR activation to tyrosine phosphorylation of c-*src* [174,175] and increased G protein activity [176,177]. Other growth factors transmodulate EGFR activity. In the transcription activation of the proto-oncogenes *fos* and *myc*, the various growth factors seem to induce via the same serum responsive element [178]. Recently, EGF has been shown to stimulate the transcription of c-*jun*, itself a transcriptional activator [179]. Other oncogenes can supplant EGF activation [180]. These various factors converge in one pathway. However, not all

Table 2. Cell types in which EGF is mitogenic

Adipocyte precursors [197]	Explanted tumors [173, 198]
Epithelial cells [199]	Fibroblast [200–202]
Passaged hepatocytes [203]	Neural crest cells [204]
Normal kidney cells [205]	Postnephrectomy tubule cells [206]
Embryonic tooth buds [105]	Keratinocytes [207]

Table 3. Differentiation-associated effects of EGF

Inhibition of cell growth
Transformed kidney cells [208]
Maturation of urothelium [209]
Early-passage hepatocytes [183]
Multidrug-resistant CHO cells [210]
Syncytiotrophoblasts [211, 212]

Differentiation-related factor production
Prolactin synthesis and secretion [213]
Increased T-cell suppressor activity [91]
Surfactant-associated protein [216]
Interferon production [214]
MHC class II expression [215]
Tyrosine hydroxylase [217]
Cell adhesion molecules in breast cancer lines [218]
Hyaluronic acid and proteoglycan [204]

Table 4. Pleiotropic EGF effects

Precocious eyelid opening [107]
Prevention of spontaneous abortion [108]
Increased rate of wound healing with decreased cellularity [219, 220]
Pregnancy-related mammary gland growth and milk production [221]
Maintenance of epidermal growth and maturation [222]

proliferative programs play upon this lead. *ras* acts independently of EGFR status [181]. The PI/calcium mitogenic response works via a distinct cAMP-responsive element to initiate de novo transcription.

Proliferation and differentiation responses

While EGF and TGF are generally viewed as mitogens (table 2), in a number of in vivo systems the effect of ligand–receptor interaction can be best described as subsuming a differentiation function (table 3). In other organ systems, both proliferation and differentiation are effected by this hormone system (table 4). Additionally, EGFR activation varies with the age of the target. Senescent fibroblasts present a weaker response and lower kinase activity in the face of equal numbers of receptors [182]. Early-passage rat hepatocytes are growth-inhibited by EGF [183], whereas this hormone serves as a mitogen in later passages [184,185].

EGF induces proliferation of normal epithelial and fibroblastic cells and most explanted tumors. However, ligand elicits differentiation markers in many postmitotic cells (see table 3 for a listing). It also is associated with a reversion of the transformed phenotype in multidrug-resistant CHO cells and transformed rat kidney cells.

A number of animal organ systems present a dual nature of the ligand–receptor interaction (table 4). EGF is necessary for maintaining adequate epidermis development. It induces proliferation of the basal layer of cells and migration of keratinocytes. However, the same factor is linked to terminal maturation of more mature cells. In wound healing, topical EGF treatment speeds both fibroblast invasion and proliferation, and organization of the wound. The fact that one ligand–receptor system achieves both programs suggests that the effect of activation is determined, at least in part, by the keyboard upon which the signaling plays.

Carcinogenesis and tumor progression

Since EGF is a mitogen and confers a transformed phenotype upon tissue culture cells (see above), searching for the activation of this system in human neoplasias is obvious. A number of tumors produce TGF, but aberrant EGF production has not been noted. With the discovery that the EGFR gene is transduced as the *erb*B oncogene, focus shifted to the receptor. A large number of carcinomas present increased numbers of binding sites or amplified genes (table 5). Furthermore, the association is more striking when one looks at tumor grade: the more advanced the neoplasia, the greater the association. Gene amplification is noted in about half of glioblastomas but is absent in gliomas. In a series of bladder carcinomas, 21 of 24 invasive neoplasias presented increased staining, while only 7 of 24 superficial tumors marked similarly. More stringent restriction of increased EGFR was seen between early and late gastric carcinomas. Lastly, EGF binding level can be utilized as a prognostic indicator in estrogen receptor-negative breast cancer.

A few caveats need be mentioned. In the situations of *erb*B and experimental models with *neu* [186], the gene directly induces cancerous formation. The association of the EGFR with human tumors is reminiscent more of that of *myc* and N-*myc* [187]. Namely, EGFR enhancement is linked to tumor aggressiveness, not the initial neoplastic change. In light of the emerging interest in emerogenes (also referred to as recessive oncogenes or anti-oncogenes) [188], this implies a sequence of changes taking a normal cell through immortalization to frank malignancy.

Implication of EGFR in the neoplastic process is not universal. Pituitary cells, which normally present average numbers of receptors, lose all EGF binding sites when seen as adenocarcinomas. The relationship between EGFR level and tumor stage is lacking in esophageal squamous tumors, precisely those tumors that have yielded some of the highest EGFR concentrations. SF268, a glioblastoma cell line that expresses increased levels of

Table 5. Neoplastic processes associated with increased EGFR

Neoplasia	Method[a]	Frequency[b]	Reference
Psoriasis	EGF binding		223
Squamous carcinoma lines	Gene amplification	10/12	18
Squamous carcinomas	Gene amplification	1/6	18
Squamous carcinoma lines	EGF binding	6/8	224
Glioblastoma multiformes	Gene amplification	4/9	225
Glioblastoma multiformes	Autophosphorylation	11/21	226
Meningiomas	Autophosphorylation	3/5	226
Bladder carcinomas	Immunostaining	21/24 invsv 7/24 spfcl	227
Non-small-cell lung carcinoma	Immunostanding	45/77	228
Primary breast carcinomas	Gene amplification	3/21	229
Primary breast carcinomas	EGF binding	57/135	230
Thyroid carcinomas	EGF binding	5/8	231
Pancreatic carcinoma lines	EGF binding Gene amplification	4/4	231 232
Gastric carcinomas	Immunostaining	38/130 advncd 0/26 early	233
Esophageal carcinomas[c]	EGF binding	22/31	17
Pituitary adenomas[d]	EGF binding	22/22	234

[a]Parameter utilized to determine aberrant expression.
[b]Number of cases showing overexpression/number of cases examined.
[c]In this series there was no relationship between EGF binding and prognosis.
[d]In the pituitary adenomas, EGF binding was absent.

binding and gene amplification [189], fails to respond to EGF in vitro [190]. The kinase activity of this overexpressed receptor cannot be elicited.

The weight of circumstantial evidence does favor a positive role for the EGFR in tumor aggressiveness. In two series of tumor cell variants presenting differing levels of receptors, those subclones with the highest levels grew best when implanted in animals [191–193]. Thus, enhanced EGFR expression may present a growth advantage by either increased responsiveness to circulating ligand or density-dependent autoactivation of the mitogenic cascade. Reversion of the transformed phenotype induced by *neu* can be accomplished through down regulation of the *neu* protein by antibodies directed against this oncogene [83]. Immunologically targeting this growth factor receptor prevented tumors in transplanted animals [194]. The presence of this receptor family can be linked to tumor development, and its absence to the abrogation of such phenomena.

Denouement

In sum, we have a receptor–ligand system that is utilized in a number of tissues to control normal growth and differentiation. Two cell-encoded ligands activate this receptor indistinguishably. The prohormal structure of these ligands and their relationship to lineage-determining genes in lower forms suggest that they subsume a receptor role in addition to their endocrine functions. Their relationship to each other and the separate roles they may play have yet to be determined.

In their interaction with the EGFR, these two ligands seem to be interchangeable. Upon binding, the receptor aggregates and its kinase activity is unleashed. A cascade of events follows. However, these initial stages may be elicited without final alteration of the genetic program. For this to occur, constant activation with internalization must be accomplished. Intriguing observations hint at the possibility of activated EGFR abutting or even entering the nucleus to transmit its signal. However, the outcome of such signaling depends on the genetic keyboard of the target cell as similar sequences lead to either proliferation or differentiation.

The working of the EGFR in normal signaling allows for subtle alterations to produce phenotypic changes. Already, transduced oncogenes and naturally occurring mutations have hinted at the mechanisms involved in the fine-tuned control and its breakdown. The EGFR system has been associated with a number of human epithelial tumors. Obvious hypotheses can be constructed invoking increased mitogenic responsiveness of the amplified protein. However, in a number of instances the system induces terminal differentiation. Herein, abrogation of the EGF response may be necessary to maintain uncontrolled growth. This may be occurring in those neoplasias in which the receptor is aberrantly absent or inactivated. Much further work is necessary, but there is reason to believe that elucidation of the role of this receptor system may lead to better and more specific diagnostic and treatment modalities.

References

1. Downward J, Yarden Y, Mayes E, Scrace G, Totty N, Stockwell P, Ullrich A, Schlessinger J, Waterfield MD: Close similarity of epidermal growth factor receptor and v-erb-B oncogene protein sequences. Nature 307:521–527.
2. Ullrich A, Coussens L, Hayflick JS, Dull TJ, Tam AW, Lee J, Yarden Y, Libermann TA, Schlessinger J, Downward J, Mayes ELV, Whittle N, Waterfield MD, Seeburg PH: Human epidermal growth factor receptor cDNA sequence and aberrant expression of the amplified gene in A431 epidermoid carcinoma cells. Nature 309:418–425, 1984.
3. Lin CR, WS Chen, Kruiger W, Stolarsky LS, Weber W, Evans RM, Verma IM, Gill GN, Rosenfeld MG: Expression cloning of human EGF receptor complementary DNA: gene amplification and three related messenger RNA products in A431 cells. Science 224: 843–848,1984.
4. Xu Y, Ishii S, Clark AJL, Sullivan M, Wilson RK, Ma DP, Roe BA, Merlino GT, Pastan I: Human epidermal growth factor receptor cDNA is homologous to a variety of RNAs overproduced in A431 carcinoma cells. Nature 309:806–810, 1984.
5. Fung Y-K Lewis WG, Crittenden LB, Kung H-J: Activation of the cellular oncogene c-erbB by LTR insertion: molecular basis for induction of erythroblastosis by avian leukosis virus. Cell 33:357–368, 1983.
6. Goustin AS, Leof EB, Shipley GD, Moses HL: Growth factors and cancer. Cancer Res

46:1015–1029, 1986.
7. Heldin C, Westermark B: Growth factor: mechanism of action and relation to oncogenes. Cell 37:9–20, 1984.
8. Carpenter G: Properties of the receptor for epidermal growth factor. Cell 37:357–358, 1984.
9. Carpenter G: Receptors for epidermal growth factor and other polypeptide mitogens. Annu Rev Biochem 56:881–914, 1987.
10. King CS, Cooper JA, Moss B Twardzik DR: Vaccinia virus growth factor stimulates tyrosine protein kinase activity of A431 cell epidermal growth factor receptors. Mol Cell Biol 6:332–336, 1986.
11. Nilsen TW, Maroney PA, Goodwin RG, Rottman FM, Crittenden LB, Raines MA Kung H-J: C-*erb*B activation in ALV-induced erythroblastosis: novel RNA processing and promoter insertion results in expression of an amino-truncated EGF-receptor. Cell 41:719–726,1985.
12. Goodwin RG, Rottman FM, Callaghan T, Kung H-J, Maroney PA, Nilsen T: C-*erb*B activation in avian leukosis virus-induced erythroblastosis: multiple epidermal growth factor receptor mRNAs are generated by alternative RNA processing. Mol Cell Biol 6:3128–3133, 1986.
13. Miles BD, Robinson HL: High-frequency transduction of c-*erb*B in avian leukosis virus-induced erythroblastosis. J Virol 54:295–303, 1985.
14. Carpenter G, Cohen S: Epidermal growth factor. Annu Rev Biochem 48:193–216, 1979.
15. Carpenter G, Zendegui JG: Epidermal growth factor, its receptor, and related proteins. Exp Cell Res 164:1–10, 1986.
16. Xu Y, Richert N, Ito S, Merlino GT, Pastan I: Characterization of epidermal growth factor receptor gene expression in malignant and normal human cell lines. Proc Natl Acad Sci USA 81:7308–7312, 1984.
17. Ozawa S, Ueda M, Ando N, Abe O, Shimizu N: High incidence of EGF receptor hyperproduction in esophageal squamous-cell carcinomas. Int J Cancer 39:333–337, 1987.
18. Yamamoto T, Kamata N, Kawano H, Shimizu S, Kuroki T, Toyoshima K, Rikimaru K, Normura N, Ishizaki R, Pastan I, Gamou S, Shimizu N: High incidence of amplification of the epidermal growth factor receptor gene in human squamous carcinoma cell lines. Cancer Res 46:414–416, 1986.
19. Giard DJ, Aaronson SA, Todaro GJ, Arnstein P, Kersey JH, Dosik H, Parks WP: In vitro cultivation of human tumors: establishment of cell lines derived from a series of solid tumors. J Natl Cancer Inst 51:1417–1423 (A431), 1973.
20. Rees AR, Gregoriou M, Johnson P, Garland PB: High affinity epidermal growth factor receptors on the surface of A431 cells have restricted lateral diffusion. EMBO J 3:1843–1847, 1984.
21. Gregoriou M, Rees AR: Properties of a monoclonal antibody to epidermal growth factor receptor with implications for the mechanisms of action of EGF. EMBO J 3:929–937, 1984.
22. Schlessinger J: Allsoteric regulation of the epidermal growth factor receptor kinase. J Cell Biol 103:2067–2072, 1986.
23. Biswas R, Basu M, Sen-Majumdar A, Das M: Intrapeptide autophosphorylation of the epidermal growth factor receptor: regulation of kinase catalytic function by receptor dimerization. Biochemistry 24:3795–3802, 1985.
24. Fanger BO, Austin KS, Earp HS, Cidlowski JA: Cross-linking of epidermal growth factor receptors in intact cells: detection of initial stages of receptor clustering and determination of molecular weight of high-affinity receptors, 1986. Biochemistry 25:6414–6420, 1986.
25. Yarden Y, Schlessinger J: Epidermal growth factor induces rapid, reversible aggregation of the purified epidermal growth factor receptor. Biochemistry 26:1443–1451, 1987.
26. Boni-Schnetzler M, Pilch PF: Mechanism of epidermal growth factor receptor autophosphorylation and high-affinity binding. Proc Natl Acad Sci USA 84:7832–7836, 1987.
27. Zidovetzki R, Yarden Y, Schlessinger J, Jovin TM: Microaggregation of hormone-occupied epidermal growth factor receptors on plasma membrane preparations. EMBO J 5:247–250, 1986.
28. Carlin CR, Knowles BB: Biosynthesis and glycosylation of the epidermal growth factor

receptor in human tumor-derived cell lines A431 and Hep 3B. Mol Cell Biol 6:257–264, 1986.
29. Soderquist AM, G Carpenter: Glycosylation of the epidermal growth factor receptor in A431 cells: the contribution of carbohydrate to receptor function. J Biol Chem 259:12586–12594, 1984.
30. Mayes ELV, Waterfield MD: Biosynthesis of the epidermal growth factor receptor in A431 cells. EMBO J3:531–537, 1984.
31. Slieker LJ, Lane MD: Post-translational processing of the epidermal growth factor receptor: glycosylation-dependent acquisition of ligand-binding capacity. J Biol Chem 260:687–690, 1985.
32. Slieker LJ, Martensen TM, Lane MD: Synthesis of epidermal growth factor receptor in human A431 cells. J Biol Chem 261:15233–15241, 1986.
33. Hunter T, Ling N Cooper JA: Protein kinase C phosphorylation of the EGF receptor at a threonine residue close to the cytoplasmic face of the plasma membrane. Nature 311:480–483, 1984.
34. Davis RJ, Czech MP: Stimulation of epidermal growth factor receptor threonine 654 phosphorylation bby platelet-derived growth factor in protein kinase C-deficient human fibroblasts. J Biol Chem 262:6832–6841, 1987.
35. Lin CR, Chen WS, Lazar CS, Carpenter CD, Gill GN, Evans RM, Rosenfeld MG: Protein kinase C phosphorylation at Thr 654 of the unoccupied EGF receptor and EGF binding regulate functional receptor loss by independent mechanisms. Cell 44:839–848, 1986.
36. Downward J, Parker P Waterfield MD: Autophosphorylation sites on the epidermal growth factor receptor. Nature 311:483–485, 1984.
37. Gullick WJ, Downward J Waterfield MD: Antibodies to the autophosphorylation sites of the epidermal growth factor receptor protein-tyrosine kinase as probes of structure and function. EMBO J 4:2869–2877, 1985.
38. Yarden Y, Escobedo JA, Kuang W, Yang-Feng TL, Daniel TO, Tremble PM, Chen EY, Ando ME, Harkins RN, Franke U, Fried VA, Ullrich A, Williams LT. Structure of the receptor for platelet-derived growth factor helps define a family of closely related growth factor receptors. Nature 323:226–232, 1986.
39. Ross R, Raines EW, Bowen-Pope DF. The biology of platelet-derived growth factor. Cell 46:155–169, 1986.
40. Bargmann CI, Hung M, Weinberg RA: The *neu* oncogene encodes an epidermal growth factor receptor-related protein. Nature 319:226–230, 1986.
41. Coussens L, Yang-Feng TL, Liao Y, Chen E, Gray A, McGrath J, Seeburg PH, Libermann T, Schlessinger J, Francke U, Levinson A, Ullrich A: Tyrosine kinase receptor with extensive homology to EGF receptor shares chromosomal location with *neu* oncogene. Science 230:1132–1139, 1985.
42. Ullrich A, Bell J, Chen E, Herrera R, Petruzzelli L, Dull TJ, Gray A, Coussens L, Liao Y, Tsubokawa M, Mason A, Seeburg PH, Grunfeld C, Rosen OM, Ramachandran J: Human insulin receptor and its relationship to the tyrosine kinase family of oncogenes. Nature 313:756–761, 1985.
43. Ebina Y, Ellis L, Jarnagin K, Edery M, Graf L, Clauser E, Ou J, Masiarz F, Kan YW, Goldfine ID, Roth R, Rutter WJ: The human insulin receptor cDNA: the structural basis for hormone-activated transmembrane signalling. Cell 40:747–758, 1985.
44. Russo MW, Lukas TJ, Cohen S, Staros JV: Identification of residues in the nucleotide binding site of the epidermal growth factor receptor/kinase. J Biol Chem 260:5205–5208, 1985.
45. Scherr CJ, Rettenmier C, Sacca R, Roussel M, Look At, Stanley ER: The c-*fms* proto-oncogene product is related to the receptor for the mononuclear phagocyte growth factor, CSF-1. Cell 41:665–676, 1985.
46. Coussens L, van Beveren C, Smith D, Chen E, Mitchell R, Isacke C, Verma IM, Ullrich A: Structural alteration of viral homologue of receptor protooncogene *fms* at carboxyl terminus. Nature 320:277–280, 1986.

47. Ullrich A, Riedel H, Yarden Y, Coussens L, Gray A, Dull T, Schlessinger J, Waterfield MD. Parker PJ: Protein kinases in cellular signal transduction: tyrosine kinase growth factor receptors and protein kinase C. CSH Symp Quant Biol 51:713–724, 1986.
48. Downward J, Waterfield MD, Parker PJ: Autophosphorylation annd protein kinase C phosphorylation of the epidermal growth factor receptor: effect on tyrosine kinase activity and ligand binding affinity. J Biol Chem 260:14538–14546, 1985.
49. Bertics PJ, Gill GN: Self-phosphorylation enhances the protein-tyrosine kinase activity of the epidermal growth factor receptors on plasma membrane preparations. EMBO J 5:247–50, 1986.
50. Chinkers M, Garbers DL: Suppression of protein tyrosine kinase activity of the epidermal growth factor receptor by epidermal growth factor. J Biol Chem 261:8295–8297, 1986.
51. Jansson M, Philipson L, Vennstrom B: Isolation and characterization of multiple human genes homologous to the oncogenes of avian erythroblastosis virus. EMBO J 2:561–565, 1983.
52. Haley J, Whittle N, Bennett P, Kinchington K, Ullrich A, Waterfield M: The human EGF receptor gene: Structure of the 110kb locus and identification of sequences regulating its transcription. Oncogene Res 1:375–396, 1987.
53. Ishii S, Xu Y, Stratton RH, Roe BA, Merlino GT, Pastan I: Characterization and sequence of the promoter region of the human epidermal growth factor receptor gene. Proc Natl Acad Sci USA 82: 4920–4924, 1985.
54. Ishii S, Merlino GT, Pastan I: Promoter region of the human Harvey *ras* proto-oncogene: similarly to the EGF receptor proto-oncogene promoter. Science 230:1378–1381, 1985.
55. Dynan WS, Tjian R: Control of eukaryotic messenger RNA synthesis by sequence-specific DNA-binding protein. Nature 316:774–778, 1985.
56. Hung M, Thompson KL, Chiu I, Rosner MR: Characterization of rodent epidermal growth factor receptor transcripts using a mouse genomic probe. Biochem Biophys Res Comm 141: 1109–1115, 1986.
57. Weber W, Gill GN, Spiess J: Production of an epidermal growth factor receptor-related protein. Science 224:294–297, 1984.
58. Engelbreth-Holm J, Rothe Meyer A: On the connection between erythroblastosis (Haemocytoblastosis), myelosis, and sarcoma in chicken. Acta Pathol Microbiol Scand 12:352–377, 1935.
59. Yamamoto T, Nishida Y, Miyajimi N, Kawai S, Ooi T, Toyoshima K: The *erb*B gene of avian erythroblastosis virus is a member of the *src* gene family. Cell 35:71–78, 1983.
60. Privalsky ML, Ralston R, Bishop JM: The membrane glycoprotein encoded by the retroviral oncogene v-*erb*B is structurally related to tyrosine-specific protein kinases. Proc Natl Acad Sci USA 81:704–707, 1984.
61. Tracey SE, Woda BA, Robinson HL: Induction of angiosarcoma by a c-*erb*B transducing virus. J Virol 54:304–310, 1985.
62. Gamett DC, Tracy SE, Robinson HL: Differences in sequences encoding the carboxyl-terminal domain of the epidermal growth factor receptor correlate with differences in the disease potential of viral *erb*B genes. Proc Natl Acad Sci USA 83:6053–6057, 1986.
63. Wells A, Bishop JM: Genetic determinants of neoplastic transformation by the retroviral oncogene v-*erb*-B. Proc Natl Acad Sci USA 85:7597–7601, 1988.
64. Henry C, Coquillaud M, Saule S, Stehelin D, Debuuirre B: The four C-terminal amino acids of the v-*erb*A polypeptide are encoded by an intronic sequence of the v-*erb*B oncogene. Virol 140:179–182, 1985.
65. Schatzman RC, Evans GI, Privalsky ML, Bishop JM: Orientation of the ve-*erb*B gene product in the plasma membrane. Mol Cell Biol 6:1329–1333, 1986.
66. Mize NK, Andrews DW, Lingappa VR: A stop transfer sequence recognizes receptors for nascent chain translocation across the endoplamsic reticulum membrane. Cell 47:711–719, 1986.
67. Privalsky ML, Sealy L, Bishop JM, McGrath JP, Levinson AD: The product of the Avian Erythroblastosis virus *erb*B locus is a glycoprotein. Cell 32:1257–1267, 1983.

68. Schmidt JA, Beug H, Hayman MJ: Effects of inhibitors of glycoprotein processing on the synthesis and biological activity of the erbB oncogene. EMBO J 4:105–112, 1985.
69. Beug H, Hayman MJ: Temperature-sensitive mutants of avian erythroblastosis virus: surface expression of the erbB product correlates with transformation. Cell 36:963–972, 1984.
70. Hayman MJ, Kitchener G, Knight J, McMahon J, Watson R, Beug H: Analysis of the autophosphorylation activity of transformation defective mutants of avian erythroblastosis virus. Virology 150:270–275, 1986.
71. Decker SJ: Phosphorylation of the erbB gene product from an avian erythro-blastosis virus-transformed chick fibroblast cell line. J Biol Chem 260:2003–2006, 1985.
72. Kris RM, Lax I, Gullick W, Waterfield MD, Fridkin M Schlessinger J: Anti-bodies against a synthetic peptide as a probe for the kinase activity of the avian EGF receptor and v-erbB protein. Cell 40:619–625, 1985.
73. Semba K, Kamata N, Toyoshima K, Yamamoto T: A v-erbB-related proto-oncogene, c-erbB-2, is distinct from thhe c-erbB-1/epidermal growth factor-receptor gene and is amplified in a human salivary gland adenocarcinoma. Proc Natl Acad Sci USA 82: 6497–6501, 1985.
74. Shih C, Paddy LC, Murray M, Weinberg RA: Transforming genes of carcinomas and neuroblastomas introduced into mouse fibroblasts. Nature 290:261–264, 1981.
75. Fukushige S, Matsubara K, Yoshida M, Sasaki M, Suzuki T, Semba K, Toyoshima K, Yamamoto T: Localization of a novel v-erbB-related gene, c-erbB-2, on human chromosome 17 and its amplification in a gastric cancer cell line. Mol Cell Biol 6:955–958, 1986.
76. Kaneko Y, Homma C, Maseki N, Sakurai M, Toyoshima K, Yamamoto T: Human c-erbB-2 reamins on chromosome 17 in band q21 in the 15;17 translocation associated with acute promyelocytic leukemia. Jpn J Cancer Res 78:16–19, 1987.
77. Toyoshima K, Semba K, Akiyama T, Ikawa S, Yamamoto T: The c-erbB-2 gene encodes a receptor-like protein withh tyrosine kinase activity. CSH Symp Quant Biol 51:977–982, 1986.
78. Ishii S, Imamoto F, Yamanashi Y, Toyoshima K, Yamamoto T: Characterization of the promoter region of the human c-erbB-2 protooncogene. Proc Natl Acad Sci USA 84:4374–4378, 1987.
79. Tal M, King CR, Kraus MH, Ullrich A, Schlessinger J Givol D: Human HER2 (neu) promoter: evidence for multiple mechanisms for transcriptional initiation. Mol Cell Biol 7:2597–2601, 1987.
80. Yamamoto T, Ikawa S, Akiyama T, Semba K, Nomura N, Miyajima N, Saito T Toyoshima K: Similarity of protein encoded by the human c-erbB-2 gene to epidermal growth factor receptor. Nature 319:230–234, 1986.
81. Kraus MH, Popescu NC, Amsbaugh SC, King CR: Overexpression of the EGF receptor-related proto-oncogene erbB-2 in human mammary tumor cel lines by different molecular mechanisms. EMBO J 6:605–610, 1987.
82. Stern DF, Heffernan PA, Weinberg RA: p185, a product of the neu protooncogene, is a receptorlike protein associated with tyrosine kinase activity. Mol Cell Biol 6:1729–1740, 1986.
83. Drebin JA, Link VC, Stern DF, Weinberg RA, Greene MI: Down-modulation of an oncogene protein product and reversion of the transformed phenotype by monoclonal antibodies. Cell 41:695–706, 1985.
84. Bargmann CI, Hung M, Weinberg RA: Multiple independent activations of the neu oncogene by a point mutation altering the transmembrane domain of p 185. Cell 45:649–657 1986.
85. Kokai Y, Cohen JA, Drebin JA, Greene MI: Stage- and tissue-specific expression of the neu oncogene in rat development. Proc Natl Acad Sci USA 84:8498–8501, 1987.
86. Gullick WJ, Berger MS, Bennett PLP, Rothbard JB, Waterfield MD: Expression of the c-erbB-2 protein in normal and transformed cells. Int J Cancer 40:246–254, 1987.

87. Cooke RM, Wilkinson AJ, Baron M, Pastore A, Tappin MJ, Campbell ID, Gregory H, Sheard B: The solution structure of human epidermal growth factor. Nature 327:339–341, 1987.
88. Montelione GT, K Wuthrich, Nice EC, Burgess AW, Scheraga HA: Solution structure of murine epidermal growth factor: determination of the polypeptide backbone chain-fold by nuclear magnetic resonance and distance geometry. Proc Natl Acad Sci USA 84:5226–5230, 1987.
89. Makino K, Morimoto M, Nishi M, Sakamoto S, Tamura A, Inooka H, Akasaka K: Proton nuclear magnetic resonance study on the solution conformation of human epidermal growth factor. Proc Natl Acad Sci USA 84:7841–7845, 1987.
90. Koch JH, Fifis T, Bender VJ, Moss BA: Molecular species of epidermal growth factor carrying immunosuppressive activity. J Cell Biochem 25:45–59, 1984.
91. Pesonen K, Viinikka L, Koskimies A, Banks AR, Nicolson M, Perheentupa J: Size heterogeneity of epidermal growth factor in human body fluids. Life Sci 40:2489–2494, 1987.
92. Tsukumo K, Nakamura H, Sakamoto S. Purification and characterization of high molecular weight human epidermal growth factor from human urine. Biochem Biophys Res Comm 145:126–133, 1987.
93. Stromberg K, Hudgins Wr, Dorman LS, Henderson LE, Sowder Rc, Sherrell BJ, Mount CD, Orth DN: Human brain tumor-associated urinary high molecular weight transforming growth factor: a high molecular weight form of epidermal growth factor. Cancer Res 47:1190–1196, 1987.
94. Bell GI, Fong NM, Stempien MM, Wormsted MA, Caput D, Ku L, Urdea MS, Rall LB, Sanchez-Pescador R. Human epidermal growth factor precursor: cDNA sequence, expression in vitro and gene organization. Nucleic Acids Res 14:8427–8446, 1986.
95. Scott J, Urdea M, Quiroga M, Sanchez-Pescador R, Fong N, Selby M, Rutter WJ, Bell GI: Structure of a mouse submaxillary messenger RNA encoding epidermal growth factor and seven related proteins. Science 221:236–240, 1983.
96. Gray A, Dull TJ, Ullrich A: Nucleotide sequence of epidermal growth factor cDNA predicts a 128,000-molecular weight protein precursor. Nature 303:722–725, 1983.
97. Russell DW, Schneider WJ, Yamamoto T, Luskey KL, Brown MS, Goldstein JL: Domain map of the LDL receptor: sequence homology with the epidermal growth factor precursor. Cell 37:577–585, 1984.
98. Davis CG, goldstein JL, Sudhof TC, Anderson RGW, Russell DW, Brown MS: Acid-dependent ligand dissociation and recycling of LDL receptor mediated by growth factor homology region. Nature 326:760–765, 1987.
99. Wharton KA, Johansen KM, Xu T, Artavanis-Tsakonas S: Nucleotide sequence from the neurogenic locus notch implies a gene product that shares homology with proteins containing EGF-like repeats. Cell 43:567–581, 1985.
100. Knust E, Dietrich U, Tepass U, Bremer KA, Weigel D, Vassin H, Campos-Ortega JA: EGF homologous sequences encoded in the genome of Drosophila melanogaster, and their relation ot neurogenic genes. EMBO J 6:761–766, 1987.
101. Greenwald I: *lin*-12, a nematode homeotic gene, is homologous to a set of mammalian proteins that includes epidermal growth factor. Cell 43:583–590, 1985.
102. Baldwin G: Epidermal growth factor precursor is related to the translation product of the Moloney sarcoma virus oncogene *mos*. Proc Natl Acad Sci USA 82:1921–1925, 1985.
103. Rall LB, Scott J, Bell GI, Crawford RJ, Penschow JD, Niall HD, Coghlan JP: Mouse prepro-epidermal growth factor synthesis by the kidney and other tissues. Nature 313:228–231, 1985.
104. Partanen A, Thesleff I: Localization and quantitation of ^{125}I-epidermal growth factor binding in mouse embryonic tooth and other embryonic tissues at different developmental stages. Dev Biol 120:186–197, 1987.
105. Popliker M, Shatz A, Avivi A, Ullrich A, Schlessinger J, Webb CG: Onset of endogenous synthesis of epidermal growth factor in neonatal mice. Dev Biol 119:38–44, 1987.

106. Tsutsumi O, Tsutsumi A, Oka T: A possible physiological role of milk epidermal growth factor in neonatal eyelid opening. Am J Physiol 252:R376–379, 1987.
107. Tsutsumi O, Oka T: Epidermal growth factor deficiency during pregancy causes abortion in mice. Am J Obstet Gynecol 156:241–244, 1987.
108. Smith JM, Sporn MB, Roberts AB, Derynck R, Winkler ME, Gregory H: Human transforming growth factor-a causes precocious eyelid opening in newborn mice. Nature 315:515–516, 1985.
109. Marquardt H, Hunkapiller M, Hood L, Todaro G: Rat transforming growth factor type I: structure and relation to epidermal growth factor. Science 223:1079–1082, 1984.
110. Derynck R, Roberts A, Winkler M, Chen E, Goeddel D: Human transforming growth factor: precursor structure and expression in E. coli. Cell 38:287–297, 1984.
111. Lee DC, Rose TM, Webb NR, Todaro GJ: Cloning and sequence analysis of a cDNA for rat transforming growth factor-a. Nature 313:489–491, 1985.
112. Carpenter G, Stoscheck CM, Preston YA, DeLarco JE: Antibodies to the epidermal growth factor receptor block the biological activities of sarcoma growth factor. Proc Natl Acad Sci USA 80:5627–5630, 1983.
113. Gan BS, Hollenberg MD, MacCannell KL, Lederis K, Winkler ME, Derynck R: Distinct vascular actions of epidermal growth factor-urogastrone and transforming factor-a. J Pharm Exp Therap 242:331–337, 1987.
114. Pike L, Marquardt H, Todaro G, Gallis B, Casnellie J, Bornstein P, Krebs E: Tranforming growth factor and epidermal growth factor stimulate the phosphorylation of a synthetic, tyrosine-containing peptide in a similar manner. J Biol Chem 257:14628–14631, 1982.
115. Bringman TS, Lindquist PB, Derynck R: Different transforming growth factor-a species are derived from a glycosylated and palmitoylated transmembrane precursor. Cell 48:429–440, 1987.
116. Francke U, Yang-Feng TL, Brissenden JE, Ullrich A: Chromosomal mapping of genes involved in growth control. CSH Symp Quant Biol 51:855–866, 1986.
117. Derynck R, Goeddel DV, Ullrich A, Gutterman JU, Williams RD, Bringman TS, Berger WH: Synthesis of messinger RNAs for transforming growth factors a and b and the epidermal growth factor receptor by human tumors. Cancer Res 47:707–712, 1987.
118. Han VKM, Hunter ES, Pratt RM, Zendegui JG, Lee DC: Expression of rat transforming growth factor alpha mRNA during development occurs predominantly in the maternal decidua. Mol Cell Biol 7:2335–2343, 1987.
119. Brown JP, Twardzik DR, Marquardt H, Todaro GJ: Vaccinia virus encodes a polypeptide homologous to epidermal growth factor and transforming growth factor. Nature 313:491–492, 1985.
120. Zaslavsky V, Hofschneider PH: Host involvement in vaccinia virus replication. Intervipology 26:93–103, 1986.
121. Strayer DS, Leibowitz JL: Inhibition of epidermal growth factor-induced cellular proliferation. Am J Pathol 128:203–209, 1987.
122. King CS, Cooper JA: Effects of protein kinase C activation after epidermal growthh factor binding on epidermal growth factor receptor phosphorylation. J Biol Chem 261:10073–10078, 1986.
123. McCaffrey PG, Friedman B, Rosner MR: Diacylglycerol modulates binding and phosphorylation of the epidermal growth factor receptor. J Biol Chem 259:12502–12507, 1984.
124. Beguinot L, Hanover JA, Ito S, Richert ND, Willingham MC, Pastan I: Phorbol esters induce transient internalization without degradation of unoccupied epidermal growth factor receptors. Proc Natl Acad Sci USA 82:2774–2778, 1985.
125. Whitely B, Glaser L: Epidermal growth factor (EGF) promotes phosphorylation at threonine-654 of the EGF receptor: possible role of protein kinase C in homologous regulation of the EGF receptor. J Cell Biol 103:1355–1362, 1986.
126. Gill GN, Bertics PJ, Santon JB: Epidermal growth factor and its receptor. Mol Cell Endocrinol 51:169–186, 1987.
127. Gorman RM, Poretz RD: Resolution of multiple endosomal compartments associated with

the internalization of epidermal growth factor and transferrin. J Cell Physiol 131:158–164, 1987.
128. Schaudies RP, Gorman RM, Savage CR, Poretz RD: Proteolytic processing of epidermal growth factor within endosomes. Biochem Biophys Res Comm 143:710–715, 1987.
129. Stoscheck CM, Carpenter G: Down regulation of epidermal growth factor receptors: direct demonstration of receptor degradation in human fibroblasts. J Cell Biol 98:1048–1053, 1984.
130. Erneux C, Cohen S, Garbers DL: The kinetics of tyrosine phosphorylation by the purified epidermal growth factor receptor kinase of A431 cells. J Biol Chem 258:4137–4142, 1983.
131. Hertel C, Coulter SJ, Perkins JP: The involvement of cellular aTP in receptor-mediated internalization of epidermal growth factor and hormone-induced internalization of β-adrenergic receptors. J Biol Chem 261:5974–5980, 1986.
132. Weber W, Bertics PJ, Gill GN: Immunoaffinity purification of the epidermal growth factor receptor: stoichiometry of binding and kinetics of self-phosporylation. J Biol Chem 259:14631–14636, 1984.
133. Forsayeth JR, Caro JF, Sinha MK, Maddus BA, Goldfine ID: Monoclonal antibodies to the human insulin receptor that activate glucose transport but not insulin receptor kinase activity. Proc Natl Acad Sci USA 84:3448–3451, 1987.
134. Bernard O, de St Groth BF, Ullrich A, Green W, Schlessinger J. High-affinity interleukin 2 binding by an oncogenic hybrid interleukin 2-epidermal growth factor receptor molecule. Proc Natl Acad Sci USA 84:2125–2129, 1987.
135. Riedel H, Dull TJ, Schlessinger J, Ullrich A: A chimaeric receptor allows insulin to stimulate tyrosine kinase activity of epidermal growth factor receptor. Nature 324:68–70, 1986.
136. Mathey-Prevot B, Baltimore D: Recombinants within the tyrosine kinase region of v-*abl* and v-*src* identify a v-*abl* segment that confers lymphoid specificity. Mol Cell Biol 8:234–240 1988.
137. Ellis L, Morgan DO, Koshland DE, Clauser E, Moe GR, Bollag G, Roth RA, Rutter WJ: Linking functional domains of the human insulin receptor with the bacterial aspartate receptor. Proc Natl Acad Sci USA 83:8137–8141, 1986.
138. Privalsky ML: Creation of a chimeric oncogene: analysis of the biochemical and biological properties of a v-*erbB*/*src* frusion polypeptide. J Virol 61:1938–1948, 1987.
139. Davis RJ, Czech MP: Stimulation of epidermal growth factor receptor threonine 654 phosphorylation by platelet-derived growth factor in protein kinase C-deficient human fibroblasts. J Biol Chem 262:6832–6841, 1987.
140. Olashaw NE, O'Keefe EJ, Pledger WJ: Platelet-derived growth factor modulates epidermal growth factor receptors by a mechanism distinct from that of phorbol esters. Proc Natl Acad Sci USA 83:3834–3838, 1986.
141. Honegger AM, Dull TJ, Felder S, van Obberghen E, Bellot F, Szapary D, Schmidt A, Ullrich A Schlessinger J: Point mutation at the ATP binding site of EGF receptor abolishes protein-tyrosine kinase activity and alters cellular routing. Cell 51:199–209, 1987.
142. Gates RE, King LE: Different forms of the epidermal growth factor receptor kinases have different autophosphorylation sites. Biochem 24:5209–5215, 1985.
143. Hunter T, Cooper JA: Protein-tyrosine kinases. Ann Rev Bochem 54:897–930, 1985.
144. Basu M, Biswas R, Das M: 42,000-molecular weight EGF receptor has protein kinase activity. Nature 311:477–480, 1984.
145. Murthy U, Basu M, Sen-Majumdar A, Das M. Perinuclear location and recycling of epidermal growth factor receptor kinase: immunofluorescent visualization using antibodies directed to kinase and extracellular domains. J Cell Biol 103:33–342, 1986.
146. Kaneko Y: Tumor promoter teleocidin inhibits internalization and nuclear accumulation of epidermal growth factor in cultured human hepatoma cells. FEBS Let 143:5–8, 1982.
147. Raper SE, Burwen SJ, Barker ME, Jones AL: Translocation of epidermal growth factor to the hepatocyte nucleus during rat liver regeneration. Gastroenterology, 92:1243–1250, 1987.
148. Kaneko Y: Epidermal growth factor enhances acetylation of nuclear proteins in cultured

human liver cells. Biochim Biophys Acta 762:111–118, 1983.
149. Marti U, Burwen S, Wells A, Barker M, Huling S, Feren A, Jones AL: Localization of epidermal growth factor receptor in hepatocyte nuclei. Submitted.
150. Green MR, Mycock C, Smith CG, Couchman JR: Biochemical and ultrastructural processing of [^{125}I]epidermal growth factor in rat epidermis and hair follicles: accumulation of nuclear label. J Invest Dermatol 88:259–265, 1987.
151. Mroczkowski B, Mosig G, Cohen S: ATP-stimulated interaction between epidermal growth factor receptor and supercoiled DNA. Nature 309:270–273, 1984.
152. Basu M, Frick K, Sen-Majumdar A, Scher CD, Das M: EGF receptor-associated DNA-nicking activity is due to a M_r-100,000 dissociable protein. Nature 316:640–641, 1985.
153. Stoscheck CM, King LE: Functional and structural characteristics of EGF and its receptor and their relationship to transforming proteins. J Cell Biochem 31:135–152, 1986.
154. Huang K, Wallner BP, Mattaliano RJ, Tizard R, Burne C, Frey A, Hession C, McGray P, Sinclair LK, Chow EP, Browning JL, Ramachandran KL, Tang J, Smart JE Pepinsky RB: Two human 35 kd inhibitors of phospholipase A_2 are related to substrates of pp60^{v-src} and of the epidermal growth factor receptor/kinase. Cell 46:191–199, 1986.
155. Haigler HT, Schlaepfer DD, Burgess WH: Characterization of lipocortin I and an immunologically unrelated 33-kDa protein as epidermal growth factor receptor/kinase substrates and phospholipase A_2 inhibitors. J Biol Chem 262:6921–6930, 1987.
156. Prywes R, Livneh E, Ullrich A, Schlessinger J: Mutations in the cytoplasmic domain of EGF receptor affect EGF binding and receptor internalization. EMBO J 5:2179–2190, 1986.
157. Sunada H, Magun BE, Mendelsohn J MacLeod CL: Monoclonal antibody against epidermal growth factor receptor is internalized without stimulating receptor phosphorylation. Proc Natl Acad Sci USA 83:3825–3829, 1986.
158. Chen W, Lazar C, Poenie M, Tsien R, Gill GN, Rosenfeld MG: Requirement for intrinsic protein tyrosine kinase in the immediate and late actions of the EGF receptor. Nature 328:820–823, 1987.
159. Wahl MI, Sweatt D, Carpenter G: Epidermal growth factor (EGF) stimulates inositol triphosphate formation in cells which overexpress the EGF receptor. Biochem Biophys Res Comm 142:688–695, 1987.
160. Walker DH, Pike LJ: Phosphotidylinositol kinase is activated in membranes derived from cells treated with epidermal growth factor. Proc Natl Acad Sci USA 84:7513–7517.
161. Pandiella A, Malgaroli A, Meldolesi J, Vicentini LM: EGF raises cytosolic Ca^{2+} in A431 and Swiss 3T3 cells by a dual mechanism: redistribution from intracellular stores and stimulated influx. Exp Cell Res 170:175–185, 1987.
162. Blenis J, Erikson RL: Stimulation of ribosomal protein S6 kinase activity by pp60^{v-src} or by serum: dissociation from phorbol ester-stimulated activity. Proc Natl Acad Sci USA 83:1733–1737, 1986.
163. McCaffrey P, Ran W, Campis J, Rosner MR: Two independent growth factor-generated signals regulate c-*fos* and c-*myc* mRNA levels in Swiss 3T3 cells. J Biol Chem 262:1442–1445, 1987.
164. Filmus J, Benchimol S, Buick RN: Comparative analysis of the involvement of p53, c-*myc* and c-*fos* in epidermal growth factor-mediated signal transduction. Exp Cell Res 169:554–559, 1987.
165. Earp HS, Austin KS, Blaisdell J, Rubin RA, Nelson KG, Lee LW, Grisham JW: Epidermal growth factor (EGF) stimulates EGF receptor synthesis. J Biol Chem 261:4777–4780, 1986.
166. Bjorge JD, Kudlow JE: Epidermal growth factor receptor synthesis is stimulated by phorbol ester and epidermal growth factor. J Biol Chem 262:6615–6622, 1987.
167. Wakshull EM, Wharton W: Stabilized complexes of epidermal growth factor and its receptor on the cell surface stimulate RNA synthesis but not mitogenesis. Proc Natl Acad Sci USA 82:8513–8517, 1985.
168. Besterman JM, Watson SP, Cuatrecasas P: Lack of association of epidermal growth factor-, insulin-, and serum-induced mitogenesis with stimulation of phospho-inositide degradation

in BALB/c 3T3 fibroblasts. J Biol Chem 261:723–727, 1986.
169. Velu TJ, L Beguinot, Vass WC, Willingham MC, Merlino GT, Pastan I, Lowy DR: Epidermal growth factor-dependent transformation by a human EGF receptor protooncogene. Science 238:1408–1410, 1987.
170. di Fiore PP, Pierce JH, Fleming TP, Hazan R, Ullrich A, King CR, Schlessinger J, Aaronson SA: Overexpression of the human EGF receptor confers an EGF-dependent transformed phenotype to NIH 3T3 cells. Cell 51:1063–1070, 1987.
171. Sand T, Christoffersen T: Temporal requirement for epidermal growth factor and insulin in the stimulation of hepatocyte DNA synthesis. J Cell Physiol 131:141–148, 1987.
172. Hamburger AW, White CP, Brown RW: Effect of epidermal growth factor on proliferation of human tumor cells in soft agar. J Natl Cancer Inst 67:825–830, 1981.
173. Gebhardt A, Bell JC, Foulkes JG: Abelson transformed fibroblasts lacking the EGF receptor are not tumorigenic in nude mice. EMBO J 5:2191–2195, 1986.
174. Luttrell DK, Luttrell LM, Parsons SJ: Augmented mitogenic responsiveness to epidermal growth factor in murine fibroblasts that overexpress pp60^{c-src}. Mol Cell Biol 8:497–501, 1988.
175. David-Pfeuty T, Guesdon F: Epidermal growth factor stimulates serine and tyrosine phsophorylation in a 59-kD protein in purified plasma membranes from rat liver. Biochem Biophys Res Comm 145:982–988, 1987.
176. Kamata T, Feramisco JR: Epidermal growth factor stimulates guanine nucleotide binding activity and phosphorylation of *ras* oncogene proteins. Nature 310:147–150, 1984.
177. Valentine-Braun KA, Northup JK, Hollenberg MD: Epidermal growth factor (Urogastrone)-mediated phosphorylation of a 35-kDa substrate in human placental membranes: relationship to the b subunit of the guanine nucleotide regulatory complex. Proc Natl Acad Sci USA 83:236–240, 1986.
178. Stern DF, Roberts AB, Roche NS, Sporn MB, Weinberg RA: Differential responsiveness of *myc*- and *ras*- tranfected cells to growth factors: selective stimulation of *myc*-transfected cells by epidermal growth factor. Mol Cell Biol 6:870–877, 1986.
179. Quantin B, Breathnach R: Epidermal growth factor stimulates transcription of the c-*jun* proto-oncogene in rat fibroblasts. Nature 334:538–539, 1988.
180. Weissman B, Aaronson SA: Members of the *src* and *ras* oncogene families supplant the epidermal growth factor requirement of BALB/MK-2 keratinocytes and induce distinct alterations in their terminal differentiation program. Mol Cell Biol 5:3386–3396, 1985.
181. McKay IA, Malone P, Marshall CJ, Hall A: Malignant transformation of murine fibroblasts by a human c-Ha-*ras*-1 oncogene does not require a functional epidermal growth factor receptor. Mol Cell Biol 6:3382–3387, 1986.
182. Carlin CR, Phillips PD, Knowles BB, Cristofalo VJ: Diminished in vitro tyrosine kinase activity of the EGF receptor of senescent human fibroblasts. Nature 306:617–620, 1983.
183. Tsao MS, Liu C: Inhibition of growth of early passage normal rat liver epithelial cell lines by epidermal growth factor. Lab Invest 58:636–642, 1988.
184. Francavilla A, Ove P, Polimeno L, Sciascia C, Coetzee ML, Stanzl TE: Epidermal growth factor and proliferation in rat hepatocyte in primary culture isolated at different times after partial hepatectomy. Cancer Res 46:1318–1323, 1986.
185. Rush GF, Alberts D: The hepatic binding and uptake kinetics of epidermal growth factor: studies with isolated rat hepatocytes. Life Sci 40:679–685, 1987.
186. Muller W, Pattengale P, Wallace R, Leder P: Single-step induction of mammary adenocarcinoma in transgenic mice bearing the activated *neu* oncogene. Cell 54:105–115, 1988.
187. Makela TP, Alitalo K: Proto-oncogene amplification: role in tumor progression. Ann Clin Res 18:290–296, 1986.
188. Klein G: The approaching era of the tumor suppressor genes. Science 238:1539–1545, 1987.
189. Wells A, Bishop JM, Helmeste D: Amplified gene for EGF receptor in a human glioblastoma cell line presenting an enzymatically inactive protein. Mol Cell Biol 8:4561–4565, 1988.

190. Westphal M, Harsh GR, Rosenblum ML, Hammonds RG: Epidermal growth factor receptors in the human glioblastoma cell line SF268 differ from those in epider-moid carcinoma cell line A431. Biochem Biophys Res Comm 132:284–289, 1985.
191. Gill GN, Weber W, Thompson DM, Lin C, Evans RM, Rosenfeld MG, Gamou S, Shimizu N: Relationship between production of epidermal growth factor receptors, gene amplification, and chromosome 7 translocation in variant A431 cells. Som Cell Mol Genet 11:309–318, 1984.
192. Ginsburg E, Vonderhaar BK: Epidermal growth factor stimulates the growth of A431 tumors in athymic mice. Cancer Lett 28:143–150, 1985.
193. Filmus J, Trent JM, Pollak MN, Buick RN: Epidermal growth factor receptor gene-amplified MDA-468 breast cancer cell line and its nonamplified variants. Mol Cell Biol 7:251–257, 1987.
194. Drebin JA, Link VC, Weinberg RA, Greene MI: Inhibition of tumor growth by a monoclonal antibody reactive with an oncogene-encoded tumor antigen. Proc Natl Acad Sci USA 83:9129–9133, 1986.
195. Chang W, Upton C, Hu S, Purchio AF, McFadden G: The genome of shope fibroma virus, a tumorigenic poxvirus, contains a growth factor gene with sequence similarity to those encoding epidermal growth factor and transforming growth factor alpha. Mol Cell Biol 7:535–540, 1987.
196. Upton C, Macen JL, McFadden G: Mapping and sequencing of a gene from myxoma virus that is related to those encoding epidermal growth factor and transforming growth factor alpha. J Virol 61:1271–1275, 1987.
197. Serrero G: EGF inhibits the differentiation of adipocyte precursors in primary culture. Biochem Biophys Res Comm 146:194–202, 1987.
198. Singletary SE, Baker FL, Spitzer G, Tomasovic B, Brock WA, Ajani JA, Kelly AM: Biological effects of epidermal growth factor on the in vitro growth of human tumors. Cancer Res 47:403–406, 1987.
199. Pruss RM, Herschman HR: Variants of 3T3 cells lacking mitogenic response to epidermal growth factor. Proc Natl Acad Sci USA 74:3918–3921, 1977.
200. Liboi E, Pelosi E, Testa U, Peschle C, Rossi GB: Proliferative response and oncogene expression induced by epidermal growth factor in EL2 rat fibroblasts. Mol Cell Biol 6:2275–2278, 1986.
201. Carpenter G, Cohen S: Human epidermal growth factor and the proliferation of human fibroblasts. J Cell Physiol 88:227–238, 1976.
202. Palombella VJ, Yamashiro DJ, Maxfield FR, Decker SJ, Vilcek J: Tumor necrosis factor increases the number of epidermal growth factor receptors on human fibroblasts. J Biol Chem 262:1950–1954, 1987.
203. Francavilla A, Ove P, Polimeno L, Sciascia C, Coetzee M, Pellici R, Todo S, Kam I, Starz TE: Different response to epidermal growth factor of hepatocytes in cultures isolated from male or female rat liver: inhibitor effect of estrogen on binding and mitogenic effect of epidermal growth factor. Gastroenterology 93:597–605, 1987.
204. Erickson CA, Turley EA: The effects of epidermal growth factor on neural crest cells in tissue culture. Exp Cell Res 169:267–279, 1987.
205. van Zoelen EJJ, van Oostwaard TMJ, de Laat SW: The role of polypeptide growth factors in phenotypic transformation of normal rat kidney cells. J Biol Chem 263:64–68, 1988.
206. Jennische E, Andersson G, Hansson H: Epidermal growth factor is expressed by cells in the distal tubules during postnephrectomy renal growth. Acta Physiol Scand 129:449–450, 1987.
207. Barrandon Y, Green H: Cell migration is essential for sustained growth of keratinocyte colonies: the roles of transforming growth factor-a and epidermal growth factor. Cell 50:1131–1137, 1987.
208. Lin MC, Darfler FJ, Beckner SK: Induction of glucagon sensitivity in a transformed kidney cell line by prostaglandin E_2 and its inhibition by epidermal growth factor. Mol Cell Biol 7:4324–4328, 1987.

209. Dubeau L, Jones PA: Growth of normal and neoplastic urothelium and response to epidermal growth factor in a defined serum-free medium. Cancer Res 47:2107–2112, 1987.
210. Meyers MB, Merluzzi VJ, Spengler BA, Biedler JL: Epidermal growth factor receptor is increased in multidrug-resistant Chinese hamster and mouse tumor cells. Proc Natl Acad Sci USA 83:5521–5525, 1986.
211. Maruo T, Matsuo H, Oishi T, Hayashi M, Nishino R, Mochizuki M: Induction of differentiated trophoblast function by epidermal growth factor: relation of immunohistochemically detected cellular epidermal growth factor receptor levels. J Clin Endocrinol Metab 64:744, 1987.
212. Maruo T, Mochizuki M: Immunohistochemical localization of epidermal growth factor receptor and myc oncogene product in human placenta: implication for trophoblast proliferation and differentiation. Am J Obstet Gynecol 156:721–727, 1987.
213. Hapgood J, Libermann TA, Lax I, Yarden Y, Schreiber AB, Naor Z, Schlessinger J: Monoclonal antibodies against epidermal growth factor receptor induce prolactin synthesis in cultured rat pituitary cells (GH_3). Proc Natl Acad Sci USA 80:6451–6455, 1983.
214. Johnson HM, torres BA: Peptide growth factors PDGF, EGF, and FGF regulate interferon-g production. J Immunol 134:2824–2826, 1985.
215. Acres RB, Land JR, Feldman M: Effects of platelet-derived growth factor and epidermal growth factor on antigen-induced proliferation of human T-cell lines. Immunology 54:9–16, 1985.
216. Whisett JA, Weaver TE, Lieberman MA, Clark JC, Daugherty C: Differential effects of epidermal growth factor and transforming growth factor-b on synthesis of $M_r = 35,000$ surfactant-associated protein in fetal lung. J Biol Chem 262:7908–7913, 1987.
217. Lewis EJ, Chikarishi DM: Regulated expression of the tyrosine hydroxylase gene by epidermal growth factor. Mol Cell Biol 7:3332–3336, 1987.
218. Thorne HJ, DG Jose, H Zhang, PJ Dempsey RH Whitehead: Epidermal growth factor stimulates the synthesis of cell-attachment proteins in the human breast cancer cell line PMC42. Int J Cancer 40:207–212, 1987.
219. Sporn MB, Roberts AB, Shule JH, Smith JM, Ward JM, Sodek J: Polypeptide transforming growth factors isolated from bovine sources and used for wound healing in vivo. Science 219: 1329–1331, 1983.
220. Singh G, Foster CS: Epidermal growth factor in alkali-burned corneal epithelial wound healing. Am J Ophth 103:802–807, 1987.
221. Okamoto S, Oka T: Evidence for physiological function of epidermal growth factor: pregestational sialoadenectomy of mice decreases milk production and increases offspring mortality during lactation period. Proc Natl Acad Sci USA 81:6059–6063, 1984.
222. Tsutsumi O, Kubota Y, Oka T: Effect of sialoadenectomy, treatment with epidermal growth factor (EGF) antiserum and replacement of EGF on the epidermis in mice. J Endocrinol 113:193–197, 1987.
223. Nanney LB, Stoscheck CM, Magid M, King LE: Altered [^{125}I]epidermal growth factor binding and receptor distribution in psoriasis. J Invest Dermatol 86:260–265, 1986.
224. Cowley G, Smith JA, Gusterson B, Hendler F, Ozanne B: The amount of EGF receptor is elevated on squamous cell carcinomas. Cancer Cells 1:5–10, 1984.
225. Libermann TA, Nusbaum HR, Razon N, Kris R, Lax I, Soreq H, Whittle N, Waterfield MD, Ullrich A, Schlessinger J: Amplification, enhanced expression and possible rearrangemnt of EGF receptor gene in primary human brain tumours of glial origin. Nature 313:144–147, 1985.
226. Libermann TA, Razon N, Bartal AD, Yarden Y, Schlessinger J, Soreq H: Expression of epidermal growth factor receptors in human brain tumors. Cancer Res 44:753–760, 1984.
227. Neal DE, Marsh C, Bennett MK, Abel PD, Hall RR, Sainsbury JRC, Harris AL: Epidermal-growth-factor receptors in human bladder cancer: comparison of invasive and superficial tumours. Lancet 1:366–368, 1985.
228. Veale D, Ashcroft T, Marsh C, Gibson GJ, Harris AL: Epidermal growth factor receptors in non-small cell lung cancer. Br J Cancer 55:513–516, 1987.

229. Ro J, North SM, Gallick GE, Hortobagyi GN, Gutterman JU, Blick M: Amplified and overexpressed epidermal growth factor receptor gene in uncultured primary human breast carcinoma. Cancer Res 48:161–164, 1988.
230. Sainsbury JRC, Farndon JR, Needham GK, Malcolm AJ, Harris AL: Epidermal-growth-factor receptor status as predictor of early recurrence of and death from breast cancer. Lancet 1:1398–1402, 1987.
231. Duh Q, Gum ET, Gerend PL, Raper SE, Clark OH: Epidermal growth factor receptors in normal and neoplastic thyroid tissue. Surgery 98:1000–1006, 1985.
232. Korc M, Meltzer P, Trent J: Enhanced expresion of epidermal growth factor recepttor correlates with alterations of chromosome 7 in human pancreatic cancer. Proc Natl Acad Sci USA 83:5141–5144, 1986.
233. Yasui W, Sumiyoshi H, Hata J, Kameda T, Ochiai A, Ito H, Tahara E: Expression of epidermal growth factor receptor in human gastric and colonic carcinomas. Cancer Res 48:137–141, 1988.
234. Birman P, Michard M, Li JY Peillon F, Bression D: Epidermal growth factor-binding sites, present in normal human and rat pituitaries, are absent in human pituitary adenomas. J Clin Endocrinol Metab 65:275–281, 1987.

7. The platelet-derived growth factor system

Shaun R. Coughlin and Mark T. Keating

Platelet-derived growth factor (PDGF) is a potent mitogen for mesenchymal cells in culture. PDGF was first recognized as a regulator of mesenchymal cell proliferation in the setting of vascular injury and wound healing [1,2]. It has become clear, however, that PDGF and its receptors (the PDGF system) play equally important roles in normal developmental and pathological processes, as well as in the genesis of certain neoplasms. In this respect, the PDGF system is appropriately considered within the broader context of human oncogenes.

The discovery that PDGF is structurally related to the product encoded by the v-*sis* oncogene of the simian sarcoma virus has led to the study of the PDGF system as a model for autocrine activation of cell proliferation [3–14]. Additional striking connections between the PDGF system and oncogenes have surfaced. The receptor for PDGF is a tyrosine kinase, an unusual enzyme activity shared by certain growth factor receptors and by one class of oncogene products. The structure of the PDGF receptor is similar to that of the hematopoietic colony stimulating factor-1 (CSF-1) receptor, which is encoded by the proto-oncogene c-*fms* [15]. Activation of the PDGF receptor leads to tyrosine phosphorylation of c-*src* [16], another tyrosine kinase, and c-*raf* [17], a serine/threonine kinase. Furthermore, in a variety of mammalian systems, activation of the PDGF receptor leads to increased expression of other proto-oncogenes, including c-*myc* and c-*fos* [18–22].

Molecular structure and function

PDGF was discovered 15 years ago as a serum component having growth-promoting activity for cultured vascular smooth muscle cells [2]. Ross and colleagues noted that serum prepared from plasma from which platelets had been removed would not support the proliferation of smooth muscle cells in culture. Addition of a platelet extract to this preparation reconstituted its mitogenic activity. This became the basis for the assay subsequently used to purify PDGF [23–26]. PDGF purified from human platelets was found to be a disulfide-linked heterodimer composed of polypeptide chains denoted A

Benz, C. and Liu, E., (eds.), Oncogenes. © *1989 Kluwer Academic Publishers.*
ISBN 0-7923-0237-0. All rights reserved.

and B. These two chains are distinct gene products, but they are 60% identical at the amino acid level. In addition to the heterodimeric AB form of PDGF, two homodimeric forms, denoted AA and BB, have been discovered [27–30]. The existence of multiple isoforms of PDGF and the finding that PDGF is not only released by platelets but is produced by endothelial cells, monocyte/macrophages, smooth muscle cells, malignant cells, and normal embryonic tissues [31–48] has expanded the view of the potential in vivo roles of PDGF.

PDGF elicits cell proliferation by binding to and activating a specific cell surface receptor. One form of PDGF receptor has been purified from Balb/c 3T3 cells, and a cDNA encoding this receptor has been cloned [15]. Transfection of this receptor cDNA was found to confer PDGF-responsiveness upon cells normally unresponsive to PDGF [49]; and the behavior of the transfected cells suggested that the cloned receptor accounted for all the known cellular responses to the PDGF AB heterodimer [50]. Interestingly, the affinity of this cloned receptor for the BB form of PDGF is much higher than its affinity for the AA form [50]. Recent studies have suggested that some cells may express a different form of PDGF receptor that binds AA with high affinity [51,52]. Characterization of this receptor and its role in determining the relative responsiveness of cells to various isoforms of PDGF is an area of active investigation.

Several aspects of the structure of the cloned PDGF receptor are noteworthy. It is a single polypeptide chain divided approximately in half by a lone transmembrane domain. The extracellular portion of the receptor is made up of five immunoglobulin-like domains, making the receptor a member of the immunoglobulin superfamily [53]. The cytoplasmic portion of the receptor contains a tyrosine kinase domain. The enzymatic activity of this domain is normally regulated by PDGF binding to the extracellular domain, and this is necessary for signal transduction by the PDGF receptor [54]. Activation of the receptor's tyrosine kinase leads to autophosphorylation of the receptor at tyrosine residues, and this is associated with induction of a conformational change in the receptor molecule [55]. The importance of this conformational change in signal transduction is under study.

The PDGF receptor's tyrosine kinase domain, defined by homology with c-*src* and other tyrosine kinases, possesses an unusual feature in that it is split into two portions by a 100-amino-acid stretch called the kinase insert. The sequence of the PDGF receptor's kinase insert is highly conserved from mouse to human, and this structure has been shown to be critical for mitogenic signaling by the PDGF receptor [56]. The general structure of the PDGF receptor, with five extracellular immunoglobulinlike domains and a cytoplasmic tyrosine kinase domain split by a large kinase insert, is shared by the c-*fms* gene product [15]. The c-*fms* proto-oncogene encodes a membrane receptor for the homodimeric growth factor, colony stimulating factor-1 (CSF-1). It is likely that the human genes for the PDGF receptor and c-*fms* arose by duplication of a common ancestral gene, given their extreme proximity on chromosome 5 [15,57]. It is not known, however, if the structural similarities between PDGF and CSF-1 and their corresponding receptors have additional implications in terms of signal transduction. It may be that each of the dimeric ligands leads to receptor dimerization upon binding, and that the common structural features shared by these two systems are necessary for this specific mode of receptor activation and transmission of the mitogenic signal to the cell's interior.

Autocrine stimulation and malignant transformation

As mentioned earlier, PDGF itself is structurally related to the protein product encoded by the v-*sis* oncogene of the simian sarcoma virus [6–10], an acutely transforming retrovirus initially isolated from a fibrosarcoma that arose spontaneously in a pet wooly monkey. The gene responsible for the transforming activity of the simian sarcoma virus, v-*sis*, represents the PDGF B-chain (c-*sis*) gene coopted by the virus [10–11]. The v-*sis* gene encodes a protein product $p28^{sis}$ that is processed to a 56-kDa disulfide-linked homodimer that is then proteolytically cleaved [58]. The mature form of this protein is essentially identical to the human PDGF BB homodimer, and is functionally indistinguishable from platelet PDGF when added to cells in culture [59–62]. The fact that the oncogene responsible for the transforming activity of the simian sarcoma virus encodes a PDGF-like molecule, coupled with the finding that only cells that express the PDGF receptor can be transformed by the v-*sis* gene [63], suggests that autocrine activation of the PDGF receptor may be responsible for malignant transformation. However, addition of exogenous PDGF to cells in culture is not sufficient to elicit the transformed phenotype. This simple autocrine model of transformation thus raises an important question: Is endogenous cellular expression of the v-*sis* gene product qualitatively different from cellular exposure to exogenous PDGF?

One possible difference between the addition of exogenous PDGF and v-*sis* expression is the mechanism by which the PDGF receptor becomes activated. Some studies have suggested that the v-*sis* protein is secreted from cells and is then able to act back upon the extracellular ligand-binding domain of the PDGF receptor in a manner identical to PDGF [59,61,64,65]. The only difference between a v-*sis*-transformed cell and a normal cell in this model is that the PDGF receptor is continuously stimulated by constitutive expression of v-*sis* in the transformed cells. Other studies have asked whether the PDGF receptor might be activated in a novel fashion in v-*sis*-tranformed cells. A signal sequence is required for the transforming activity of the v-*sis* gene [65]. Like other proteins designed for export, the v-*sis* gene product is inserted into the rough endoplasmic reticulum (ER) and processed through the smooth ER and Golgi. The PDGF receptor is a transmembrane cell surface protein; thus its ligand-binding domain is inserted into the ER and is potentially available to bind to a v-*sis* gene product that is being processed through the same intracellular compartments. Several recent studies addressed the possibility that PDGF receptor might be activated intracellularly, and found that most of the receptor produced in v-*sis*-transformed cells actually did become activated before export to the cell surface [66,67]. This intracellular activation probably occurred when sufficiently mature receptors and v-*sis*-encoded protein came together in the Golgi compartment. Autocrine activation of the PDGF receptor within this intracellular compartment appeared to shunt the activated receptor into a novel degradative pathway, resulting in a markedly shortened PDGF receptor half-life.

Thus intracellular activation of the PDGF receptor in v-*sis* transformed cells represents a distinctly different route of receptor activation from that used by exogenous exposure to PDGF, and this may have important implications for therapeutic strategies aimed at blocking the autocrine growth stimulation of transformed cells. However, it is not yet known if the intracellular activation of the PDGF receptor stimulates any novel second messenger pathways or has other functionally important consequences that may explain why the simian sarcoma virus can elicit a transformed phenotype while PDGF cannot. One recent study is provocative in this regard. Most studies of v-*sis* transformation have utilized murine cell lines, such as NIH3T3 cells, that are burdened by endogenous retroviruses and may already possess *second events* necessary for transformation [8,9]. In contrast to murine cells, infection of normal human fibroblasts with simian sarcoma virus led to no greater growth in soft agar than did treatment with exogenous PDGF, nor did viral infection immortalize these normal mesenchymal cells [68]. This study suggested that infection with simian sarcoma virus may lead to activation of PDGF receptors in a manner that is functionally indistinguishable from PDGF.

How can this possibility be reconciled with the fact that simian sarcoma virus produces fibrosarcomas or malignant gliomas in animals? Some features of tumor formation after infection with simian sarcoma virus are noteworthy. This retrovirus is much less oncogenic than other sarcoma viruses, such as the Rous sarcoma virus. Intramuscular inoculation of newborn marmosets with large numbers of virions led to tumor formation in only 50% of animals after latent periods of 4 to 6 weeks; these tumors were either indolent fibrosarcomas or fibromas that eventually regressed [69]. Such observations are consistent with the model that autocrine activation of the PDGF receptor by the v-*sis* gene product leads only to cell proliferation but not to the fully transformed phenotype. These proliferating cells might then be at increased risk for accumulating second events, which would ultimately lead to the fully transformed and malignant phenotype.

Conclusions

There is no doubt that autocrine activation of the PDGF receptor occurs in a number of model systems. However, the exact role of the PDGF system in human malignancy remains unclear. A number of cell lines derived from human gliomas and osteosarcomas express one or more of the PDGF isoforms along with the PDGF receptor [41,42,70]. Whether the actual tumors depend upon PDGF receptor activation for maintenance of their malignant phenotype is a matter for future investigation. Because PDGF-neutralizing antibody would not be expected to block intracellular activation of the PDGF receptor, definitive in vitro studies await the application of antisense approaches to specifically block expression of either PDGF or its receptor, while definitive in vivo approaches await the development of specific PDGF receptor antagonists.

Acknowledgment

The authors wish to thank L.T. Williams for helpful discussions.

References

1. Ross R, Glomset JA: Atherosclerosis and the arterial smooth muscle cell. Science 180: 1332–1339, 1973.
2. Ross R, Glomset J, Kariya B, Harker CA: Platelet-dependent serum factor that stimulates the proliferation of arterial smooth muscle cells in vitro. Proc Natl Acad Sci USA 71:1207–1210, 1974.
3. Robbins KC, Antoniades HN, Devare SG, Hunkapiller MW, Aaronson SA: Structural and immunological similarities between simian sarcoma virus gene product(s) and human platelet-derived growth factor. Nature 305:605–608, 1983.
4. Josephs SF, Dalla-Favera R, Gelmann EP, Gallo RC, Wong-staal F: 5' viral and human cellular sequences corresponding to the transforming gene of simian sarcoma virus. Science 219:503–505, 1983.
5. Josephs SF, Guo C, Ratner L, Wong-Staal F: Human proto-oncogene nucleotide sequences corresponding to the transforming region of simian sarcoma virus. Science 223:487–491, 1984.
6. Waterfield MD, Scrace GT, et al.: Platelet-derived growth factor is structurally related to the putative transforming protein $p28^{sis}$ of simian sarcoma virus. Nature 304:35–39, 1983.
7. Aaronson SA: Nucleotide sequence analysis identifies the human c-sis proto-oncogene as a structural gene for platelet-derived growth factor. Cell 37:123–129, 1984.
8. Devare SG, Reddy EP, Law DJ, Robbins KC, Aaronson SA: Nucleotide sequence of the simian sarcoma virus genome: demonstration that its acquired cellular sequences encode transforming gene product $p28^{sis}$. Proc Natl Acad Sci USA 80:731–735, 1983.
9. Devare SG, Reddy, EP, et al.: Nucleotide sequence of the transforming gene of simian sarcoma virus. Proc Natl Acad Sci USA 79:3179–3182, 1982.
10. Doolittle RF, Hunkapiller WM, et al.: Simian sarcoma virus oncogene, v-sis, is derived from the gene (or genes) encoding a platelet-derived growth factor. Science 221:275–277, 1983.
11. Chiu I-M, Reddy EP, et al.: Nucleotide sequence analysis identifies the human c-sis proto-oncogene as a structural gene for platelet-derived growth factor. Cell 37:123–129, 1984.
12. Gazit A, Igarashi H, et al.: Expression of the normal human sis/PDGF-2 coding sequence induces cellular transformation. Cell 39:89–97, 1984.
13. Johnsson A, Betsholtz C, von der Helm K, Heldin C-H, Westermark B: Platelet-derived growth factor agonist activates a secreted form of the v-sis oncogene product. Proc Natl Acad Sci USA 82:1721–1725, 1985.

14. Heldin C-H, Hammacher A, Wister M, Westermark B: Structural and functional aspects of platelet-derived growth factor. Br J Cancer 57:591–593, 1988.
15. Yarden Y, Escobedo JA, et al.: Structure of the receptor from platelet-derived growth factor receptors. Nature 323:226–232, 1986.
16. Ralston R, Bishop JM: The product of the proto-oncogene c-*src* is modified during the cellular response to PDGF. Proc Natl Acad Sci USA 82:7845–7849, 1985.
17. Morrison DK, Kaplan DR, Rapp NJ, Roberts RM: Signal transduction from membrane to cytoplasm: Growth factors and membrane-bound oncogene products increase Raf-1 phosphorylation and associated protein kinase activity. Proc Natl Acad Sci USA, in press.
18. Greenberg ME, Ziff EM: Stimulation of 3T3 cells induces transcription of the c-*fos* proto-oncogene. Nature 311:433–438, 1984.
19. Kruijer W, Cooper JA, Hunter T, Verma IM: Platelet-derived growth factor induces rapid but transient expression of the c-*fos* gene and protein. Nature 312:711–716, 1984.
20. Muller R, Bravo R, Burckhardt J, Curran T: Induction of c-*fos* gene and protein by growth factors precedes activation of c-*myc*. Nature 312:716–720, 1984.
21. Curran T, Miller AD, Zokas L, Verma IM: Viral and cellular *fos* proteins: a comparative analysis. Cell 36:259–268, 1984.
22. Kelly K, Cocharan BH, Stiles CD, Leder P: Cell-specific regulation of the c-*myc* gene by lymphocyte mitogens and platelet-derived growth factor. Cell 35:603–610, 1983.
23. Antoniades HN: Human platelet-derived growth factor (PDGF): purification of PDGF-I and PDGF-II and separation of their reduced subunits. Proc Natl Acad Sci USA 78:7314–7317, 1981.
24. Deule TF, Huang JS: Platelet-derived growth factor: purification, properties, and biological activities. Prog Hematol 13:201–221, 1983.
25. Heldin C-H, Westermark B, Wasteson A: Platelet-derived growth factor: purification and partial characterization. Proc Natl Acad Sci USA 76:3722–3726, 1979.
26. Raines E, Ross R: Platelet-derived growth factor: High yield purification and evidence for multiple forms. J Biol Chem 257:5154–5160, 1982.
27. Heldin C-H, Johnsson A, et al.: A human osteosarcoma cell line secretes a growth factor structurally related to a homodimer of PDGF A-chains. Nature 319:511–514, 1986.
28. Heldin C-H, Westermark B, Wasteson A: Chemical and biological properties of a growth factor from human-cultured osteosarcoma cells: resemblance with platelet-derived growth factor. J Cell Physiol 105:235–246, 1980.
29. Betsholtz C, Johnson A, et al.: cDNA sequence and chromosomal localization of human platelet-derived growth factor A-chain and its expression in tumor cell lines. Nature 320:695–699, 1986.
30. van Zoelen EJJ, van de Ven WJM, et al.: Neuroblastoma cells express c-*sis* and produce a transforming growth factor antigenically related to the platelet-derived growth factor. Mol Cell Biol 5:2289–2297, 1985.
31. Martinet Y, Bitterman PB, et al.: Activated human monocytes express the c-*sis* proto-oncogene and release a mediator showing PDGF-like activity. Nature 319:158–160, 1986.
32. Niman HL, Houghten RA, Bown-Pope DF: Detection of high molecular weight forms of platelet-derived growth factor by sequence-specific antisera. Science 226:701–703, 1984.
33. Niman HL, Thompson AMH, et al.: Anti-peptide antibodies detect oncogene-related proteins in urine. Proc Natl Acad Sci USA 82:7924–7928, 1985.
34. Owen AJ, Pantazis P, Antoniades HN: Simian sarcoma virus-transformed cells secrete a mitogen identical to platelet-derived growth factor. Science 225:54–56, 1984.
35. Rizzino A, Bowen-Pope DE: Production of PDGF-like factors by embryonal carcinoma cells and response to PDGF by endoderm-like cells. Dev Biol 110:15–22, 1985.
36. Seifert RA, Schwartz SM, Bowen-Pope DE: Developmentally regulated production of platelet-derived growth factor-like molecules. Nature 311:669–671, 1984.
37. Shimokado K, Raines EW, et al.: A significant part of macrophage-derived growth factor consists of at least two forms of PDGF. Cell 43:277–286, 1985.
38. Walker LN, Bowen-Pope DF, Ross R, Reidy MA: Production of PDGF-like molecules by

cultured arterial smooth muscle cells accompanies proliferation after arterial injury. Proc Natl Acad Sci USA 83:7311–7315, 1986.
39. Westin EH, Wong-Staal F, et al.: Expression of cellular homologues of retroviral oncogenes in human hematopoietic cells. Proc Natl Acad Sci USA 79:2490–2494, 1982.
40. Barrett TB, Gajdusek CM, Schwartz SM, McDougal JK Benditt EP: Expression of the *sis* gene by endothelial cells in culture and in vivo. Proc Natl Acad Sci USA 81:6772–6774, 1984.
41. Betsholtz C, Westermark B, Ek B, Heldin C-H: Coexpression of a PDGF-like factor and PDGF receptors in a human osteosarcoma cell line: Implications for autocrine receptor activation. Cell 39:447–457, 1984.
42. Bowen-Pope DF, Vogel A, Ross R: Production of platelet-derived growth factor-like molecules and reduced expression of platelet-derived growth factor receptors accompany transformation by a wide spectrum of agents. Proc Natl Acad Sci USA 81:2396–2400, 1984.
43. Collins T, Ginsburg D, Boss JM, Orkin SH, Pober JS: Cultured human endothelial cells express platelet-derived growth factor chain 2: cDNA cloning and structural analysis. Nature 316:748–750, 1985.
44. Dicorleto PE, Bowen-Pope DF: Cultured endothelial cells produce a platelet-derived growth factor-like protein. Proc Natl Acad Sci USA 80:1919–1923, 1983.
45. Fox PL, Dicorleto PE: Regulation of production of a platelet-derived growth factor-like protein by cultured bovine aortic endothelial cells. J Cell Physiol 121:298–308, 1984.
46. Goustin AS, Betsholtz C, et al.: Coexpression of the *sis* and *myc* proto-oncogenes in developing human placenta suggests autocrine control of trophoblast growth. Cell 41:301–312, 1985.
47. Graves DT, Owen AJ, et al.: Detection of c-*sis* transcripts and synthesis of PDGF-like proteins by human osteosarcoma cells. Science 226:972–974, 1984.
48. Slamon DJ, Cline MJ: Expression of cellular oncogenes during embryonic and fetal development of the mouse. Proc Natl Acad Sci USA 81:7141–7145, 1984.
49. Escobedo JA, Keating MT, Ives HE, Williams LT: Platelet-derived growth factor receptors expressed by cDNA transfection couple to a diverse group of cellular responses associated with cell proliferation. J Biol Chem 263:1482–1487, 1988.
50. Escobedo JA, et al.: A common PDGF receptor is activated by homodimeric A and B forms of PDGF. Science 240:1532–1534, 1988.
51. Hart CE, et al.: Two classes of PDGF receptor recognize different isoforms of PDGF. Science 240:1529–1531, 1988.
52. Heldin C-H, et al.: Binding of different dimeric forms of PDGF to human fibroblasts: evidence for two separate receptor types. EMBO J 7:1387–1392, 1988.
53. Bazen JF, Fletterick RJ, Escobedo JA, Williams LT: The PDGF receptor is a member of the immunoglobulin gene superfamily. In preparation.
54. Excobedo JA, Barr PJ, Williams LT: The role of the tyrosine kinase and membrane spanning domains in PDGF receptor signal transduction. Mol Cell Biol in press.
55. Keating MT, Escobedo JA, Williams LT: Ligand activation causes a phosphylation-dependent change in platelet-derived growth factor receptor conformation J Biol Chem 263:12805–12808, 1988.
56. Escobedo JA, Williams LT: A PDGF receptor domain essential for mitogenesis but not for many other responses to PDGF. Nature 335:85–87, 1988.
57. Roberts WM, Loo AT, Rousse MF, Sherr CJ: Tandem linkage of human CSF-1 receptor (c-*fms*) and PDGF receptor genes. Cell 55:655–661, 1988.
58. Robbins KC, Leal F, Pierce JH, Aaronson SA: Biosynthetic pathway of the v-*sis*/PDGF-2 gene product in SSV-transformed cells. EMBO J 4:1783–1786, 1985.
59. Garrett JSG, Coughlin SR, et al.: Blockage of autocrine stimulation in SSV-transformed cells reverses down regulation of PDGF receptors. Proc Natl Acad Sci USA 81:7466–7470, 1984.
60. Huang JS, Huang SS, Deuel TF: Transforming protein simian sarcoma virus stimulates autocrine growth of SSV-transformed cells through PDGF cell-surface receptors. Cell 39:79–87, 1984.

61. Johnson A, Betsholtz C, Heldin C-H, Westermark B: Antibodies against platelet-derived growth factor inhibit acute transformation by simian sarcoma virus. Nature 317:438–440, 1985.
62. Johnsson A, Bethsholtz C, von der Heim K, Heldin C-H. Westermark B: Platelet-derived growth factor agonist activity of a secreted form of the v-*sis* oncogene product. Proc Natl Acad Sci USA 82:1721–1725.
63. Leal F, Williams LT, Robbins KC, Aaronson SA? Evidence that the v-*sis* gene product transforms by interaction with the receptor for platelet-derived growth factor. Science 230:327–330, 1985.
64. Betsholtz C, Johnsson A, Helding C-H, Westermark B: Efficient reversion of simian sarcoma virus-transformation and inhibition of growth factor-induced mitogenesis by suramin. Proc Natl Acad Sci USA 83:6440–6444, 1986.
65. Donoghue DJ, Hannink M: Requirement for signal sequence in biological expression of the v-*sis* oncogene. Science 226:1197–1199, 1984.
66. Keating MT, Williams LT: Autocrine stimulation of intracellular PDGF receptors in v-*sis*-transformed cells. Science 239:914–916, 1988.
67. Huang SS, Huang JS: Rapid turnover of the platelet-derived growth factor receptor in sis-transformed cells and reversal by suramin. Implications for the mechanism of autocrine transformation. J Biol Chem 263:12608–12618, 1988.
68. Johnsson A, Betsholtz C, Heldin C-H, Westermark B: The phenotypic characteristics of simian sarcoma virus-transformed human fibroblasts suggests that the v-*sis* gene product acts solely as a PDGF receptor agonist in cell transformation, EMBO J 5:1535–1541, 1986.
69. Deinhardt F: Biology of primate retroviruses. In Klein G (ed): Viral Oncology. New York, Raven Press, 1980, pp 357–398.
70. Harsh GR, Rosenblum ML, Williams LT: Oncogene-related growth factors and growth factor receptors in human malignant glioma-derived cell lines. J Neuro-Oncol, in press.

8. Transforming growth factors-α and -β and their potential roles in neoplastic transformation

Rik Derynck

Two types of growth factors have been termed transforming growth factors (TGFs) because they were discovered for their ability to elicit cellular transformation when added to an immortalized nonneoplastic cell line. One of these, TGF-α, is structurally related to epidermal growth factor (EGF) and competes for binding to the same receptor, while the other one, TGF-β, is a structurally unrelated protein with distinct receptors.

The initial observation that led to the identification of TGF-α was that several retrovirus-transformed rodent cells had a strongly reduced number of EGF binding sites on their surface [1]. It was postulated that these cells release a factor that is able to bind to the EGF receptor and, in turn, makes it unavailable for binding of the externally added ligand. Such an EGF receptor-binding factor was subsequently identified in the medium of sarcoma virus-transformed cells and was therefore called sarcoma growth factor (SGF) [2]. Further examination of a variety of cell sources showed that this same factor was made by many other transformed cells, but not by adult normal cells [3–5], leading to the assumption that it was somehow involved in the establishment or maintenance of the transformed phenotype.

SGF preparations are able to induce profound morphological changes in rat fibroblasts when added to the medium. These changes result in a phenotype similar to that of virally transformed cells. Removal of these preparations results in a reversion of cell phenotype back toward the normal. In other experiments it was shown that these preparations enable normal, anchorage-dependent rat fibroblasts to grow in soft agar. However, when these anchorage-independent soft agar colonies are selected and subsequently plated in the absence of these preparations, they grow as normal, contact-inhibited, growth-arrested fibroblasts [2,6]. The fact that preparations of this factor were able to convert normal rat kidney (NRK) cells into phenotypically transformed cells and that this factor was synthesized by many different transformed cells led to the name *transforming growth factor*.

Initially its was assumed that SGF to TGF was a single peptide [2], but we know now that the preparations consisted of the structurally unrelated pepitdes TGF-α and TGF-β. Although the binding to the EGF receptor is due solely to the presence of TGF-α, the profound morphological changes

Benz, C. and Liu, E., (eds.), Oncogenes. © *1989 Kluwer Academic Publishers.*
ISBN 0-7923-0237-0. All rights reserved.

observed with the rat fibroblasts are due to the cooperative effect of TGF-α and TGF-β [7,8]. TGF-β by itself will not induce colony formation by NRK cells in soft agar, while pure TGF-α preparations will have only a minimal effect in this assay system. In contrast, the simultaneous presence of both TGF-α and TGF-β will result in the acquisition of the transformed phenotype by the NRK cells, as shown by the appearance of a high number of large colonies in the soft agar assay. It should be stressed that the need for both growth factors to promote phenotypic transformation is dependent upon the cell system used. TGF-α and -β are indeed both needed in the NRK system [7,8]. However, in some other systems TGF-α (or EGF) and -β can function as antagonists [9], and in the AKR-2B cell system, TGF-β alone can induce anchorage-independent colony formation [10]. It is also important to realize that some other combinations of growth factors may be able to induce a phenotypic transformation of some cell lines. These assays should thus not be considered as specific for either TGF-α or -β.

Transforming growth factor-α

TGF-α is derived from a transmembrane precursor

Analyses of supernatants and extracts from rodent and human cells indicate that there exists a size heterogeneity of several possibly different TGF-α species [2,3,11]. The molecular weights, estimated on the basis of gel filtration, range from the 6-kDa species secreted by several tumor cell lines [11] to the 34-kDa TGF-α detected in the urine of cancer patients [12]. The low-molecular-weight TGF-α species has been purified to homogeneity from several cell sources [11,13,14,15]. Subsequent amino acid sequencing led to the establishment of the complete amino acid sequence of the 50-amino-acid-long rat TGF-α [15] and of the amino terminus of the low-molecular-weight TGF-α from human sources [11]. These data on the structure of TGF-α have now been confirmed and extended by the analysis of TGF-α cDNA clones.

cDNA characterization has revealed that the 50-amino-acid from of TGF-α is synthesized as an internal part of a 160- (human) [16] or 159- (rat) [17] amino-acid precursor. Remarkably, this short coding sequence is carried within an mRNA of 4.5–4.8 kb, which, at least in the human case, corresponds to 6 exons in a gene at least 70 to 100 kb long [18]. The deduced amino acid sequence of the TGF-α precursor reveals the presence of a potential membrane-spanning, hydrophobic domain, suggesting that the TGF-α precursor may be a transmembrane protein (figure 1) [16,17,19]. The extracellular precursor domain is about 100 amino acids long and includes the N-terminal signal sequence and the 50-amino-acid TGF-α. To generate the 50-amino-acid TGF-α, proteolytic cleavage of the precursor must occur at both the amino and carboxyl terminus between an alanine residue and valine dipeptide. This Ala-Val-Val trimer is located within the sequence Val-Ala-

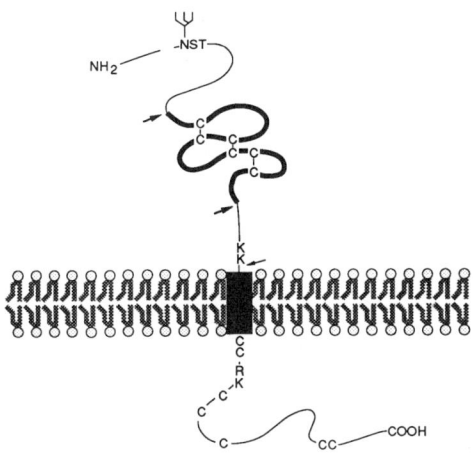

Figure 1. Schematic diagram of the TGF-α precursor and its processing. The N-terminal sequence is shown as already cleaved from the precursor (from [19]).

Ala-Ala-Val-Val at the amino terminus and within the similar sequence Ala-Val-Val-Ala-Ala at the carboxyl end [16,17]. Proteolytic processing of a precursor protein by a protease with such specificity has not been described for any other polypeptide, but this type of processing is reminiscent of the cleavage specificity of the elastases [20]. In contrast, cleavage of many precursors of polypeptide hormones takes place at dibasic residues [21–24]. Such a sequence, a Lys-lys, is located 8 amino acids downstream of the C-terminus of the 50-amino-acid TGF-α (figure 1).

The 50-amino-acid TGF-α is about 30% identical to the 53-residue-long EGF [15]. This identity includes all six similarly spaced cysteines and several other residues that may be important in the determination of the confirmation. This sequence relationship and the presumed formation of three similar disulfide bridges in both molecules provide a molecular explanation for the interaction of the two growth factors with the same cellular receptor [25].

We have mentioned above that besides the 50-amino-acid TGF-α, several larger forms of the TGF-α can be detected in the medium of transformed cells. Genomic Southern hybridization using the human TGF-α cDNA as a probe did not reveal any evidence for more than one TGF-α gene [16]. These data suggested that the larger forms may be derived from the same gene and thus from the same precursor.

Subsequent experimental evidence indicates that the size heterogeneity of the TGF-α species can be explained by differential processing of the extracellular domain of the transmembrane precursor and by glycosylation of the larger forms. The sequence of the 50-amino-acid TGF-α is preceded by an Asn-Ser-Thr triplet that is a potential N-glycosylation site [16,17], and it has been established that the larger forms derived from the same precursor are indeed N-glycosylated [19,26,27]. The presence of this sequence at the

N-terminus thus indicates that these forms have not undergone a cleavage at the site immediately preceding the 50-amino-acid TGF-α sequence. Besides this N-terminal sequence heterogeneity, there exists also a C-terminal heterogenity, due to the presence of the two potential cleavage sites [9] (figure 1). In addition, it has also been shown that the larger TGF-α forms are O-glycosylated [27]. The type and extent of proteolytic cleavage and glycosylations may depend on the cell source, thus explaining differences in the sizes of the TGF-α species secreted from various cell sources.

Analysis of the processing of the TGF-α precursor has shown that the precursor is anchored in the membrane as a transmembrane protein [19,26,27]. The C-terminus, about 35 residues long, is thus a cytoplasmic domain. This region contains seven cysteines and undergoes covalent palmitate attachment at one or more cysteines [19]. These peculiar structural features and the extreme sequence conservation between species suggest that this segment has a biological function, which still remains unresolved.

Some observations indicate that the TGF-α precursor is not cleaved in certain cell types and is exposed as a transmembrane protein on the cell surface, raising the possibility that the uncleaved precursor functions as some type of receptor or that it can interact with the receptor on a neighboring cell. The latter possible function is currently under investigation, but makes it conceivable that a TGF-α-expressing cell can exert an autocrine or paracrine mitogenic effect without releasing the soluble ligand.

TGF-α synthesis by normal and tumor cells

The initial detection of TGF-α activity in culture supernatants of rodent fibroblasts transformed with Moloney or Kirsten murine sarcoma viruses [3–5,28] was followed by a survey of various transformed cell lines. This indicated that this activity could be found predominantly in the medium of retrovirally transformed cells and to a much lesser extent in cells transformed with DNA viruses or chemical carcinogens [28]. However, it has been reported that transformation by SV40 [29] or polyoma [30] will induce TGF-α secretion. In the latter case, transfection of rat cells with the DNA segment coding for middle T is sufficient to induce both the transformed phenotype and TGF-α production. The close correlation between TGF-α synthesis and transformation is also illustrated by experiments with rat cells transformed with a Kirsten murine sarcoma virus; these cells secrete TGF-α only when phenotypic transformation occurs at the permissive temperature [5].

We examined a large variety of human tumor cell lines and surgically removed tumors for the presence of TGF-α mRNA [31]. This study showed that TGF-α mRNA could not be detected in the hemopoietic tumor cell lines that were examined. On the other hand, it was detectable in many solid tumors or cell lines from such origin. While TGF-α mRNA is present in several sarcomas or sarcoma cell lines, its occurrence is biased towards carcinomas and tumors of neuroectodermal origin. TGF-α mRNA is most consistently synthesized in renal carcinomas and in squamous carcinomas, but can also be frequently found in mammary carcinomas and in tumors of neuronal origin. It is possible that TGF-α is also consistently synthesized by some other tumor types, but the low number of tumor samples of some types precludes generalizations. The occurrence of TGF-α mRNA in such a large variety of solid tumors suggests that the synthesis of TGF-α may play a biological role in malignant transformation and tumor development in vivo. The synthesis of TGF-α by these tumors could also explain the presence of a high-molecular-weight EGF receptor binding factor that reacts with anti-TGF-α antibodies in the urine of some cancer patients and not in the urine of normal controls [12,32].

The detection of TGF-α expression by the tumor cells could have a correlation with the expression of this growth factor during fetal development. We therefore analyzed by in situ hybridization the localization of TGF-α mRNA in the developing mouse fetus [33]. This indicated that TGF-α expression peaks at days 12 to 13 of the 21-day fetal development and then gradually declines to a nondetectable level. TGF-α expression is localized in the fetal compartment of the placenta and also in the otic vesicle, oral cavity, nasopharyngeal pouch, first and second branchial arch, and developing mesonephric tubules of the kidney in the fetus [33].

TGF-α exerts its mitogenic effect through the EGF receptors at the cell surface. These receptors are expressed in mouse embryos as early as day 11 and continue to be detected through day 17 of the gestation [34]. It is thus likely that TGF-α can display a mitogenic effect on several fetal cell populations in an autocrine, paracrine, or endocrine fashion. The presence of TGF-α in the oral cavity and the pharyngeal pouch suggests that it plays a role in the development of tissues in this area. This would be consistent with the findings that EGF or TGF-α are mitogenic for the palate [35].

We also investigated the synthesis of TGF-α in the adult mouse brain using in situ hybridization [36]. This analysis revealed that several structures in the brain have a low yet significant expression of the TGF-α gene. It is also possible that the glial cells make TGF-α mRNA. This would not be surprising, since many glioblastomas derived from these cells express the TGF-α gene [31,37]. The possible role of TGF-α in the physiology of the brain is unknown, although a neurotrophic activity for EGF has been documented [38].

The observation that TGF-α is consistently expressed in squamous carcinomas that are of epithelial origin led us to investigate the synthesis of TGF-α by normal human keratinocytes in vitro and in vivo [39]. Northern analysis and measurements of secreted TGF-α in the medium indicate that cultured keratinocytes derived from human neonatal foreskin and adult skin secrete TGF-α. Immunohistochemistry and in situ hybridization also showed TGF-α expression in the skin in vivo. The presence of EGF receptors on the surface keratinocytes in culture and in vivo and the strong mitogenic effect of TGF-α on keratinocytes suggests that TGF-α synthesized by the keratinocytes can exert an autocrine or paracrine stimulation in the skin. Therefore, endogenous TGF-α production could contribute to the in vivo proliferation of the normal keratinocytes in the skin [39].

Studies of normal keratinocytes cultured under serum-free conditions have indicated that the TGF-α expression can be induced by TGF-α or EGF, growth factors which are structurally related and interact with the same receptor. It is thus possible for a growth factor to induce its own expression [39]. This mechanism of autoregulation of cell proliferation could be responsible for amplification of the growth factor response. Such autostimulation has now also been found in the case of several other growth factors [39–42] and may be a general amplification mechanism among growth modulators.

Given the recent localization of TGF-α expression in embryonic development, in the adult brain, and in keratinocytes, it is not surprising that TGF-α expression can be detected in several tumor types, especially the carcinomas [31]. Squamous carcinomas are from epithelial origin, and keratinocytes, and several other epithelial cell populations, have the capacity to express TGF-α. Similarly, the expression of TGF-α in renal carcinomas is consistent with the localization of TGF-α mRNA in the developing kidney, while it is also possible that adult kidney epithelial cells synthesis TGF-α. Finally, the synthesis of TGF-α in the embryonic otic vesicle, which is in part formed as an extension of the brain, and in the normal adult brain may correlate with TGF-α expression in gliomas and other tumors from neuroectodermal origin [31,37]. It is not known how the levels of TGF-α expression in the tumor cells relate to the matched normal counterpart cells.

The presence of TGF-α expression in normal skin prompted us to evaluate the TGF-α expression in psoriasis, a common skin disease in which non-malignant epidermal hyperproliferation is prominent [43]. Since human skin and cultured normal human keratinocytes produce TGF-α, and since TGF-α is strongly mitogenic for keratinocytes [44], the overexpression of TGF-α could be responsible at least in part for the initiation and/or the maintenance of epidermal hyperproliferation in a psoriatic lesion. Expression of TGF-α in epidermal biopsies was evaluated by Northern analysis and by analysis of protein levels using a specific antibody assay [45]. These analyses demonstrated that TGF-α is strongly overexpressed in psoriatic skin, in comparison to the normal skin either from normal volunteers or from psoriatic patients. It is therefore possible that TGF-α may be a prime mediator of the epidermal hyperproliferative response in psoriasis [45].

A variety of factors are capable of altering epidermal growth and perturbing the homeostasis of skin. Perhaps the best-characterized factors are the phorbol esters, which are potent tumor promoters in mammalian skin and are hyperplastic agents that cause rapid proliferation and pronounced thickening of the epidermis [46]. The most potent tumor promoter, 12-0-tetradecanoyl phorbol-13-acetate (TPA) exerts a highly pleiotropic response in vitro and in vivo and is able to induce the expression of a variety of genes. TPA mediates many of its effects via protein kinase C, a Ca^{2+}-activated and phospholipid-dependent enzyme that serves as the high-affinity receptor for this phorbol ester [47,48]. Treatment of normal human keratinocytes in culture showed that TPA induces TGF-α mRNA expression and secretion of TGF-α [49]. This induction of TGF-α gene expression was significantly greater than the effect elicited by EGF or TGF-α. This action of the phorbol ester is presumably mediated through activation of kinase C, since dioctanoylglycerol, a membrane-permeable synthetic diacylglycerol and a physiological activator of protein kinase C, is also able to induce TGF-α expression. In addition, this effect can be blocked by pretreatment with the isoquinoline sulfonamide H7, a potent inhibitor of kinase C. It is thus likely that treatment of skin with TPA results in the enhanced synthesis of TGF-α. Therefore, it is conceivable that the benign, hyperplastic proliferation of epidermis resulting from TPA treatment is due in part to the mitogenic response of keratinocytes to TGF-α [49].

It thus becomes clear that TGF-α may play a role in normal physiology and that its expression is not just restricted to tumor cells. TGF-α could normally play a role in wound healing, considering its expression by activated macrophages and by skin keratinocytes. An EGF-receptor-binding peptide, which may be EGF or TGF-α (or yet another factor) has also been detected in platelets [50]. The synthesis of TGF-α and the corresponding receptors by skin keratinocytes and the mitogenic effect of TGF-α on keratinocytes also suggest a role of TGF-α in the normal physiology of the skin and in the development of psoriasis.

A potential role of TGF-α in cellular transformation

Now that it has been established that TGF-α is a polypeptide hormone that may play a role under normal physiological conditions, it should not be assumed that it cannot play a role in malignant transformation. Earlier studies have shown that transformation by the *ras* oncogene results in an induction of the TGF-α gene expression both in immortalized fibroblasts and in epithelial cells [5,51]. In addition, transformation of fibroblasts by SV40 or polyoma virus [29,30] and perhaps by several other oncogenes can also result in TGF-α secretion. The observation that a transforming factor was secreted by some retrovirus-transformed cell lines led to the hypothesis that the secreted growth factors could interact with the producer cells in an 'autocrine' fashion [52]. Such autocrine interaction of TGF-α with the tumor cells could be important in the establishment and maintenance of the transformed phenotype. A variety of studies have addressed the possibilities that expression of a growth factor would be sufficient to induce malignant transformation in an autocrine fashion. We can now conclude that these autocrine interactions may play a crucial role in several experimental systems of growth-factor-induced transformation in cell culture, but it is still unclear how relevant they are in the clinical development of human tumors.

Several groups have studied whether TGF-α or EGF expression could be sufficient to induce transformation of fibroblasts. High-level expression of

EGF in rat 3T3 fibroblasts [53] and of TGF-α in the immortalized rat-1 [54] and NRK [55] fibroblasts can induce transformation and tumorigenicity in an autocrine fashion. TGF-α expression in these cells results in a 'transformed' morphology, soft agar colony formation, and formation of tumors in nude mice. TGF-α-induced transformation is much weaker than *ras*- or *sis*-induced transformations of the same cells, which result in unambiguous focus formation, larger colonies in soft agar, and much more aggressive tumor formation in nude mice. Also, a relatively high level of TGF-α synthesis in excess of the endogenous TGF-α synthesis of most tumor cells is needed before transformation or tumorigenicity is seen. It was also shown that TGF-α expression in NIH-3T3 fibroblasts results in an altered growth and lack of contact inhibition, yet there was no efficient growth of transformed colonies [56]. These apparent differences with the results in other cell lines mentioned above could be due at least in part to the use of different cell populations, as is often observed in biological experiments. In addition, the assay for colony formation of the transfected NIH 3T3 cells [56] is different from the anchorage-independence assay in soft agar used for the other cell systems. The former assay evaluates the growth of single transfected cells on a monolayer of non-transformed fibroblasts. The presence of these nontransformed fibroblasts could suppress the transformed characteristics of the transfected cells, as has been observed with *ras*-transformed cells [57]. However, suppression of transformation by nontransformed cells cannot take place in the anchorage-independence assays in soft agar, in which only transfected cells were seeded in physical separation from each other. In conclusion, a high level of endogenous TGF-α expression may induce transformation in immortalized rodent fibroblast cell lines, but the resulting transformation is certainly not as drastic as with the *ras*- or *sis*-oncogenes. Such weak transformation and the fact that immortalized cell lines are already close to transformation makes it unlikely that TGF-α expression alone can induce transformation of primary cells.

On the other hand, it is certainly possible that TGF-α expression gives the transformed cells growth advantages. Indeed, epithelial cells transfected with TGF-α expression vector developed larger benign tumors in vivo than their counterparts that did not express TGF-α [58]. Similarly, the increased proliferation of hormone-dependent breast carcinoma cells following estrogen treatment may be due at least in part to the estrogen-induced TGF-α expression [59]. A role for TGF-α in the proliferation of the tumor cells does not necessarily imply a higher level of endogenous TGF-α expression. It is certainly conceivable that the transformed cells have acquired an increased responsiveness to TGF-α, either due to an increased number of receptors at the cell surface or to other factors that play a role in signal transduction and are independent of the number of surface receptors. It has been observed that tumor cells that express the TGF-α gene often have a relatively high level of EGF/TGF-α receptor expression [31]. This correlation is especially striking in the case of the squamous, renal, and mammary carcinomas. It has also been shown that fibroblasts overexpressing the receptor can acquire the transformed phenotype when exposed to either EGF or TGF-α [60,61]. It is thus possible that a combined expression of sufficiently high levels of TGF-α and its receptor is of crucial and clinical importance in malignant transformation in vivo.

Transforming growth factor-β

Different structurally related TGF-β species

In spite of its name, TGF-β is structurally unrelated to TGF-α, has very different biological activities, and binds to different receptors (for review see [62,63]). Most cells in culture, whether they are normal or transformed, secrete TGF-β and have receptors. While for a long time it was thought that there was only one type of TGF-β, it has recently become evident that we are dealing with a small family of related molecules. Human platelets have provided the major source for purification for TGF-β [64,65]. This type of TGF-β which we now call TGF-β1, has served as the basis for the vast majority of the biological studies and is therefore by far the best-characterized TGF-β species. TGF-β1 is also present in relatively high concentrations in bone [66,67] and is the TGF-β species secreted by most cells in culture. Characterization of the protein [65] and corresponding cDNAs [68,69] indicates that mature active TGF-β1 is a disulfide-linked dimer of two identical 112-amino-acid-long polypeptide chains, each of which contains nine cysteines. The TGF-β monomer constitutes the C-terminal part of a 390-amino-acid precursor. Proteolytic cleavage of the precursor takes place following four basic residues that immediately precede the mature TGF-β monomer sequence. Most cells synthesize their TGF-β1 in an inactive or 'latent' form. Also, the TGF-β1 stored in the platelets is in an inactive complex [70,71]. Biochemical characterization of this complex has indicated that the mature TGF-β homodimer interacts in a noncovalent way with a dimer of the precursor segments from which the signal peptides are removed. In addition, a 135-kDa polypeptide that is unrelated to the TGF-β precursor is associated with this complex [72,73]. Activation, which is usually done by acid treatment, results in the removal of these interactions with the other polypeptides and exposes the TGF-β such that it can then interact with the surface receptors. While such drastic acid treatment is certainly effective, it is unlikely that this takes place under physiological conditions. Rather, it is more plausible that activation in vivo occurs through the action of proteases, since it has been shown that plasmin and cathepsin are able to activate the inactive TGF-β complex [74]. It is as yet unclear under what conditions in vivo this protease-mediated activation of the TGF-β takes place.

A second and distinct form of TGF-β has recently been isolated. This TGF-β2 has been found in porcine platelets [75], in bovine bone [76], and in the medium of several cell lines [77–79]. Also, the growth inhibitor originally described by Holley et al. from the medium of the monkey cell line BSC-1 is identical to TGF-β2 [78]. Finally, the existence of a third type of TGF-β, TGF-β3, has recently been demonstrated by the isolation of specific cDNAs [80,81]. It is possible that this type of TGF-β is made primarily by cells from mesodermal origin [80].

The isolation of human cDNAs for the three TGF-β species allows a detailed comparison of the polypeptide sequences for all three TGF-β precursors [80,81], shown in figure 2. The three mature TGF-β monomer sequences constitute the C-terminal segments of their respective precursors. All three TGF-β monomers are 112 amino acids long, including their nine conserved cysteines which determine the disulfide bridge formation. TGF-β3 is about 80% similar to TGF-β1 and TGF-β2, while TGF-β2 is 72% similar to TGF-β1. In contrast, the precursor sequences for the three TGF-β species are remarkably dissimilar. Indeed, relatively large gaps have to be introduced in order to achieve maximal similarity. However, some structural features are conserved in all three precursors, presumably due to their biological significance. Both TGF-β1 and β2 contain three potential N-glycosylation sites, in contrast to the TGF-β3 precursor which has four sites. Two of these sites are conserved in all three precursors. In the case of the TGF-β1 precursor, it has been shown that these two sites have N-linked carbohydrate moieties to which a mannose-6-phosphate group is attached [82]. Also conserved in the TGF-β1 and TGF-β3 precursors is the tetrapeptide RGDL, which has been detected in several extracellular matrix proteins that are involved in interactions with the cell surface [83]. This tetrapeptide is absent in the TGF-β2 precursor. A major difference between the three precursor sequences is their number of cysteine residues. The TGF-β3 precursor segment contains five cysteines versus three in the corresponding TGF-β1 precursor sequence and six in the TGF-β2 precursor segment. Three of these are in corresponding positions in all three precursors. Considering the structural differences among the three types of TGF-β and their precursors, it will be important to explore their differential expression and their regulation in cell populations in vivo. In analogy with TGF-β1, it can be assumed that TGF-β2 and -β3 are also made as latent or inactive complexes due to an interaction of the mature TGF-β dimers with their corresponding precursor dimers. However, the major structural differences in the precursor segments make it possible that there are major biological or biochemical differences between the latent complexes.

Cellular sources of TGF-β synthesis and biological activities

TGF-β has its own specific cell surface receptors, which can be found on most cell types. TGF-β receptors are present in normal and transformed cells of fibroblastic, epithelial, and hematopoietic origin [84,85]. Thus the capability of the cells to make TGF-β and the TGF-β receptors is ubiquitous. There are no major differences in the abundance of receptors between cells of different

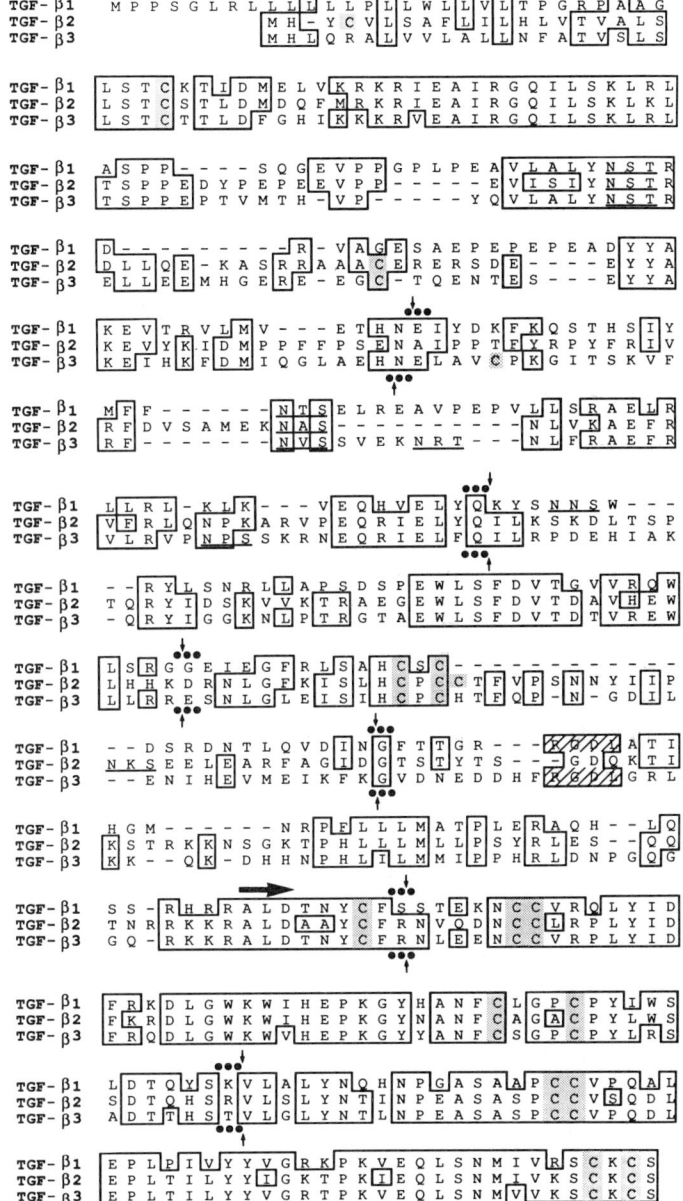

Figure 2. Polypeptide sequence similarity between the human TGF-β1, -β2, and -β3 precursors at the amino acid level. The three dots represent the nucleotides of the codon for the corresponding amino acid, and the arrow marks the insertion point of the intron (from [80]).

origin, be it normal or transformed. Three types of TGF-β receptors have been identified by cross-linking studies. The three receptor types are glycosylated surface molecules that are structurally different from each other. They have been classified as type I (60–70 kDa), type II (85–95 kDa), and type III (80–330 kDa) receptors [75,86]. The latter type of receptors form a disulfide-linked complex of 560 to 600 kDa and appear to be the predominant form of TGF-β receptor in most mammalian cells. However, some cell types such as myoblasts do not contain the type III receptors. It has not been demonstrated that all three receptors are able to mediate ligand-induced signal transduction, and there is some evidence that only the smallest receptor species is involved in mediating the major biological activities of TGF-β.

The biological activities of TGF-β are very diverse [63] and depend upon the cell type and the culture conditions, such as the presence of other growth factors. The capability of TGF-β to induce anchorage independence in the presence or absence of EGF appears to be restricted to several fibroblast cell lines [87] in culture. In addition, TGF-β stimulates DNA synthesis and mitosis in fibroblasts. The mitogenic effect of TGF-β on fibroblast cultures may in part be due to an indirect stimulation, since TGF-β can induce in these cells the expression of c-sis mRNA, which encodes the B chain of platelet-derived growth factor [88]. In contrast to the mitogenic effect on fibroblasts, TGF-β is also a potent inhibitor of proliferation for many normal and transformed cell lines [89]. The normal cell types include keratinocytes [90], endothelial cells [91], hepatocytes [92], and lymphocytes [93]. The basis for the growth inhibition induced by TGF-β is as yet unclear. TGF-β is also a potent chemotactic agent for macrophages [94] and dermal fibroblasts [95].

A major effect of TGF-β is the regulation of the cellular interaction with the extracellular matrix. TGF-β has been shown to induce the synthesis of collagen [96,97], fibronectin [96,98], the fibronectin receptors [99], and matrix proteoglycans [100]. In addition, the synthesis of plasminogen activator inhibitor type I [101] and collagenase inhibitors [102] are increased. As a net result of all these effects, TGF-β may induce an increased deposition and a decreased degradation of the extracellular matrix. It is possible that the stimulation of anchorage-independent growth of fibroblasts is a secondary effect of the increased extracellular matrix deposition, induced by TGF-β [96].

The mitogenic and chemotactic activities of TGF-β, together with the effects on extracellular matrix, are presumably the basis for the ability of TGF-β to stimulate connective tissue formation and to enhance wound healing in vivo [97,103]. It is conceivable that TGF-β is naturally involved in normal wound healing, since it is present in high levels in the α-granules of blood platelets [65].

Both TGF-β1 and TGF-β2 have many similar biological activities [75], although there are some striking differences in their relative potencies in some systems. This is shown by their differential effect on multipotential hematopoietic progenitor cells [104] and on mesoderm induction in *Xenopus laevis* embryos [105]. It is not yet known how similar or different TGF-β3 is in its biological activities in comparison to TGF-β1 and -β2.

Is there a role for TGF-β *in malignant transformation?*

Several studies have compared normal and transformed cells for their level of TGF-β synthesis and their sensitivity to TGF-β. Determination of TGF-β levels secreted by retrovirus-transformed fibroblasts and the nontransformed, immortalized counterparts has led to the conclusion that malignant transformation increased TGF-β synthesis [106]. Additional studies in other laboratories have not been able to confirm this result for other cell lines. Thus an induction of TGF-β synthesis following transformation should probably not be considered as a general phenomenon, but may occur in some cases. Another comparative study observed the development of a markedly increased sensitivity to stimulation of growth in soft agar by TGF-β in the chemically transformed AKR-2B and C3H/10T1/2 cells relative to their nontransformed counterparts [10,107]. This change in responsiveness to TGF-β was not due to differences in receptor levels, since there was only a very slight reduction in numbers of receptors on the chemically transformed cells relative to the nontransformed parents with no detectable change in affinity. This suggested that a postreceptor mechanism was responsible for the increased sensitivity observed in the chemically tranformed cells. Using the C3H/10T1/2 cells, which are completely unresponsive to TGF-β stimulation of soft agar growth, it was shown that c-*myc* expression controls at least in part the responsiveness to TGF-β [108]. Transfection with an activated *ras* induces a similar phenotype to that induced by TGF-β but without the requirement for added TGF-β, suggesting that *ras* p21 may enhance autocrine stimulation by endogeneous TGF-β or may be involved in the transduction of the TGF-β signal [108,109].

It is likely that the involvement of TGF-β in malignant transformation is very different in nonfibroblastic cells, such as epithelial cells. Normal epithelial cells and keratinocytes in culture are very sensitive to the growth-inhibitory activity of TGF-β. They are also inhibited in their growth by serum, which contains high levels of latent TGF-β, suggesting that these cells are able to activate the inactive TGF-β complexes. Studies on squamous carcinoma cell lines, derived from bronchial epithelial cells or keratinocytes, have revealed a loss of the inhibitory response to TGF-β exhibited by the normal cells [90]. The loss of the normal inhibitory response to TGF-β in epithelial cells could result in an enhanced proliferative potential of the neoplastic cells [109].

Many other carcinoma cell lines grow well in serum but are inhibited by pure, active TGF-β [110], suggesting that these cells have lost the capability of activating the inactive form of TGF-β present in serum. Since most cells, including carcinoma cells, produce TGF-β in the inactive form, it is possible that a loss of the ability to activate TGF-β may be one change that can occur in carcinoma cells. The resulting loss of a normal inhibitory response could have the same effect as the acquisition of an abnormal stimulatory effect and may thus also result in a growth advantage. This change in response to TGF-β may represent one of the multiple changes required for the conversion of certain normal cells to fully neoplastic cells [109].

The synthesis of TGF-β by transformed cells could not only confer an advantage to proliferation of the producing cells at the cellular level, but could also give a growth advantage to the developing tumor in vivo. The induction by TGF-β of a variety of proteins that constitute the extracellular matrix [96,97,99] could result in an increased stroma formation, which could support the increased proliferation of the cells and the resulting tumor growth. TGF-β secretion by the tumor cells could also result in a local suppression of the immune system, since it has been shown that TGF-β can suppress the growth and functionality of lymphocytes [93,111,112]. Such potential advantages of the tumor cells in vivo due to TGF-β secretion would imply that there is a certain level of activation of the latent TGF-β complexes either by the tumor cells themselves or by factors in the local environment. Yet, there is currently no unambiguous evidence to support this hypothesis. Therefore, it is evident that a lot more work will be needed to obtain an insight into the complex biology of TGF-β and its roles in the physiology of normal and tumor cells.

References

1. Todaro GJ, De Larco JE, Cohen S: Transformation by murine and feline sarcoma viruses specifically blocks binding of epidermal growth factor to cells. Nature 264:26–31, 1976.
2. De Larco JE, Todaro GJ: Growth factors from murine sarcoma virus transformed cells. Proc. Natl Acad Sci USA 75:4001–4005, 1978.
3. Todaro GJ, Fryling C, De Larco JE: Transforming growth factors produced by certain human tumor cells: polypeptides that interact with epidermal growth factor receptors. Proc. Natl Acad Sci USA 77:5258–5262, 1980.
4. Roberts AB, Lamb LC, Newton DL, Sporn MB, De Larco JE, Todaro GJ: Transforming growth factors: isolation of polypeptides from virally and chemically transformed cells by acid/ethanol extraction. Proc. Natl Acad Sci USA 77:3494–3498, 1980.
5. Ozanne B, Fulton RJ, Kaplan PL: Kirsten murine sarcoma virus transformed cell and a spontaneously transformed rat cell line produce transforming factors. J Cell Physiol 105: 163–180, 1980.
6. Roberts AB, Frolik CA, Anzano MA, Sporn MB: Transforming growth factors from neoplastic and non-neoplastic tissues. Fed Proc 42:2621–2625, 1983.
7. Anzano MA, Roberts AB, Meyers CA, Komoriya A, Lamb LC, Smith JM Sporn MB: Synergistic interaction of two classes of transforming growth factors from murine sarcoma cells. Cancer Res 42:4776–4778, 1982.
8. Anzano, MA, Roberts AB, Smith JM, Sporn MB, De Larco JE: Sarcoma growth factor from conditioned medium of virally transformed cells is composed of both type α and β transforming growth factors. Proc. Natl Acad Sci USA 80:6264–6268, 1983.
9. Roberts AB, Anzano MA, Wakefield LM, Roche NS, Stern DF, Sporn MB: Type β transforming growth factor: a bifunctional regulation of cellular growth. Proc. Natl Acad Sci USA 82:119–123, 1985.
10. Tucker RF, Volkenant ME, Branum EL, Moses HL: Comparison of intra- and extracellular transforming growth factors from nontransformed and chemically transformed mouse embryo cells. Cancer Res 43:1581–1586, 1983.
11. Marquardt H, Hunkapiller MW, Hood LE, Twardzik DR, De Larco JE, Stephenson JR, Todaro GJ: Transforming growth factors produced by retrovirus-transformed rodent cells and human melanoma cells: amino acid sequence homology with epidermal growth factor.

Proc. Natl Acad Sci USA 80:4684–4688, 1983.
12. Sherwin SA, Twardzik DR, Bohn WH, Cockley KD, Todaro GJ: High molecular weight transforming growth factor activity in the urine of patients with disseminated cancer. Cancer Res 43:403–407, 1983.
13. Marquardt H, Todaro GJ: Human transforming growth factor. Production by a melanoma cell line, purification and initial characterization. J Biol Chem 257:5220–5225, 1982.
14. Massagué, J: Epidermal growth factor-like transforming growth factor. I. Isolation, chemical characterization and potentiation by other transforming growth factors from feline sarcoma virus-transformed rat cells. J Biol chem 258:13606–13613, 1983.
15. Marquardt H, Hunkapiller MW, Hood LE, Todaro GJ: Rat transforming growth factor type 1: structure and relation to epidermal growth factor. Science 223:1079–1082, 1984.
16. Derynck R, Roberts AB, Winkler ME, Chen EY, Goeddel DV: Human transforming growth factor-α: precursor structure and expression in *E. coli*. Cell 38:287–297, 1984.
17. Lee DC, Rose TM, Webb NR, Todaro GJ: Cloning and sequence analysis of a cDNA for rat transforming growth factor-α. Nature 313:489–491, 1985.
18. Derynck R: Human transforming growth factor-α; precursor sequence, gene structure and heterologous expression. Cancer Cells 3:79–86, 1985.
19. Bringman TS, Lindquist PB, Derynck R: Different transforming growth factor-α species are derived from a glycosylated and palmitoylated transmembrane precursor. Cell 48: 429–440, 1987.
20. Naughton MA, Sanger F: Purification and specificity of pancreatic elastase. Biochem J 78:156–163, 1961.
21. Noda M, Furatani Y, Takahashi H, Toyosato M, Hirose T, Imayama S, Nakanishi S, Numa S: Cloning and sequence analysis of bovine adrenal preproenkephalin. Nature 295:202–206, 1982.
22. Gübler U, Seeburg P, Hoffman BJ, Gage LP, Udenfriend S: Molecular cloning establishes pro-enkephalin as a precursor of enkephalin-containing peptides. Nature 295:206–208, 1982.
23. Amara SG, Jonas V, Rosenfeld MG, Ong ES, Evans RM: Alternative RNA processing in calcitonin gene expression generates mRNAs encoding different polypeptide products. Nature 298:240–244, 1982.
24. Nakanishi S, Inoue E, Nakamura M, Change ACY, Cohen SN, Numa S: Nucleotide sequence of cloned cDNA for bovine corticotropin-β-lipotropin precursor. Nature 278:423–427, 1979.
25. Massagué J: Epidermal growth factor like transforming growth factor. II. Interaction with epidermal growth factor receptors in human placenta membranes and A431 cells. J Biol Chem: 13614–13620, 1983.
26. Gentry LE, Twardzik DR, Lim GJ, Ranchalis JE, Lee DC: Expression and characterization of transforming growth factor-α precursor protein in transfected mammalian cells. Mol Cell Biol 7:1585–1591, 1987.
27. Teixido J, Gilmore R, Lee DC, Massagué J: Integral membrane glycoprotein properties of the prohormone pro-transforming growth factor-α. Nature 326:883–885, 1987.
28. Todaro GJ, Lee DC, Webb NR, Rose TM, Brown JP: Rat type α transforming growth factor: structure and possible function as a membrane receptor. Cancer Cells 3:51–58, 1985.
29. Kaplan PL, Topp WC, Ozanne B: Simian virus 40 induces the production of a polypeptide transforming growth factor(s). Virology 108:484–490, 1981.
30. Kaplan PL, Ozanne B: Polyoma virus-transformed cells produce transforming growth factor(s) and grow in serum-free medium. Virology 123:372–380, 1982.
31. Derynck R, Goeddel DV, Ullrich A, Gutterman JU, Williams R, Bringman TS, Berger WH: Synthesis of mRNAs for transforming growth factors-α and -β and the epidermal growth factor receptor by human tumors. Cancer Res 47:707–712, 1987.
32. Twardzik DR, Limball ES, Sherwin SA, Ranchalis JE, Todaro GJ: Comparison of growth factors functionally related to epidermal growth factor in the urine of normal and human

tumor bearing athymic mice. Cancer Res 45:1934–1939, 1985.
33. Wilcox JN, Derynck R: Developmental expression of transforming growth factor-α and -β in mouse fetus. Mol Cell Biol 8:3415–3422, 1988.
34. Nexo E, Hollenberg MD, Figueroa A, Pratt RM: Detection of epidermal growth factor-urogastrone and its receptor during fetal mouse development. Proc Natl Acad Sci USA 77:2782–2785, 1980.
35. Pratt RM: Role of epidermal growth factor in embryonic development. In: Sawyer R (ed): The Molecular and Developmental Biology of Keratins. Current Topics in Developmental Biology, volume 22. 1987, pp 175–192.
36. Wilcox JN, Derynck R: Localization of cells synthesizing transforming growth factor-α in the mouse brain. J Neurosc. 8:1901–1904, 1988.
37. Nistér M, Libermann TA, Betsholz C, Petterson M, Claesson-Welsh L, Heldin CH, Schlessinger J Westermark B: Expression of messenger RNAs for platelet-derived growth factor and transforming growth factor-α in human malignant glioma cell lines. Cancer Res 48:3910–3918, 1988.
38. Morrison RS, Kornblum HI, Leslie FM, Bradshaw RA: Trophic stimulation of cultured neurons from neonatal rat brain by epidermal growth factor. Science 238:72–75, 1987.
39. Coffey RJ, Derynck R, Wilcox JN, Bringman TS, Goustin TS, Moses HL, Pittelkow MR: Production and auto-induction of transforming growth factor-α in human keratinocytes. Nature 328:817–820 (1987).
40. Paulsson Y, Hammacher A, Heldin C-H, Westermark B: Possible positive autocrine feedback in the prereplicative phase of human fibroblasts. Nature 328:714–717, 1987.
41. Warner SJC, Auger KR, Libby P: Human interleukin 1 induces interleukin 1 gene expression in human vascular smooth muscle cells. J Exp Med 165:1316–1331, 1987.
42. Van Obberghen-Shilling E, Roche NS, Flanders KC, Sporn MB, Roberts AB: Transforming growth factor-β 1 positively regulates its own expression in normal and transformed cells. J Biol Chem 263:7741–7746, 1988.
43. Weinstein GD, McCullough JL, Ross PA: Cell kinetic basis for pathophysiology of psoriasis. J Invest Dermatol 85:597–583, 1985.
44. Barrandon Y, Green H: Cell migration is essential for sustained growth of keratinocyte colonies: the roles of transforming growth factor-α and epidermal growth factor. Cell 50:1131–1137, 1987.
45. Elder JT, Fisher GJ, Lindquist PB, Bennett GL: Pittelkow M, Coffey RJ, Ellingsworth J, Derynck R, Voorhees JJ: Overexpression of TGF-α in psoriatic skin. Science, 243:811–814, 1989.
46. Argyris TS: The regulation of epidermal hyperplastic growth. CRC Critical Rev Toxicol 9:152–200, 1981.
47. Nishizuke Y: The role of protein kinase C in cell surface signal transduction and tumour production. Nature 308:693–698, 1984.
48. Nishizuka Y: Studies and perspective of protein kinase C. Science 233:305–312, 1986.
49. Pittelkow MR, Lindquist PB, Derynck R, Abraham R, Graves-Deal R, Coffey RJ: Induction of transforming growth factor-α expression in human keratinocytes by phorbol esters. J Biol Chem 264:5164–5171, 1989.
50. Oka, Orth: Human plasma epidermal growth factor/β-urogastrone is associated with blood platelets. J Clin Invest 72:249–259, 1983.
51. Salomon DS, Perroteau I, Kidwell WR, Tam J, Derynck R: Loss of growth responsiveness to epidermal growth factor and enhanced production of alpha-transforming growth factor in *ras*-transformed mammary epithelial cells. J Cell Physiol 130:297–409, 1987.
52. Sporn MBN, Todaro GJ: Autocrine secretion and malignant transformation of cells. N Engl J Med 303:878–880, 1980.
53. Stern DF, Hare DA, Cecchini MA, Weinberg RA: Construction of a novel oncogene based on synthetic sequences encoding epidermal growth factor. Science 235:321–324, 1987.
54. Rosenthal A, Lindquist PB, Bringman TS, Goeddel DV, Derynck R: Expression in rat fibroblasts of a transforming growth factor-α cDNA results in transformation. Cell 46:301–309, 1986.

55. Watanabe S, Lazar E, Sporn MB: Transfection of normal rat kidney (NRK) cells by an infectious retrovirus carrying a synthetic rat type α transforming growth factor gene. Proc Natl Acad Sci USA 84:1258–1262, 1987.
56. Finzi E, Fleming T, Segatto O, Pennington C, Bringman TS, Derynck R, Aaronson SA: The human TGF-α coding sequence is not a direct acting oncogene when overexpressed in NIH/3T3 cells. Proc Natl Acad Sci USA 84:3733–3737, 1987.
57. Land H, Chen AC, Morgenstern JP, Parada LF, Weinberg RA: Behavior of *myc* and *ras* oncogenes in transformation of rat embryo fibroblasts. Mol Cell Biol 6:1917–1925, 1986.
58. Finzi E, Kilkenny A, Strickland JE, Balashak M, Bringman TS, Derynck R, Aaronson SA, Yuspa SH: TGF-α stimulates growth of skin papillomas by autocrine and paracrine mechanisms but does not cause neoplastic progression. Mol Carcinogenesis 1:7–12, 1988.
59. Dickson RB, Kasid A, Huff KK, Bates SE, Knabbe C, Bronzertt D, Gellman EP, Lippman ME: Activation of growth factor secretion in tumorigenic states of breast cancer induced by 17 β-estradiol or c-Ha-*ras* oncogene. Proc Natl Acad Sci USA 84:837–841, 1987.
60. DiFiore PP, Pierce JH, Fleming TA, Hazan R, Ullrich A, King CR, Schlessinger J, Aaronson SA: Overexpression of the human EGF receptor confers an EGF-dependent transformed phenotype to NIH3T3 cells. Cell 51:1063–1070, 1987.
61. Riedel H, Massoglia S, Schlessinger J, Ullrich A: Ligand activation of overexpressed epidermal growth factor receptors transforms NIH 3T3 mouse fibroblasts. Proc Natl Acad Sci USA 85:1477–1481, 1988.
62. Sporn MB, Roberts AB, Wakefield LM, Assoian RK: Transforming growth factor-β: biological function and chemical structure. Science 233:532–534, 1987.
63. Sporn MB, Roberts AB, Wakefield LM, de Crombrugghe B: Some recent advances in the chemistry and biology of transforming growth factor-beta. J Cell Biol 105:1039–1045, 1987.
64. Childs CB, Proper JA, Tucker RF, Moses HL: Serum contains a platelet-derived transforming growth factor. Proc Natl Acad Sci USA 79:5312–5316, 1982.
65. Assoian RK, Komoriya A, Meyers CA, Miller DM, Sporn MB: Transforming growth factor-β in human platelets. Identification of a major storage site, purification, and characterization. J Biol Chem 258:7155–7160, 1983.
66. Seyedin SM, Thomas TC, Thompson AY, Rosen DM, Piez KA: Purification and characterization of two cartilage-inducing factors from bovine demineralized bone. Proc Natl Acad Sci USA 82:2267–2271, 1985.
67. Seyedin SM, Thompson AY, Bentz H, Rosen DM, McPherson M, Conti A, Siegel NR, Galluppi GR, Piez KA: Cartilage-inducing factor-A: apparent identity to transforming growth factor-beta. J Biol Chem 261:5693–5695, 1986.
68. Derynck R, Jarrett JA, Chen EY, Eaton DH, Bell JR, Assoian RK, Roberts AB, Sporn MB, Goeddel DV: Human transforming growth factor-beta complimentary DNA sequence and expression in normal and transformed cells. Nature 316:701–705, 1985.
69. Derynck R, Jarrett JA, Chen EY, Goeddel DV: The murine transforming growth factor-beta precursor. J Biol Chem 261:4377–4379, 1986.
70. Lawrence DA, Pircher R, Kryceve-Martinerie C, Jullien P: Normal embryo fibroblasts release transforming growth factors in a latent form. J Cell Physiol 121:184–188, 1984.
71. Pircher DA, Lawrence DA and Jullien P: Latent beta-transforming growth factor in non-transformed and Kirsten sarcoma virus-transformed normal rat kidney cells, clone 49F. Cancer Res 44:5538–5543, 1984.
72. Miyazono K, Hellman U, Wernstedt C, Heldin C-H: Latent high molecular weight complex of transforming growth factor-β. Purification from human platelets and structural characterization. J Biol Chem 263:6407–6415, 1988.
73. Wakefield LM, Smith DM, Flanders KC, Sporn MB: Latent transforming growth factor-β. A high molecular weight complex containing precursor sequences. J Biol Chem 263:7646–7654, 1988.
74. Lyons RM, Keski-Oja J, Moses HL: Proteolytic activation of latent transforming growth factor-β from fibroblast-conditioned medium. J Cell Biol 106:1659–1665, 1988.
75. Cheifetz S, Weatherbee JA, Tsang ML, Anderson JK, Mole JE, Lucas R, Massagué J: The transforming growth factor-β system, a complex pattern of cross-reactive ligands and

receptors. Cell 48:409–415, 1987.
76. Seyedin SM, Segarini PR, Rosen DM, Thompson AY, Bentz H, Graycar J: Cartilage-inducing factor-B is a unique protein structurally and functionally related to transforming growth factor β. J Biol Chem 262:1946–1949, 1987.
77. de Martin R, Haendler B, Hofer-Warbinek R, Gaugitsch H, Wrann M, Schlüsener H, Seifert JM, Bodmer S, Fontana A, Hofer E: Complimentary DNA for human glioblastoma-derived T cell expressor factor, a novel member of the transforming growth factor β family. EMBO J 6:3673–3677, 1987.
78. Hanks SK, Armour R, Baldwin JH, Maldonado F, Spiess J, Holley RW: Amino acid sequence of the BSC-1 cell growth inhibitor (polyergin) deduced from the nucleotide sequence of the cDNA. Proc Natl Acad Sci USA 85:79–82, 1988.
79. Madisen L, Webb NR, Rose TM, Marquardt H, Ikeda T, Twardzik D, Seyedin SM, Purchio AF: Transforming growth factor-β_2: cDNA cloning and sequence analysis. DNA 7:1–8, 1988.
80. Derynck R, Lindquist PB, Lee A, Wen D, Tamm J Graycar JL, Rhee L, Mason AJ, Miller DA, Coffey RJ, Moses HL, Chen EY: A new type of transforming growth factor-β, TGF-β3. EMBO J 7:3737–3743, 1988.
81. ten Dijke P, Hansen P, Iwata KK, Pieler C, Foulkes JG: Identification of another member of the transforming growth factor type β gene family. Proc Natl Acad Sci USA 85:4715–4719, 1988.
82. Purchio AF, Cooper JA, Brunner AM, Liwbin MN, Gentry LE, Koracina KS, Roth RA, Marquardt M: Identification of mannose-6-phosphate in two asparagine-linked sugar chains of recombinant transforming growth factor-β1 precursor. J Biol Chem 263:14211–14215, 1988.
83. Ruoslahti E, Pierschbacher MD: New perspectives in cell adhesion: RGD and integrins. Science 238:491–497, 1987.
84. Massagué J, Like B: Cellular receptors for type beta transforming growth factor. Ligand binding and affinity labeling in human and rodent cell lines. J Biol Chem 260:2636–2645, 1985.
85. Wakefield LM, Smith DM, Masui T Harris CC, Sporn MB: Distribution and modulation of the cellular receptor for transforming growth factor-β. J Cell Biol 105:965–975, 1987.
86. Cheifetz S, Like B, Massagué J: Cellular distribution of type I and type II receptors for transforming growth factor-beta. J Biol Chem 261:9972–9978, 1986.
87. Shipley GD, Tucker RF, Moses HL: Type β transforming growth factor/growth inhibitor stimulates entry of monolayer cultures of AKR-2B cells into S phase after a prolonged prereplicative interval. Proc Natl Acad Sci USA 82:4147–4151, 1985.
88. Leof EB, Proper JA, Goustin AS, Shipley GD, DiCorleto PE, Moses HL: Induction of c-*sis* mRNA and activity similar to platelet-derived growth factor by transforming growth factor-beta: a proposed model for indirect mitogenesis involving autocrine activity. Proc Natl Acad Sci USA 83:2453–2457, 1986.
89. Tucker RF, Shipley, GD, Moses HL, Holley RW: Growth inhibitor from BSC-1 cells closely related to platelet type beta transforming growth factor. Science 226:705–707, 1984.
90. Shipley GD, Pittelkow MR, Wille JJ, Jr Scott RE, Moses HL: Reversible inhibition of human prokeratinocyte proliferation by type beta transforming growth factor–growth inhibitor in serum-free medium. Cancer Res 46:2068–2971, 1986.
91. Takehara K, LeRoy EC, Grotendorst GR: TGF-β inhibition of endothelial cell proliferaton: alteration of EGF binding and EGF-induced growth regulatory (competence) gene expression. Cell 149:415–422, 1987.
92. Carr BJ, Hayashi I, Branum EL, Moses HL: Inhibition of DNA synthesis in rat hepatocytes by platelet-derived type beta transforming growth factor. Cancer Res. 46:2330–2334, 1986.
93. Kehrl JH, Wakefield LM, Roberts AB, Jakowlew S, Alvarez-Mon M, Derynck R, Sporn MB, Fauci AS: Production of transforming growth factor-beta by human T lymphocytes and its potential role in the regulation of T cell growth. J Exp Med 163:1037–1050, 1986.
94. Wahl SM, Hunt DA, Wakefield LM, McCartney-Francis, N, Wahl LM, Roberts AB,

Sporn MB: Transforming growth factor-beta (TGF-β) induces monocyte chemotaxis and growth factor production. Proc Natl Acad Sci USA 84:5788–5792, 1987.
95. Postlethwaite AE, Keski-Oja J, Moses HL, Kang AH: Stimulation of the chemotactic migration of human fibroblasts by transforming growth factor-β. J Exp Med 165:251–256, 1987.
96. Ignotz RA, Massagué J: Transforming growth factor-beta stimulates the expression of fibronectin and collagen and their incorporation into the extracellular matrix. J Biol Chem 261:4337–4345, 1986.
97. Roberts AB, Sporn, MB, Assoian RK, Smith JM, Roche NS, Wakefield LM, Heine UI, Liotta LA, Falanga V, Kehrl JH, Fauci AS: Transforming growth factor type-beta: rapid induction of fibrosis and angiogenesis in vivo and stimulation of collagen formation in vitro. Proc Natl Acad Sci USA 83:4167–4171, 1986.
98. Ignotz RA, Endo T, Massagué J, Regulation of fibronectin and type I collagen mRNA levels by transforming growth factor-β. J Biol Chem 262:6443–6447, 1987.
99. Ignotz RA, Massagué J: Cell adhesion protein receptors as targets for transforming growth factor-β action. Cell 51:189–197, 1987.
100. Bassols A, Massagué J: Transforming growth factor-β regulates the expression and structure of extracellular matrix chondroitin/dermatan sulfate proteoglycans. J Biol Chem 263:3039–3045, 1988.
101. Laiho M, Saksela O, Andreasen PA, Keski-Oja J: Enhanced production and extracellular deposition of the endothelial type plasminogen activator inhibitor in cultured human lung fibroblasts by transforming growth factor-beta. J Cell Biol 103:2403–2410, 1986.
102. Edwards DR, Murphy G, Reynolds JJ, Whitham SE, Docherty AJP, Angel P, Health JK: Transforming growth factor beta modulates the expression of collagenase and metalloproteinase inhibitors. EMBO J 6:1899–1904, 19817.
103. Mustoe TA, Pierce GF, Thomason A, Gramates P, Sporn MB, Deuel TF: Accelerated healing of incisional wounds in rats induced by transforming growth factor-β. Science 237:1333–1335, 1987.
104. Ohta M, Greenberger JS, Anklesaria P, Bassols A, Massagué J: Two forms of transforming growth factor-β distinguished by multipotential hematopoietic progenitor cells. Nature 329:539–541, 1987.
105. Rosa F, Roberts AB, Danielpour D, Dart LL, Sporn MB, Dawid I: Mesoderm induction in amphibians: the role of TGF-β2-like factors. Science 239:783–785, 1988.
106. Anzano MA, Roberts AB, deLarco JE, Wakefield LM, Assocan RK, Roche NS, Smith JM, Lazarus JE, Sporn MB: Increased secretion of type β transforming growth factor accompanies viral transformation of cells. Mol Cell Biol 5:242–247, 1985.
107. Moses HL, Childs CB, Halper J, Shipley GD, Tucker RF: Role of transforming growth factors in neoplastic transformation. In: Veneziale CM (ed): Control of Cell Growth and Proliferation. New York, Van Nostrand Reinhold Co., 1984, pp 147–167.
108. Leof EB, Proper JA, Moses HL: Modulation of transforming growth factor beta action by activated *ras* and c-*myc*. Mol Cell Biol 7:2649–2652, 1987.
109. Moses HL, Coffey RJ, Leof EB, Lyons RM, Keski-Oja J: Transforming growth factor-β regulation of cell proliferation. J Cell Physiol 5 (Suppl).1–7, 1987.
110. Moses HL, Tucker RF, Leof EB, Coffey RJ, Halper J, Shipley GD: Type beta transforming growth factor is a growth stimulator and a growth inhibitor. Cancer Cells 3:65–71, 1985.
111. Kehrl JH, Roberts AB, Wakefield LM, Jakowlew S, Sporn MB, Fauci AS: Transforming growth factor-β is an important immunomodulatory protein for human B lymphocytes. J Immunol 137:3855–3860, 1986.
112. Rook AH, Kehrl JH, Wakefield LM, Roberts AB, Sporn MB, Burlington, DB, Lane HC, Fauci AS: Effects of transforming growth factor-β on the functions of natural killer cells: depressed cytolytic activity and blunting of interferon-responsiveness. J Immunol 136:3916–3920, 1986.

Clinical Aspects of Oncogenes in Human Neoplasia

9. Oncogenes in human solid tumors

Christoph F. Rochlitz and Christopher C. Benz

Introduction

The past decade has witnessed great changes in our understanding of the molecular origins of cancer. Toward this end, major contributions have come from the identification of oncogenes and their cellular counterparts, proto-oncogenes, as well as recessive anti-oncogenes, or tumor-suppressor genes. These general topics have been extensively reviewed [1–16]. The purpose of this chapter is to address what is known about oncogene abnormalities in specific human solid tumors, including the incidence and mode of oncogene activation, its putative role in tumor formation and metastasis, and the clinical significance of oncogene abnormalities relating to tumor behavior and patient prognosis. Before focusing on specific tumor types, it is useful to summarize those concepts pertinent to oncogene activation that might help in understanding the present evidence supporting a role for oncogenes in the development or progression of naturally occurring human tumors.

Mechanisms of oncogene activation

Proto-oncogenes become activated and can contribute to tumor development or progression either by abnormal expression of a normal proto-oncogene product (RNA or protein) or by the expression of an abnormal oncogene product. Expression may be altered either by proviral DNA insertion, gene amplification, or chromosomal translocation and subsequent disruption of normal transcriptional and posttranscriptional regulatory mechanisms. Alternatively, expression of an altered oncogene product may result from DNA mutation, gene deletion, or chromosomal rearrangement. All of these potential oncogene-activating mechanisms have been detected in human solid tumors. For example, Durst et al. [17] described the integration of papilloma viral sequences near normal proto-oncogene sequences in cervical carcinomas. There are also many reports on N-*myc* amplification in advanced stage neuroblastomas [18–21], c-*erbB*-2 (HER-2/*neu*) amplification in breast cancers [22–24], and *myc* (c,N,L) or *ras* (Ki) amplifications in lung cancers [25–30]. Although DNA amplification usually results in RNA and protein over-

Benz, C. and Liu, E., (eds.), Oncogenes. © *1989 Kluwer Academic Publishers.*
ISBN 0-7923-0237-0. All rights reserved.

expression, the latter can also be observed in the absence of amplification. Overexpression is probably the most frequently reported oncogene abnormality described in human tumor specimens. In Slamon's study on 15 different oncogenes [31], multiple oncogenes were found to be transcriptionally active in all of the 54 tumor specimens analyzed (20 different types), and in nearly 80% of cases the level of oncogene expression in tumor tissue was greater than that found in normal tissue.

Chromosomal translocations and the disruption of oncogene regulatory sequences are most commonly found in lymphomas and leukemias (see chapter 10). Translocations characteristic of specific solid tumors are much less common; perhaps these are obscured by the difficulty in culturing tumor tissue for karyotype analysis, or by the tendency for human tumors to show aneuploidy and genetic instability [11]. There are nonetheless, specific translocations being detected in solid tumors with increasing frequency, such as t (11;22) (q24;q12) in Ewing's sarcomas [32–35] and t (3;8) (p14.2;q24.13) in renal cell carcinomas [36]. Whether or not oncogene activation occurs with these chromosomal translocations remains unknown.

The best-studied examples of oncogene activation are those induced by single base mutations, and this occurs most frequently in the *ras* proto-oncogenes. Rodenhuis et al. [37] reported a 50% incidence of Ki-*ras* point mutations in adenocarcinomas of the lung, and Bos et al. [38] and Forrester et al. [39] independently identified Ki-*ras* point mutations in approximately 40% of human colon carcinomas.

Chromosomal rearrangements and deletions probably occur nonspecifically as a manifestation of the genetic instability observed in solid tumors [11]; however, there are specific chromosome deletions that appear to characterize certain solid tumors. The oldest recognized abnormality of this sort is the 13q deletion found in retinoblastoma specimens [40]. Other examples of tumor-specific chromosome deletions include the 11p13 loss in Wilms' tumor and other embryonal malignancies [41], the 1p loss in neuroblastomas [42], the 17p and 18q losses in colon cancers and the additional 5q loss in colon cancers arising in patients with familial polyposis coli [43,44], the 10q loss in prostate cancers [45], the 3p loss in renal-cell carcinomas [46,47] and lung cancers [48], the 11p loss in bladder cancers [49], the 22q loss in neurofibromas and meningiomas [50], and the several different deletions known to occur with multiple endocrine neoplasia [51–54]. The implication that recessive anti-oncogenes (tumor-suppressor genes) may be lost or inactivated by these specific genetic lesions is based on the retinoblastoma model, and the detailed evidence supporting this hypothesis is presented elsewhere (see chapter 13). There are other possible influences arising from the loss of chromosomal material that can affect the function and expression of cellular oncogenes, and these will be mentioned later.

Lastly, many of the single mechanisms by which oncogenes are activated can also occur in concert [55,56]; tumors with several activated oncogenes are not only commonly recognized but also exhibit very aggressive behavior, both clinically and by in vitro assay [57]. Oncogene abnormalities described for each of the common types of human solid tumors are reviewed in this chapter and classified according to the level of their molecular analysis (DNA, RNA, protein) and in the context of either an experimental tumor model or a surgically resected specimen with clinical correlations.

Oncogene activation during carcinogenesis

In 1983, Balmain and Pragnell [58] reported that the DNA extracted from carcinogen-induced squamous-cell carcinomas in mice caused morphological transformation of NIH/3T3 fibroblasts, and the responsible transforming genes were identified as mutated forms of the Ha-*ras* proto-oncogene. Subsequent studies showed that the same Ha-*ras* mutations were present in chemically induced murine skin papillomas, which are premalignant lesions known to progress to invasive carcinomas at an incidence of 5%–7% [59]. Since 85% of papillomas exhibited the transformed Ha-*ras* oncogene, the investigators concluded that malignant progression from papilloma to carcinoma was likely determined by at least one other genetic event besides activation of Ha-*ras* [59]. Similarly, Quintanilla et al. [60] found specific A–T transversions in the second nucleotide of Ha-*ras* codon 61 in over 90% of papillomas and skin carcinomas induced by dimethylbenzanthrene (DMBA). This mutation was heterozygous in most papillomas, but was homozygous or amplified in carcinomas. These studies support the belief that Ha-*ras* activation can occur during tumor initiation but is, in itself, insufficient to produce a frank carcinoma.

Mutation of one *ras* allele and activation of the other by a second event, such as gene amplification, could potentially occur at different stages of carcinogenesis. Alternatively, it is likely that other oncogenes become activated prior to *ras* mutation and at some time during the premalignant stage of tumor development [60]. Bos and colleagues [38] and Forrester and colleagues [39], in two large studies looking at the incidence of Ki-*ras* mutations in human colon carcinomas, found that activating Ki-*ras* mutations are present in 40% of invasive primary tumors and in virtually all of the benign adenomas from which these invasive carcinomas arose. Furthermore, Reynolds et al. [61] demonstrated that 30% of premalignant hepatic adenomas and nearly 80% of murine hepatocellular carcinomas contain activated Ha-*ras* oncogenes. Finally, Sukumar et al. [62] identified single-base transversions in Ha-*ras* codon 12 in both early and late stages of all rat mammary carcinomas induced by the potent carcinogen, NMU. In summary, the number of independent genetic events sufficient to induce malignant transformation in any given tissue remains unknown, and current estimates range from two to seven [59]. The fact that activated oncogenes are not consistently found in all human solid tumors has led some investigators to suggest that oncogenes are not directly involved in carcinogenesis, but rather occur as an indirect result of the genetic instability commonly associated with spontaneous human tumors. However, the reproducible detection of individual transforming genes in animal tumor models, the concordance between *ras* mutations observed in experimental tumor models and in naturally occurring tumors, and the likely underestimates of activated oncogenes in human tumor specimens all suggest that oncogenes do play a pathophysiologic role in the tumors in which they are detected.

Tumor behavior and oncogene activation

The best evidence to date correlating oncogene activation with clinical tumor behavior comes from studies of neuroblastoma, where N-*myc* amplification is associated with advanced tumor stage, rapid disease progression, and poor patient survival [19–21]. Similar although slightly less significant correlations have been shown for L-, N-, and c-*myc* amplifications in lung cancer [63], and for c-*erb*B-2 (HER-2/*neu*) amplification in breast cancer [23]. There have also been a number of reports relating oncogene product overexpression with poor clinical outcome and/or aggressive tumor behavior, including overexpression of c-*myc* [64], c-*ras* [65,66], and c-*fos* [66] in colon carcinoma, c-*ras* in breast [67] and prostate [68] cancers and c-*myc* overexpression in cervical cancer [69]. However, several studies using these same tumor types have failed to show correlations between c-*myc* and c-*ras* expression and tumor behavior [70–72]; and the significance of oncogene overexpression occurring in association with other bad prognostic factors (e.g., tumor proliferation index) remains questionable.

Both concordant and discordant results are found when oncogene activations in primary and metastatic human tumor specimens are compared. Liu et al. [73] identified a Ki-*ras* point mutation in a terminal pleural effusion specimen from a patient with rapidly progressive breast cancer; the mutation was not found in tumor cells from two earlier metastatic effusions in the same patient. Rodenhuis found concordant Ki-*ras* mutations in early and advanced stages of lung cancer [37]; yet Heighway [30] demonstrated Ki-*ras* amplification occurring in lymph node metastases but not in primary lung cancer specimens. With regard to c-*myc* and N-*myc* gene copies, Wong found concordant results in both early and advanced tumor specimens collected from 45 patients with small-cell lung cancer [29]. Gallick [71], Hand [74], and Thor [65] all found differences in the degree of c-*ras* overexpression measured between colon cancer primary and metastatic tumors. Lastly, one study measuring N-*myc* amplification in neuroblastoma samples showed that the oncogene copy number remained consistent within a given tumor mass, between different tumor sites, and also at different points in time during diseases progression [75]. Thus, the various clinical studies suggest that tumor type, tumor stage, and the specific oncogene being analyzed are each important and dependent parameters.

Tissue-specific patterns of oncogene activation

It was once theorized that each oncogene might be expressed or activated only in specific tissues and tumors. This tissue/tumor-specific oncogene concept had to be revised when it was shown that many oncogenes could be expressed in the same tissue, and when it was proven that multiple oncogenes are involved in the normal regulation of cell growth, proliferation, and differentiation of embryonal and adult tissues. There are, nonetheless, data to suggest that a profile of activated oncogenes may correlate with specific types or subtypes of malignancy. In a recent review, Bishop enumerated seven oncogene lesions most commonly associated (20%–100% frequency) with human malignancies [15]: c-*abl* translocations in chronic myelogenous leukemia, c-*erb*B-1 amplifications in squamous-cell carcinomas and glioblastomas, c-*myc* translocations in Burkitt's and other types of lymphomas, c-*myc* amplifications in small-cell lung cancers and cancers of the breast, L-*myc* amplifications in small-cell lung cancers, N-*myc* amplifications in neuroblastomas and small-cell lung cancers, and c-*ras* (Ha,Ki,N) point mutations in a diverse set of solid tumors. It is interesting that the c-*myc*, L-*myc*, and N-*myc* amplifications occur in nonoverlapping subsets of small-cell lung cancers [63]; also, activating *ras* mutations appear to be specific for different tumor types. For example, N-*ras* mutations occur almost exclusively in several forms of leukemia (see chapter 10), while Ki-*ras* and Ha-*ras* mutations occur largely in solid tumors. In both colon and non-small cell lung adenocarcinomas, Ki-*ras* mutations predominate and are found in almost 50% of cases [37,38,39]; yet human breast adenocarcinomas at all stages of clinical progression are notably uninvolved with activating *ras* lesions [76]. In brief, more studies are necessary to define the incidence in which each of the approximately 40 known oncogenes are involved in specific types of human tumors.

Oncogenes as genetic markers of susceptibility to malignancy

With one possible exception, there are no well-established oncogene lesions that can be linked to a genetic predisposition for malignancy. That is to say, activating oncogene events appear to occur somatically rather than being transferred through germ-line DNA. The one exception involves Ha-*ras* allelic polymorphisms, first described by Capon et al. [77]. Different alleles of this gene, defined by a specific restriction enzyme and detected as different length DNA fragments on Southern analysis (polymorphisms), are genetically determined by the variable tandem reiteration of a 28 base-pair sequence adjacent to the Ha-*ras* gene locus, located in band 15 of the short arm of chromosome 11 (11p15). Krontiris et al. [78] reported that for the four common and 16 rare Ha-*ras* alleles, cancer patients possess a significantly higher frequency of rare alleles when compared to an unaffected population. Several investigators have tried to reproduce Krontiris' findings in specific tumor types. Lidereau et al. [79] found that common restriction fragments represented 91% of the allele pool in an unaffected population as opposed to 59% of breast cancer patients. Heighway et al. [80] reported similar findings in patients with non-small cell lung cancers. Ceccherini-Nelli et al. [81] found no significant correlation between any Ha-*ras* allelic pattern and predisposition to colorectal cancer; however, a difference in allelic patterns was observed when healthy donors were compared with cancer patients. There is no explanation for this apparent association between certain Ha-*ras* alleles and susceptibility to the development of cancer. It is possible that variations in the tandemly repeated nucleotide sequences might affect cancer risk by interfering with the control of Ha-*ras* expression; alternatively, these variations may reflect an unstable region involving an altogether different but closely linked 11p15 tumor-susceptibility gene.

Cooperation between activated oncogenes

Oncogenes can be broadly categorized by the intracellular localization of their protein products. For instance, nuclear oncogenes include *erb*-A, *fos*, *myc*, *myb*, p53, and *ski*, while cytoplasmic oncogenes include *abl*, *erb*B, *fes/fps*, *fms*, *mil/raf*, *mos*, *ras*, *ros*, *src*, and *yes*. In addition, there is a similarity of function within each of these groups. One general aspect of nuclear oncogenes is their ability to affect cellular proliferation; that is, the constitutive expression of these genes can often convert diploid cells with limited replicative potential into immortalized cells that can be passaged in vitro indefinitely [6]. These nuclear oncogenes have little effect on the property of anchorage-independent soft agar growth; cytoplasmic oncogenes, on the other hand, have little effect on replicative potential but are strong promotors of anchorage-independent growth [6]. Nuclear and cytoplasmic oncogenes cooperate effectively to induce normal cells such as fibroblasts to undergo complete malignant transformation. Land et al. [82] showed by DNA transfection that c-*myc* or mutated c-*ras* oncogenes alone were insufficient to transform rat embryonic fibroblasts, but together these two oncogenes could transform normal recipient fibroblasts into malignant and tumorigenic cells. There are now many report of cooperating sets of oncogenes having been identified in human tumor samples and cell lines. A mutated N-*ras* gene and an amplified c-*myc* gene were detected in the promyelocytic leukemia cell line, HL-60 [83]. Activated Ki-*ras* and an amplified c-*myc* gene were found in an aggressive giant-cell lung carcinoma sample [84] and also in a primary pancreatic cancer specimen [85]. Co-amplification of c-*myc* and c-*erb*B-1 were detected in an epidermoid carcinoma of the stomach [86]; and amplified c-*myc* and Ki-*ras* genes were found associated with a Ha-*ras* deletion in an aggression ovarian carcinoma [57]. From these reports it is evident that sets of activated and cooperating oncogenes do occur in vivo. It is still unclear, however, how commonly this phenomenon occurs and to what extent cooperating oncogenes actually modify tumor behavior in vivo.

Breast cancer

Experimental models

It has long been known that chemical carcinogens and genomic integration of viral DNA are both capable of inducing breast cancers in rodents. In mice, mammary cancers are commonly induced by the weakly oncogenic type B retrovirus, murine mammary tumor virus (MMTV). The regional insertion of MMTV DNA activates *int*-1 and/or *int*-2 proto-oncogenes, which are then constitutively expressed in mammary epithelium, leading to premalignant hyperplastic lesions and, finally, to infiltrating adenocarcinomas [87,88]. Although the MMTV retrovirus does not infect humans and is not directly involved in human breast tumorigenesis, the role of *int*-1 and *int*-2 activation may be important in humans as judged by the recent finding of amplified *int*-2 sequences detected in 15% of human breast cancer samples [89].

With regard to chemically induced models of breast cancer, Sukumar et al. [62] found that rat mammary carcinomas produced by a single injection of nitrosomethylurea (NMU) contained a transforming Ha-*ras* gene in the tumors of every animal tested. Molecular analysis revealed that codon 12 was mutated from GGA to GAA, resulting in glutamic acid being encoded instead of glycine in these tumors. This is notable in light of the fact that NMU is a potent alkylating agent that preferentially modifies deoxyguanosine residues by methylating the N^7 and O^6 positions. This causes the modified purine to base-pair with thymidine instead of deoxycytosine, leading to the generation of G-to-A transitions after DNA replication. In a similar fashion, Zarbel et al. [90] identified Ha-*ras* mutations in codon 61 of rat mammary carcinomas induced by another DNA alkylator, dimethylbenzanthrene (DMBA). Together, these results have led to an important chemical carcinogenesis tumor model that implicates the involvement of transforming *ras* mutations in the development of mammary adenocarcinomas.

There are many established human breast cancer cell lines, and a number of these have been found to contain activated oncogenes. A codon 12 Ha-*ras* mutation was found in one very aggressive carcinosarcoma cell line, HS578T [91]. A codon 12 Ki-*ras* mutation was identified in the adenocarcinoma cell line MDA-MB231 [92]; and an unusual tandem mutation in Ki-*ras* codon 12 was detected in another adenocarcinoma, H-466B [93]. Several transforming genes, including an amplified N-*ras* oncogene, were detected in MCF-7 cells [94]. Amplification and overexpression of c-*myc* were found in SKBR 3 breast cancer cells [95], and amplification of c-*erb*B-1 and c-*erb*B-2 oncogenes has also been reported [22,96].

Kasid et al. [97] transfected an activated Ha-*ras* oncogene into MCF-7 breast cancer cells and found that in contrast to the normal MCF-7 cells, the transfected cells were no longer dependent on exogenous estrogen for tumorigenic growth in nude mice. Frequently, human breast cancers that are estrogen-dependent in early clinical stages evolve to become estrogen-independent during disease progression, at which time the tumor may act more aggressively and is no longer responsive to antiestrogen therapy. The study by Kasid et al. [97] suggests that activated *ras* protein product assists in the conversion of tumor cells to a hormonally unresponsive and clinically more aggressive state.

Another interesting set of oncogene transfer studies in breast cancer was conducted by Leder and colleagues [98]. These investigators produced transgenic mice carrying the c-*erb*B-2 oncogene, activated by a point mutation, and fused to a murine mammary tumor virus long-terminal repeat sequence (MMTV-LTR), which acts as a steroid-inducible promotor/enhancer. All female founders possessed this MMTV-LTR/*erb*B-2 gene in all tissues analyzed and passed it on to progeny mice of both sexes in a Mendelian fashion. Of the few tissues found expressing this transgene in the progeny, only breast tissues developed infiltrating and metastasizing adenocarcinomas. Unlike the stochastic occurrence of solitary breast tumors found in transgenic animals carrying MMTV-LTR/c-*myc* or MMTV-LTR/v-Ha-*ras* fusion genes, mice expressing MMTV-LTR/*erb*B-2 showed rapid growth of polyclonal cancers throughout the epithelial tissue of every mammary gland. Thus, unlike the effect of constitutive overexpression of c-*myc* or activated Ha-*ras* genes in breast tissue, activated c-*erb*B-2 appears to be sufficient to induce a single-step malignant transformation of breast tissue that is not observed in other tissues in which it is also overexpressed [98].

Human breast tumors: DNA analysis

A summary of the incidence of activated oncogenes implicated in human breast cancers is shown in table 1, including the unexplained detection of amplified *int*-2 sequences as mentioned earlier [89]. Slamon et al. [23] first reported on a correlation between c-*erb*B-2 (HER-2/*neu*) amplification and clinical prognosis in 189 patients with primary breast cancer. This oncogene was amplified from 2-fold to more than 20-fold copies in about 30% of the tumors analyzed, and this finding predicted for a shorter patient survival and disease-free interval even when adjusted for other known poor prognostic factors, including lymph-node involvement and negative steroid receptor status. This oncogene was also analyzed by Van de Vijver's group [24] who demonstrated DNA amplification and overexpression in only 17% of 95 primary breast tumor samples. In this study, two thirds of the c-*erb*B-2 amplifications were accompanied by co-amplification of the syntenic oncogene, c-*erb*-A, which did not appear to be transcribed. Escot et al. [99] detected amplification of another oncogene, c-*myc*, in tumors from 38 of 121 patients (31%), but there was no correlation with tumor histology, stage, grade or steroid receptor content. Patients older than 50 years, however, had a significantly higher number of c-*myc* gene copies than did premenopausal patients; and 2 of 2 male patients analyzed were found to have c-*myc* amplifications in their breast cancers.

Table 1. Activated oncogenes in human breast cancer

Oncogene	Activation	% Incidence	Reference
c-myc	Amplification	20–30%	99,100
L-, N-myc	Amplification or rearrangement	<5%	99,100
c-myb	Rearrangement	<10%	99,100
c-mos	Rearrangement	<10%	102
Ha-ras	Allelic loss/rearrangement	27%	100,101
(Ki,Ha,N)-ras	Amplification or mutation	<5%	1,73,76, 91,100,101
c-int-2	Amplification	15%	89
c-erbB-2	Amplification	17–35%	23,24,100

Cline et al. [100] surveyed for DNA abnormalities in 16 different oncogenes in 53 patients with primary breast tumors. These investigators found at least one abnormality occurring in five different oncogenes in 58% of tumor specimens, with amplification of c-*myc* and c-*erb*B-2, and allelic deletions of Ha-*ras* and c-*myb* being most prevalent. The presence of an abnormal oncogene correlated with clinical tumor stage (86% incidence in stage III or IV tumors, and 39% incidence in stage I or II tumors), and also with the probability of tumor recurrence (18 of 19 recurring tumors had one or more oncogene abnormalities; 4 of 4 lymph node-positive tumors bearing oncogene abnormalities later recurred). Rochlitz et al. [76] and Theillet et al. [101] found no significant evidence for *ras* (Ha,Ki,N) abnormalities, including base mutations or amplifications, in their breast tumor populations. Rochlitz et al. [76], looking for codon 12, 13, or 61 mutations in any of the three *ras* oncogenes, screened 40 primaries, 7 lymph node and skin metastases, 9 metastatic effusions, and 5 established cell lines from patients with carcinoma of the breast. The results of this study demonstrated conclusively that *ras* mutations are rare events in breast cancer; but it is unclear at this point why breast adenocarcinomas are different in this respect from adenocarcinomas arising in the lung or colon. Thus, there is provocative evidence for the importance of oncogene amplifications in predicting breast cancer patient prognosis, but further studies are necessary to confirm the clinical significance of these findings.

Two studies [100,101] reported on the loss of Ha-*ras* alleles in the tumors of up to one third of patients with breast cancer; and in both studies there was a significant correlation between allelic loss and clinical outcome. In one of these studies [100], only 1 of 26 patients' tumors that did not recur and 5 of 5 recurring patients' tumors showed Ha-*ras* allelic loss. In the other study [101], allelic loss correlated with poorly differentiated tumors, the lack of tumor steroid receptors, and relapse with distant metastases. Although further investigations must confirm these results, Ha-*ras* allelic loss appears to correlate with biological aggressiveness of breast cancer.

Chromosomal rearrangement of the c-*myc* oncogene is a recognized occurrence in lymphomas (see chapter 10); of interest, Escot et al. [99] demonstrated similar c-*myc* rearrangements in the DNA from 5 of 121 primary breast cancers. A non-germ line c-*myc* fragment was detected in these samples and further analysis showed that the breakpoint occurred 3' to the c-*myc* oncogene, a situation similar to that observed in 15%–30% of patients with Burkitt's lymphoma who carrying c-*myc* translocations. Although the c-*myc* abnormalities were associated with older-aged patients, the total number of patients in this study was too small to draw further conclusions.

Restriction fragment length polymorphisms in the c-*mos* oncogene were found in tumors from 6 of 75 (8%) breast cancer patients but not in germ line DNA from a normal population, and in only 1 of 73 patients with leukemia [102]. As previously mentioned, there is an association between the occurrence of rare Ha-*ras* alleles and tumor susceptibility, including the development of breast cancer [79]; interestingly, women with two rare Ha-*ras* alleles have a much higher risk of developing breast cancer. Because of the statistical similarity between the 50% of breast cancer patients carrying at least one rare Ha-*ras* allele and the 60% of breast tumors that overexpress $p21^{ras}$ protein [103], investigators have speculated that *ras* expression might be dysregulated in patients bearing rare Ha-*ras* alleles.

Human breast tumors: RNA analysis

As with other solid tumors, interest in oncogene RNA expression in breast cancer has focused on *ras* and *myc* oncogenes. Several studies have shown that Ha-*ras* mRNA overexpression is a common if not ubiquitous occurrence in human breast carcinoma [31,99,101,104,105]. Spandidos and Agnantis [104] found relative overexpression of Ha-*ras* in infiltrating ductal carcinomas as compared to normal breast tissue. In a follow-up study, no correlation appeared between this overexpression and tumor stage in patients with primary breast cancer; however, in patients with lymph node metastases the levels of Ha-*ras* expression were significantly higher than in those tumors without lymph node metastases. Similarly, Theillet et al. [101] also reported elevated Ha-*ras* mRNA levels in 73% (16 of 22) of patients with primary infiltrating ductal carcinomas, but these investigators did not draw any clinical correlations. Several studies have reported that c-*myc* overexpression occurs in 70%–100% of breast tumors [31,99,106], but these analyses were confounded by the presence of stromal and inflammatory cells which can falsely elevate the measured level of c-*myc* mRNA. Nonetheless, these reports identified ductal adenocarcinomas as the histological subtype most frequently associated with c-*myc* overexpression.

Besides *ras* and *myc*, other oncogenes reported to be transcribed at elevated rates in breast cancer include c-*erb*B-1 [107,108], c-*erb*B-2 [24,109], and also c-*fes*, c-*fos*, and c-*fms* [31,110]. In the study by Kraus et al. [109], c-*erb*B-2 overexpression in breast cancers occurred with and without oncogene amplification, suggesting that unknown transcriptional deregulating mechanisms may also contribute to oncogene overexpression in breast cancers. It will be important to determine if c-*erb*B-2 overexpression, indepdenent of DNA amplification, has clinical prognostic value in breast cancer patients.

Human breast tumors: Protein analysis

At this writing, Cattoretti's report [111] remains the only study on breast cancer samples that has analyzed protein expression of an oncogene product other than $p21^{ras}$. These investigators detected p53 protein expression in about 50% of all breast tumors, and also correlated p53 levels with the presence of epidermal growth factor receptor (c-*erb* B-1), estrogen receptor content, histological tumor grade, and proliferation index as indicated by the nuclear proliferation antigen, Ki-67. Many past studies have focused on $p21^{ras}$, the membrane-associated protein products of Ha-, Ki-, and N-*ras* oncogenes [67,70,103,112,113]. Reports by Hand et al. [103,112] have found $p21^{ras}$ reactivity in 66%–90% of primary infiltrating ductal breast carcinomas, while no fibrocystic breast lesions and only 20% of benign fibroadenomas had detectable binding by monoclonal antibodies against $p21^{ras}$. Heterogeneity of *ras* oncogene expression has been commonly observed among cells in the same tumor specimen, suggesting that if *ras* has anything to do with human mammary epithelium transformation, continuous expression of this oncogene product in all tumor cells is not necessary to maintain the malignant phenotype. Ohuchi et al. [70] compared breast tissues in different stages of malignant transformation and came to the same conclusion. Furthermore, increasing amounts of $p21^{ras}$ were observed when comparing normal breast tissue with ductal hyperplasia, and atypical hyperplasia with carcinoma in situ and invasive carcinomas. However, no pattern was recognizable when primary and metastatic tumors were compared for differences in $p21^{ras}$ content. These investigators also concluded that enhanced $p21^{ras}$ expression may be involved in the early stages of mammary carcinogenesis but is probably not necessary for maintenance of the transformed phenotype. Lundy et al. [67] found concordance between $p21^{ras}$ expression in primary and metastatic tumors in 41 breast cancer patients. They found a strong correlation between lymph node positivity, tumor size, and intensity of $p21^{ras}$ immunohistochemical staining, but not with patient age or tumor receptor status. One other study tried to related $p21^{ras}$ expression with estrogen and progesterone receptor positivity by showing that two-thirds of receptor-positive patients had tumors with 10-fold overexpression of $p21^{ras}$, while two-thirds of receptor-negative patients had tumors with 3-fold above normal $p21^{ras}$ expression [113]. In summary, the immunohistochemical detection of $p21^{ras}$ may yet prove to be a useful clinical tool in defining breast cancer prognosis; at present, however, prospective studies are needed to analyze more tumors and tests are needed to evaluate the newer monoclonal antibodies that can distinguish normal from mutated forms of various $p21^{ras}$ proteins. Furthermore, with the recent discovery of amplified c-*erb* B-2 sequences in breast cancer specimens, studies correlating expression of this membrane oncoprotein with patient prognosis are eagerly awaited.

Lung cancer

Experimental models

Many oncogene abnormalities have been identified in human lung cancer cell lines; most of these findings, however, are limited to the *myc* (c,L,N) and *ras* (Ha,Ki,N) families of oncogenes. Early studies identified Ki-*ras* mutations in the LX-1 and Calu-1 cell lines (114,115,116), and additional Ki-*ras* mutations have since been found in other lung cancer cell lines [117,118]. While there have been no reported N-*ras* mutations, activated Ha-*ras* oncogenes have been described [119,120]. Amplification of one or more *myc* oncogenes is another frequent finding [26–28,121,122]. As summarized by Nau et al. [28], cell lines from 21 of 31 small-cell lung cancers (SCLC) possess *myc* amplifications (9 c-*myc*, 7 N-*myc*, 5 L-*myc*); and in particular, c-*myc* copy numbers are high in the variant types of SCLC but normal in the common form of SCLC. N-*myc* amplifications appear to be equally distributed in all types of SCLC. Amplifications in *myc* oncogenes are unusual in non-SCLC with only one reported exception [27]. However, overexpression of c-*myc* is common in all types of lung cancers [26,122,123], and rearrangement of this oncogene also occurs [124].

The findings related to *myc* amplification support the hypothesis that specific oncogene abnormalities might be used to define different histological tumor subtypes (e.g., SCLC vs. non-SCLC). This hypothesis is also supported by findings of abnormalities associated with the epidermal growth factor (EGF) receptor, encoded by c-*erb*B-1. Squamous-cell lung cancer (SQCLC), large-cell lung cancer (LCLC), and adenocarcinoma of the lung (ADCL) have all been shown to possess amplified and/or overexpressed EGF receptors in their respective cell lines [125–127]; however, this is not the case for SCLC [128].

Human lung cancers: DNA analysis

Miyaka et al. found 10-fold Ki-*ras* amplification in a SQCLC specimen by transplanting the tumor tissue into nude mice [55]. Taya et al. [84] found 10-fold Ki-*ras* amplification, a Ki-*ras* codon 12 mutation, and 8-fold c-*myc* amplification in a single specimen of a very aggressive giant-cell lung carcinoma. Yoshimoto et al. [124] observed that this particular subtype of non-SCLC may also possess a c-*myc* rearrangement. Lastly, Nau et al. [27] found 10-fold amplified N-*myc* in one SCLC specimen.

Larger analyses of lung cancer specimens have found *myc* amplifications in SCLC, with a variety of other oncogene abnormalities associated with non-SCLC. Johnson et al. [129] studied both treated and untreated patients with SCLC, and the cell lines that were derived from these patients' tumors. While 2 of 19 (11%) cell lines from untreated patients showed amplification of a *myc* oncogene (1 N-*myc*, 1 L-*myc*), 11 of 25 (44%) cell lines from treated patients showed *myc* amplifications (3 N-*myc*, 3-L-*myc*, 5 c-*myc*). Relapsing patients with *myc* amplifications had a median survival of 33 weeks as opposed to a 53-week survival for those without gene amplification, indicating that this oncogene abnormality has possible clinical significance. These findings are similar to those found in childhood neuroblastomas, where 33% of primary tumors and nearly 100% of established tumor cell lines have amplified N-*myc*. Further support for this clinical association in lung cancer patients comes from two other studies that found amplified c-*myc* in poor-prognosis cases of SCLC, unlike other types of lung carcinoma [25,28]. Finally, Wong et al. [29] examined the incidence of amplified c-*myc* and N-*myc* in 45 patients with SCLC; high copy numbers (>3-fold amplification) were found in the tumors of 11% of patients and intermediate copy numbers (1.5- to 3-fold amplification) were found in the tumors of 31% of patients. High *myc* copy numbers were generally caused by gene amplification, while intermediate copy numbers were often caused by a hyperdiploid chromosome number. Surprisingly, there was complete concordance in *myc* copy numbers between primary SCLC tumors and metastatic tumors in every case analyzed.

Heighway et al. [30] studied 18 SQCLC, 3 ADCL, and 3 SCLC and found that no c-*myc* or Ki-*ras* amplifications occurred in any primary tumors. There was, however, a 30-fold Ki-*ras* amplification found in a SQCLC lymph-node metastasis. In contrast to this report, Cline et al. [130] detected oncogene abnormalities in 15 of 27 (56%) non-SCLC primary tumors. Most frequent were allelic deletions of c-*myb* (60%) or Ha-*ras* (31%), which appeared to correlate with an increased probability of disease relapse and progression. In addition to these deletions, the other abnormalities included amplifications of c-*myc*, c-*erb*B-1 and c-*erb*B-2. These oncogene deletions are probably independent of the 3p chromosome deletion that is frequently observed in all major types of lung cancer, which is possibly associated with the loss of a tumor-suppressing anti-oncogene [48]. There is an association between the presence of certain Ha-*ras* alleles and the development of non-SCLC, as compared to an unaffected control population or group of patients with SCLC tumors [80]. Lastly, several reports have identified Ki-*ras* mutations in the tumors of patients with non-SCLC. Santos et al. [131] found an activating Ki-*ras* mutation in a patient with SQCLC, and Nakano et al. [132] found Ki-*ras* codon 12 mutations in two patients with ADCL. Most significantly, Rodenhuis et al. [37] found Ki-*ras* codon 12 mutations in 5 of 10 ADCL, 0 of 15 SQCLC, and 0 of 10 large-cell carcinomas of the lung. No N-*ras* or Ha-*ras* mutations were found in any of the non-SCLC samples tested.

Human lung cancers: RNA analysis

In the report by Slamon et al. [131], lung cancer was the only solid tumor that uniformly expressed the c-*fes* oncogene. Four other oncogenes, c-*fos*, c-*myc*, Ki-*ras*, and Ha-*ras* were expressed in all lung cancer samples studied. Griffin et al. [133] found RNA expression of c-*myb* in 5 of 5 common SCLC specimens, 3 of 4 variant SCLC specimens, and in 0 of 5 non-SCLC specimens. These investigators also suggested that an interaction between c-*myc* and c-*myb* nuclear oncogenes could potentially convert SCLC into non-SCLC. Nau et al. [134] reported N-*myc* overexpression in a patient with fulminant SCLC, and Funa et al. [135] correlated N-*myc* overexpression with disease activity in 15 untreated SCLC patients. There was a strong correlation between N-*myc* overexpression and poor response to subsequent chemotherapy, rapid tumor regrowth and short patient survival. Patients with N-*myc* expressing tumors had a median survival of 13 months as compared to 22 months for those with nonexpressing tumors; as well, 6 of 7 patients achieving a complete therapeutic response had no measurable N-*myc* tumor expression, whereas 6 of 8 patients without a clinical response to chemotherapy had N-*myc* tumor overexpression. These RNA findings are in accordance with the clinical correlations found with N-*myc* DNA amplification; together these studies indicate that the N-*myc* oncogene has diagnostic and prognostic importance in SCLC.

Human lung cancers: Protein analysis

Since EGF receptor levels correlated with poor prognosis in patients with breast cancer [136], investigators were interested in studying EGF receptor levels in various lung cancers. Veale et al. [137] analyzed 40 SQCLC and 37 other types of non-SCLC tumors. The EGF receptor immunohistochemical staining in tumor tissue was stronger than that observed in normal lung tissue, and SQCLC specimens were much more positive than ADCL or large-cell carcinoma of the lung. Despite the tumor specificity, however, there was no correlation between staining intensity and patient prognosis demonstrable in this study. Another study measured $p21^{ras}$ protein expression in non-SCLC tumors and found increased levels of this oncogene product in SQCLC specimens when compared to normal lung tissue and other lung tumors (LCLC and ADCL) [138]. These are no reports focusing on the nuclear $p62^{myc}$ protein in lung cancers, although this would be of interest since SCLC specimens commonly possess *myc* DNA amplifications.

Esophageal cancer

Very little is known about the role of oncogenes in esophageal cancer. Hollstein et al. [139] reported on the occurrence of a unique c-*mos* oncogene allele in 2 of 12 patients with esophageal cancer, and this same rare allele was not observed in any of the 63 healthy controls studied separately [102]. Tsuboi et al. [140] looked at concogene expression in a variety of gastrointestinal tumors and found no evidence of c-*myc* overexpression in 6 of 6 esophageal carcinomas.

Gastric cancer

Experimental models

Activated oncogenes have been detected in two well-established gastric carcinoma cell lines. In the MKN-7 cell line, c-*erb*B-2 was found amplified and rearranged [141]. In the BGC-823 cell line, a transforming gene was detected by DNA transfection into normal fibroblasts and identified as an activated Ha-*ras* oncogene bearing a point mutation in codon 12 [142].

Human gastric cancers: DNA analysis

Oncogene amplification is probably not as important a mechanism contributing to gastric cancers as it appears to be for breast cancers, small-cell lung cancers, or childhood neuroblastomas. Nakasato et al. [143] found c-*myc* amplification in 2 of 11 gastric carcinoma specimens that were transplanted into nude mice, but not in 19 other primaries that were not transplanted. Lymph-node metastases and several established cell lines were also negative for c-*myc* amplification. It is possible that the gastric cancer specimens were heterogeneous and contained only a few clones bearing amplified c-*myc* oncogenes, and these clones possessed a selective growth advantage in the nude mice tumorigenesis assay. Supporting this hypothesis, Shibuya et al. [144] detected c-*myc* amplification in 3 of 16 human gastric adenocarcinomas grown in nude mice, while Nomura et al. [86] found c-*myc* and c-*erb*B-1 amplifications in only 1 of 43 gastric carcinoma primaries. Other oncogenes found amplified in gastric cancer case reports include Ki-*ras* [145], *AKT*1 [146], and *yes*-1 [147].

There are no reports of large clinical studies examining activation of *ras* by point mutations in human gastric cancers, but isolated cases have shown mutated N-*ras* [148,149] and Ki-*ras* [145] sequences. Transforming genes with DNA sequences not homologous to other known oncogenes have been detected in some human gastric carcinoma samples. Sugimura and colleagues cloned and identified the *raf* [150] and *hst* oncogenes [151] from different tumor specimens; Koda et al. [152] confirmed that the *hst* transforming gene occurs in some gastric cancer specimens, but this observation needs to be verified in a larger study.

Human gastric cancers: RNA analysis

Reports on oncogene transcript levels in gastric cancers are limited to measurements of c-*myc* mRNA levels. Unlike one study [153] which found evidence of c-*myc* overexpression in only 1 of 14 gastric cancer primaries (with no Ha-*ras* Ki-*ras*, c-*mos*, c-*abl*, or c-*myb* overexpression), Tsuboi et al. [140] measured 2-fold to 3-fold above normal c-*myc* mRNA levels in over 50% of gastric cancers analyzed. The level of c-*myc* overexpression, however, did not correlate with clinical stage or metastatic potential of the primary tumors.

Human gastric cancers: Protein analysis

Czerniak et al. [154] assessed whether expression of p21^{ras} could be used as a tumor marker in gastric carcinoma cytology specimens. Of 20 gastric carcinoma samples analyzed, all stained positively with the RAP-5 anti-p21^{ras} monoclonal antibody, while only 1 of 13 benign gastric epithelial samples (from gastric ulcer patients) stained weakly positive. There was no correlation between staining intensity and tumor type, grade, or clinical stage. A similar study by Tahara et al. [155], on the other hand, demonstrated positive p21^{ras} staining in 3 of 27 (11%) early-stage and 63 and 144 (44%) advanced-stage gastric cancers, and this staining pattern correlated with depth of tumor invasion, likelihood of metastases, and overall patient prognosis. Further studies are needed to resolve the discrepancy between these two reports before any conclusion can be drawn regarding the clinical significance of *ras* protein expression in gastric cancer.

Yasui et al. [156] found that gastric cancer EGF receptor levels were significantly elevated as compared to normal gastric tissue levels, and this appeared to correlate with clinical stage since only 3.8% of early-stage and 34.4% of advanced-stage carcinomas showed immunoreactivity with the EGF receptor antibody. In comparison, antibody analysis of p62^{c-myc} protein demonstrated that premalignant tissue has the highest levels of this oncogene product, benign tissue has the lowest levels, and invasive cancer samples have intermediate levels, as measured by staining intensity [157]. These investigators suggested that c-*myc* may be involved in early malignant transformation, and once transformation has occurred, nuclear levels of c-*myc* protein fall and are possibly not necessary to sustain the malignant phenotype.

In summary, while protein analysis of oncogene expression in gastric cancer appears to show greater promise for clinical correlation than does DNA or RNA analysis, the independent prognostic value of these correlations has yet to be established for any particular oncogene in this malignancy.

Colorectal cancer

Experimental models

Yander et al. [158] induced mouse colonic tumors by treatment with dimethylhydrazine and used this tumor model to investigate oncogene amplification and overexpression. A 30-fold to 40-fold level of c-*myc* amplification associated with 10-fold c-*myc* overexpression was observed in these tumors without any detectable changes in structure or expression of other oncogenes including c-*mos*, c-*erb*B-1 or c-*ras*. Several human colon carcinoma cell lines have been studied and found to contain activated oncogenes. The SW-480 cell line was established from an adenocarcinoma of the large bowel and found to contain amplified and mutated Ki-*ras* sequences [115,159]; two other established cell lines were found to contain activating Ki-*ras* mutations [160]; and various colon cancer cell lines have been found to overexpress c-*myc* [123]. A neuroendocrine colon cancer line, COLO320, was also shown to possess an amplified and overexpressed c-*myc* oncogene along with cytogenetic evidence for homogeneously staining chromosome regions and double minutes bearing amplified c-*myc* DNA copies [161].

Human colorectal cancers: DNA analysis

Meltzer et al. [162] found both c-*myc* and c-*erb*B-2 gene amplifications in approximately 10% of colon cancers; Alexander et al. [163] reported over 20% incidence of c-*myc* DNA amplification without associated gene rearrangements. But others have found that amplifications of c-*myc* in colorectal cancers is uncommon, occurring in only 1 of 14 [66] or in 0 of 72 [164] primary colon cancer specimens. When it occurs, there does not appear to be any correlation between c-*myc* amplification and clinical prognosis [162]. Other oncogenes, such as N-*ras*, Ki-*ras*, c-*fos*, or N-*myc*, have not been found to be amplified in this tumor type.

While *ras* amplifications are not found in colon cancers, mutational activation of *ras*, especially Ki-*ras*, occurs in colon cancer specimens with an incidence of 40%–50% [38,39]. Furthermore, these oncogene abnormalities can be demonstrated in premalignant colonic adenomas, suggesting that Ki-*ras* mutations are involved in the early stages of colon cancer development. Forrester et al. [39] also found an interesting correlation between clinical stage and the intracodon localization of the transforming Ki-*ras* point mutation, with 4 of 8 early-stage tumors having codon 12, position 1 mutations while 16 of 18 late-stage tumors having codon 12, position 2 mutations. It is conceivable that a position 2 mutation could convey a more aggressive tumor phenotype; however, analysis of a greater number of tumors bearing Ki-*ras* mutations would be necessary to substantiate this hypothesis.

Unlike the findings in breast and lung cancer, there is no Ha-*ras* allelic loss in the tumor cells or presence of rare Ha-*ras* alleles in the germ line DNA of colon cancer patients [81]. However, certain Ha-*ras* allelic combinations may be observed more frequently in healthy donors than in colon cancer patients, and it has been suggested that this genetic population might be associated with greater resistance to the development of colon cancer. Other non-random gene defects, potentially linked to oncogenes or tumor-suppressing anti-oncogenes, have been found in human colon cancers. Soloman et al. [43] have demonstrated the loss of gene sequences localized to chromosome 5q in at least 20% of colon carcinoma primaries and in 5 of 10 colon cancer cell lines tested. It is of significance that the gene for familial polyposis coli, an autosomal dominant disease characterized by numerous adenomatous polyps occurring in the colon and rectum and predisposing to colon cancer, is also localized to this same 5q chromosome locus. Thus, it is possible that the chromosome 5q gene defect is directly involved in the etiology of colon carcinoma, perhaps representing the loss of an anti-oncogene [44]. Of the other non-random chromosomal abnormalities found in the colon cancers, some are close to known oncogene loci, and these may also become important factors in the development or progression of colon cancer [44].

Human colorectal cancers: RNA analysis

Since c-*myc* gene expression could simply reflect the number of proliferating cells in a primary tumor specimen, Calabretta et al. [166] correlated the expression of two G_1-phase-specific genes, the S-phase-specific H3 histone, and c-*myc* mRNA levels in a variety of colon cancer samples. These investigators showed that in some cases, increased c-*myc* mRNA levels simply reflect increased tumor growth fraction rather than uniform overexpression of this oncogene by every tumor cell. Controlling for this dependent variable, they were able to confirm the earlier reports of elevated c-*myc* expression in 50%–85% of primary colon cancers [64,140,164,167]. Unfortunately, the level of c-*myc* mRNA does not appear to correlate with clinical tumor behavior, and there are contradictory results relating c-*myc* levels with tumor grade and differentiation. Tsuboi et al. [140] and Augenlicht et al. [168] found no correlation, while Sikora et al. [64] and Rothberg et al. [168] found correlations between c-*myc* levels, degree of tumor differentation, and colonic localization of the tumors. Studies measuring c-*ras* mRNA are more concordant; three show a correlation between oncogene expression and tumor grade [168,169,170]. Monnat et al. [66] measured expression of four oncogenes (Ha-*ras*, Ki-*ras*, c-*fos*, and c-*myc*) in 14 colon cancer specimens and found overexpression of at least one oncogene in more than 50% of the samples. Clearly, larger and better controlled studies are required to compare expression of different oncogenes in colon cancer specimens in order to determine whether or not oncogene mRNA levels have any clinical value in patient prognosis or treatment.

Human colorectal cancers: Protein analysis

There are several reports on $p62^{c-myc}$ expression in colon cancer. Jones et al. [171] analyzed 100 samples and found significantly higher $p62^{c-myc}$ levels than that occurring in normal colon tissue controls. In normal tissues, however, the levels were higher in terminally differentiated cells as compared to proliferating basal crypt cells, and this contradicts the usual finding that c-*myc* expression is increased in proliferating cells. Although all cancer specimens stained positively, there was no correlation with tumor grade, DNA ploidy, clinical stage or patient prognosis, similar to the c-*myc* RNA studies described earlier [140,166,168]. Two other studies found that almost all colon carcinomas

(80%–100%) stained for $p62^{c-myc}$, and that staining intensity appeared to correlate with tumor grade [64,172].

Overexpression of $p21^{ras}$ in colon carcinoma is also well established [65,71, 74,103,154]. Gallick et al. [71] found $p21^{ras}$ to be overexpressed in about 50% of tumor samples; however, four other studies reported incidences of overexpression exceeding 90% [65,74,103,154]. As with $p62^{c-myc}$, however, the clinical significance of $p21^{ras}$ overexpression in colon cancers remains controversial. Thor et al. [65] found that overexpression of $p21^{ras}$ correlated with the degree of local tumor invasion. On the other hand, Czerniak et al. [154] could not detect any correlation with tumor behavior, and Gallick et al. [71] actually reported an inverse correlation, with less invasive tumors (Duke's stage B–C) showing greater expression than the more invasive tumors (Duke's stage D). Some investigators have indicated that $p21^{ras}$ expression varies considerably in both primary and metastatic tumors of individual patients [71,74], perhaps explaining some of these discrepant reports.

Yasui et al. [156] measured expression of the EGF receptor protein in normal and malignant colonic tissues. In contrast to their results in gastric cancer, they found no difference in EGF receptor levels occurring in benign or malignant colon tissue samples. In summary, the $p62^{c-myc}$ and $p21^{ras}$ data are most provocative, but there remains a great need for additional studies to clarify the importance of overexpression of these oncogene products in patients with colorectal cancers.

Pancreatic cancer

Cancer of the pancreas is another malignancy where very little has been reported with respect to oncogenes. Chester et al. [173] treated 70 female Syrian hamsters with either N-nitroso-bis(2-oxypropyl)amine or with this carcinogen in addition to the growth factor, EGF. EGF increased the incidence of pancreatic cancers from 44% to 75%, and these investigators speculated that an oncogene homologous to the EGF receptor (c-*erb*B-1) might be involved in the induction of tumors in this model. To date, no such homologous oncogene has been identified in this animal tumor model or in human samples of pancreatic cancer.

There are several established pancreatic carcinoma cell lines in which activated Ki-*ras* oncogenes have been found [148,174,175]. Of interest, studies analyzing fresh human tumor samples indicate that these same Ki-*ras* mutations also occur in vivo [85,176,177], which is in keeping with the activating *ras* mutations described in other human gastrointestinal tract tumors [38,39].

Liver cancer

Most of the studies on oncogene involvement in liver cancer have employed chemically induced rodent tumor models and have documented increased c-*myc* and Ha-*ras* RNA expression, DNA rearrangements, or mutational activation involving c-*raf*, c-*myc*, Ha-*ras*, or Ki-*ras* [178–183]. In these experimental models, the overexpression of oncogenes may have been due to either malignant cells or to proliferating and regenerating normal liver cells [183]. Wiseman et al. [182], however, documented that the various *ras* point mutations were specific for each of the different chemical carcinogens used to induce the murine hepatomas. It may be significant that similar *ras* mutations have also been found in strains of mice that have high rates of spontaneous hepatoma development [184,185].

The data on human hepatomas are scant and inconsistent. Although Huber et al. [186] reported increased c-*myc* expression in an aggressive hepatoma cell line, Su et al. [187] found no such elevation of c-*myc* mRNA in human hepatoma samples. An altogether new oncogene isolated by Ochiya et al. [188] from one human hepatocellular carcinoma specimen was named *lca*, for liver cancer; *lca* was mapped to chromosome 2 and has no sequence homology to other known oncogenes, but was subsequently found to be activated in another hepatoma sample. At present there is no information on the clinical importance of *lca*, or on the activation of any other oncogenes found involved in liver cancer.

Female reproductive tract cancers

Cancer of the vulva

One report described marked (>100-fold) overexpression of the EGF receptor (c-*erb*B-1) in a vulvar carcinoma cell line, A431 [189]; another report found a somewhat lesser degree of EGF receptor overexpression in three vulvar carcinoma specimens [188]. There is no additional information reported on oncogene abnormalities in vulvar cancers.

Cancer of the uterus

Two human choriocarcinoma cell lines have been shown to contain elevated levels of the human c-*fms* product, also known as colony stimulating factor-1 receptor [190]. However, with regard to the more common malignancies of the uterine body, endometrial carcinomas and uterine leiomyosarcomas, there are no reports relating to oncogenes.

Cancer of the ovary

Two embryonal carcinoma cell lines have been shown to contain amplified and overexpressing Ki-*ras* sequences [191]; and when several human embryonal carcinoma samples were analyzed, more than one-half possessed Ki-*ras* amplifications. Another type of ovarian carcinoma, serous cystadenocarcinomas, have also been found to contain activated Ki-*ras* sequences [192–

194], and some of these tumors also overexpressed p21^{ras} [190]. Overexpression of the EGF receptor was reported in an ovarian carcinoma cell line [195], but has not yet been shown in tumor specimens.

Cancer of the cervix

A variety of oncogenes, including the EGF receptor, have been found overexpressed in established cervical carcinoma cell lines [195] and in some primary cervical cancer specimens [196]. To date, the best studied oncogene in cervical cancer is c-*myc*. Covington et al. [197] found that 11 of 11 cervical tumors and 0 of 6 normal epithelial samples stained positive for p62^{c-myc}. In other studies, Riou et al. [69,198] correlated c-*myc* amplification and overexpression with clinical tumor stage and patient prognosis; patients with early stage tumors and elevated c-*myc* mRNA in their tumors had only one-half the probability of surviving 18 months as did patients without c-*myc* overexpression. An unusually high (>90%) incidence of c-*myc* abnormalities (gene amplification or rearrangement) was found in cervix cancer specimens by Ocadiz et al. [199], but this was not observed in a separate study by Hendy-Ibbs et al. [72].

In view of the well described association between papillomavirus infection and human cervix cancers, Durst et al. [17] discovered that this potentially oncogenic DNA virus frequently integrates adjacent to cellular oncogenes such as c-*src*, c-*raf*, c-*myc*, and Ki-*ras* in cervical carcinoma tissue samples. In tumors where the virus had integrated 5' to c-*myc*, elevated levels of c-*myc* mRNA were detected. Thus, these results suggest that human papillomavirus sequences might be involved in the in vivo development of cervix cancers by activating one or more cellular oncogenes.

Male reproductive tract cancers

Cancer of the testis

Sikora et al. [200] and Watson et al. [201] examined the significance of c-*myc* protein expression in a variety of testicular cancers. Increased p62^{c-myc} levels were found in seminomas, embryonal cell carcinoma and teratomas, and also in differentiating epithelial structures such as the yolk sac and embryoid bodies. Paradoxically, relapsing patients with lower levels of p62^{c-myc} had a worse prognosis than those with elevated oncoprotein levels, unlike the c-*myc* clinical correlations found in other malignancies such as gastric cancer [157].

Cancer of the prostate

Chromosome 10 deletions were found in 4 of 4 patients with cancer of the prostate [45], but the significance of this finding and its relevance to oncogenes or anti-oncogenes is uncertain.

Fleming et al. [202] reported elevation of c-*myc* mRNA in 7 of 7 tumor samples as compared to hypertrophied epithelium in otherwise normal prostate tissue. Older patients had lower levels than younger patients, and c-*myc* expression correlated with tumor growth fraction; from these results it appears that further study of c-*myc* expression as a prognostic indicator in prostate cancers is warranted. Viola et al. [68] compared prostate carcinomas with hypertrophied normal tissues and healthy control samples by looking at expression of $p21^{ras}$. None of the control or benign hypertrophy samples showed elevated $p21^{ras}$ levels; but 2 of 6 grade I, 4 of 6 grade II, and 17 of 17 grade IIII carcinomas had $p21^{ras}$ overexpression. This overexpression correlated with nuclear anaplasia and was inversely related to the degree of glandular differentiation in the tumors. Thus, $p21^{ras}$ levels may also represent a new clinical marker of prostate cancer aggressiveness, perhaps aiding in the determination of patient prognosis and therapy.

Renal cancer

There are case reports of Ha-*ras* activation [203] and overexpression of the EGF receptor (c-*erb*B-1) [195]; however, there are no large studies of oncogene involvement in primary cancers of the human kidney. The common finding of chromosome 3p deletions (or translocations) in renal cell carcinomas supports the hypothesis of an inactivated putative tumor-suppressor gene, or anti-oncogene [36,46,47]; this hypothesis is discussed in greater detail in chapter 13. Of interest, a translocation of c-*myc* was involved in the t(3;8) (p14.2;q24.13) chromosome abnormality described in one family with hereditary renal cell carcinoma [36]; and another reported 3p deletion was associated with relocation of the c-*raf*1 oncogene [46]. Thus, it is possible that oncogene deregulation might also be involved in the malignant transformation of renal epithelial cells in addition to the loss of a putative tumor suppressor gene.

Bladder cancer

Experimental models

It is interesting that the same codon 12 position 2 *ras* mutation (G to T transversion) produced by known bladder carcinogens is also among those detected in bladder cancer cell lines and human specimens [204]. Several groups have shown that the well studied EJ/T24 bladder cancer cell line possesses an activated Ha-*ras* oncogene bearing the same codon 12 glycine-to-valine mutation [205–208]. In addition, Ki-*ras* mutations [117,131] and Ha-*ras* amplifications [114] have been reported in human bladder cancer cell lines.

Human bladder cancers: DNA analysis

There is little evidence to indicate that oncogene amplification occurs with any significant frequency in bladder cancers. Apart from the cell line described above [114], there is only one other reported example of an amplified Ki-*ras* oncogene in a tumor sample [209]. Feinberg et al. [210] could not find evidence in human samples for the same Ha-*ras* codon 12 mutation as described in the EJ/T24 bladder cancer cell line; however, other investigators [203,209,211] have found evidence for this and other activated oncogenes in human bladder cancer DNA. Loss of Ha-*ras* alleles, not synonymous with *ras* activation, has been seen in a significant fraction of transitional cell carcinomas of the bladder; unlike breast cancer, however, the presence of rare Ha-*ras* alleles does not appear to correlate with an increased susceptibility to bladder cancer. Ishikawa et al. [212] found that Ha-*ras* allelic deletion occurred in 1 of 5 bladder cancers and 2 of 3 renal cancers. Fearon et al. [49] showed that parts of the short arm of chromosome 11 bearing the Ha-*ras* allele are deleted in more than 40% of transitional cell carcinomas of the urinary tract. While the significance of this finding and its potential relation to oncogene activation remains uncertain, the frequency of this 11p loss in bladder cancer approaches that observed in childhood Wilms' tumors and invokes speculation relating to a defect in a recessive tumor suppressor gene or anti-oncogene.

Human bladder cancers: RNA analysis

There are no available reports measuring oncogene RNA expression in human samples of bladder cancer.

Human bladder cancers: Protein analysis

Neal et al. [213] measured levels of the EGF receptor (c-*erb*B-1) in superficial and invasive transitional cell carcinomas of the bladder and were able to demonstrate a correlation between higher receptor levels and metastatic potential, tumor grade, and degree of local invasion. Viola et al. [214] looked at $p21^{ras}$ levels in tumors from 21 different patients. In all grade III tumors, and in no grade I tumors, there was overexpression of $p21^{ras}$. This oncoprotein was low in normal tissues and in benign hyperplastic tissues, but it was elevated in dysplastic specimens and in tissue bearing carcinoma in situ. Thus, measurements of EGF receptor and $p21^{ras}$ may both have some clinical utility in characterizing bladder carcinomas.

Head and neck cancers

A transforming oncogene was isolated from an untreated human laryngeal cancer after transfection of the tumor DNA into fibroblasts and implantation into nude mice [215]; however, further identification of this oncogene has not yet been reported. In radiation resistant human laryngeal cancers, there is a reported high incidence of c-*raf* activation [216], but the status of this oncogene or its protein product in untreated laryngeal cancers is unknown.

Expression of p21^{ras} has been examined in head and neck cancers. Azuma et al. [217] correlated p21^{ras} expression with tumor histology, staging, and patient outcome in 121 cases of squamous cell carcinomas occurring in the head and neck region. Nearly one-half of these tumors showed positive staining above background, which was not present in 44 cases of oral leukoplakia or 58 samples of normal oral mucosa. Elevated tumor expression of p21^{ras} correlated with poor patient prognosis, advanced tumor stage and undifferentiated grade, and previous tobacco abuse by the patient. Since similar findings were found in two smaller studies [218,219], the association of p21^{ras} overexpression with clinically aggressive tumor behavior indicates that this oncoprotein may be of prognostic utility. Contrary to results of EGF receptor correlations in squamous cell carcinomas arising in other anatomical sites, abnormalities involving this oncogene (c-*erb*B-1) do not seem to be of clinical significance in primary head and neck cancers [220].

Thyroid cancers

Lemoine et al. [221] found that codon 12, 13, or 61 mutations in any one of the three *ras* oncogenes (Ha,Ki,N) could be found in human thyroid cancer specimens, with 80% of follicular thyroid cancers involved as compared to only 20% of papillary thyroid cancers. Since follicular carcinomas are prone to hematogenous metastases and papillary carcinomas are prone to local lymphatic spread, these investigators proposed that mutational activation of *ras* contributed to the metastatic progression of thyroid cancers. Fusco et al. [222] isolated a new transforming oncogene that could be detected in 5 of 20 papillary thyroid carcinomas; this transforming oncogene was not detected in any other type of malignancy and appeared unrelated to other known oncogenes. The specificity of this new oncogene for papillary cancers and the specificity of *ras* involvement in follicular cancers supports the concept of tissue and tumor specific activation of oncogenes, as presented earlier in this chapter.

Overexpression of both c-*myc* and c-*fos* has been found in up to 60% of thyroid tumors [223], occurring in the absence of oncogene amplification or rearrangement. In benign thyroid neoplasms, c-*myc* was elevated in only 1 of 22 adenomas, but c-*fos* was elevated in 20 of 22 benign thyroid tumors. In the malignant tumors, elevated c-*myc* mRNA levels were associated with a worse patient prognosis, while c-*fos* levels had no correlation with patient outcome.

Brain cancers

Most reports on oncogene abnormalities in primary cancers of the brain or central nervous system have focused on oligodendrogliomas and glioblastomas. Lens et al. [224] analyzed ethylnitrosourea (ENU)-transformed rat glioma cells and found higher levels of c-*sis* oncogene transcripts when compared to levels found in normal or premalignant glial cells. Since the c-*sis* oncogene encodes the beta chain of platelet-derived growth factor (PDGF), and transformed glial cells synthesize functional PDGF receptor, the investigators suggested that development of these rat brain tumors was mediated by an autocrine-dependent growth factor mechanism. It remains unclear whether the c-*sis* oncogene, intact PDGF, or PDGF receptor is involved in the development of in vivo human gliomas.

There is an isolated report of a glioblastoma cell line that contains an activated c-*raf* oncogene [118]; and a human astrocytoma was found to possess both an amplified and rearranged N-*myc* oncogene [225]. Libermann et al. [226] measured amplification and overexpression of the EGF receptor in 4 of 10 glioblastoma specimens, but not in astrocytomas, oligodendrogliomas, meningiomas, neuroectodermal tumors, or cerebellar glioblastomas. Loss of gene sequences that map to chromosome 22q have also been shown in 17 of 40 (43%) meningioma samples [50], but the relationship of this abnormality to oncogenes or anti-oncogenes remains unknown at this point.

Multiple Endocrine Neoplasia

The syndromes of Multiple Endocrine Neoplasia (MEN types I,IIa,IIb) include the neoplastic involvement of parathyroid, pituitary, pancreas, thyroid, or adrenal glands, and these syndromes are usually inherited in an autosomal dominant pattern with incomplete penetrance. The cell types involved in these malignancies are postulated to have common embryologic and metabolic features, and are known as APUD (Amine Precursor Uptake and Decarboxylation) cells. Although nothing is known about oncogene involvement in the development of APUDomas, several genetic lesions commonly found in these MEN syndromes have been identified. A deletion on the short arm of chromosome 1 has been associated with one form of the MEN type II syndrome [51], yet other forms of this syndrome are linked to loci on chromosome 10 or 11 [52,53]. In all of these situations it is postulated that the malignancies develop as a result of the dysfunction or loss of putative recessive tumor anti-oncogenes, of the type discussed in chapter 13.

Skin cancers

Melanomas

Albino et al. [227] found that 4 of 30 different melanoma cell lines contained an activating mutation in a *ras* oncogene (1 Ha-*ras*, 3 N-*ras*). Similarly, Padua et al. [228,229] and Sekiya et al. [230,231] reported *ras* activation by point mutation and/or amplification occurring in four other human melanoma cell lines. Unfortunately, there are no analyses of melanoma tumor samples to assess the role of *ras* activation in the development of this most lethal form of human skin cancers. One study measured p21^{ras} overexpression in 3 of 5 melanoma specimens as compared to the lack of any staining intensity in normal skin or nevi controls [232]. The unusual occurrence of specific Ha-*ras* alleles does not appear to be associated with any enhanced susceptibility to develop melanoma [233,234].

Other skin cancers

Investigators studying the more common forms of skin cancer, squamous and basal cell carcinomas, have largely concerned themselves with the role of oncogenes in skin carcinogenesis. In experimental animal models addressing this question, there are many examples of cancer inducing agents producing activated oncogenes. In murine skin tumors induced by radiation, both Ki-*ras* point mutations and c-*myc* gene amplifications can be identified [235]. These results are also consistent with the Ki-*ras* mutations identified in mouse lymphomas induced by gamma irradiation [236]. Chemical agents, in contrast, have almost uniformly produced activated Ha-*ras* oncogenes by inducing point mutations [58,59,60,237]. It is postulated that at least two steps are necessary to complete the process of skin carcinogenesis. Most of the murine skin tumors arise from primary papillomas that contain the respective mutations, yet only a minority of the mutation containing papillomas actually evolve into skin cancers [58,59,60]. Furthermore, when the Ha-*ras* oncogene is linked to a strong heterologous promoter and this recombinant gene is transfected into rat keratinocytes, only papillomas are produced after engraftment of the transfected cells into the skin of nude mice [238]. Thus, Ha-*ras* activation must be an early step, one that is necessary but not sufficient to induce malignant transformation and conversion of papillomas to invasive skin cancers. One study suggested that the second event might be the mutation and/or amplification of the second Ha-*ras* allele, since the oncogene mutation was heterozygous in most papillomas and homozygous and/or amplified in some of the carcinomas [60]. Most of the results from these experimental models support the concept that oncogene cooperation, as discussed earlier in the chapter, is necessary to fully transform normal cells. To date, however, insufficient human cancers have been analyzed to enable extrapolation of the animal model data to the development of human squamous and basal cell skin cancers.

Bone and soft tissue cancers

Ewing's sarcoma

Analyses of Ewing's sarcoma specimens and established sarcoma cell lines indicate that a chromosomal translocation frequently occurs involving 22q12, often in association with the long arm of chromosome 11. Since c-*sis* is located at the chromosome 22q locus, the activation of this oncogene by chromosomal translocation has been suggested [32,33]. Bechet et al. [34] reported that overexpression or rearrangement of c-*sis* could not be found in human cell lines or primary sarcoma tumor samples. However, translocation of c-*sis* without gene rearrangment occurred from chromosome 22 to chromosome 11 in one established sarcoma cell line bearing this stable genetic abnormality [35]; thus, it is reasonable to consider that c-*sis* activation might be involved in Ewing's sarcoma by a process similar to the dysregulation of c-*myc* that occurs in Burkitt's lymphoma (chapter 10).

Osteogenic sarcoma

The only data involving oncogene abnormalities in this common and lethal form of adult bone cancer comes from analyses of tumor cell lines. One osteogenic sarcoma line, derived from a radiation induced mouse bone tumor, was found to contain an activated *ras* oncogene [239]. In the U-2 human osteosarcoma cells, c-*sis* was found to be amplified [240]. A new oncogene, *met*, was isolated from another chemically transformed sarcoma cell line [241]. In one report using tumor tissue from a single patient with osteogenic sarcoma, three different cell lines were established, and all showed c-*myc* gene amplification and overexpression [242]. Lastly, analysis of 14 different murine osteogenic sarcoma cell lines revealed that c-*abl*, c-*fos*, Ki-*ras*, and c-*myc* were each overexpressed in more than one cell line [243].

Other sarcomas

As with osteogenic sarcomas, data relating to oncogene involvement in other types of sarcomas are derived largely from experimental animal models and established tumor cell lines. Two human sarcoma cell lines, the rhabdomyosarcoma RD and the fibrosarcoma HT cells were found to contain activated N-*ras* oncogenes bearing point mutations [244,245]. Induction of a rat fibrosarcoma cell line by 1,8-dinitropyrene also activated a Ki-*ras* oncogene by point mutation [246]. Analysis of this fibrosarcoma cell line for 11 different oncogenes revealed that only the Ki-*ras* oncogene was activated in this tumor model.

Childhood cancers

Retinoblastomas

The importance of the retinoblastoma 13q chromosome deletion and the loss of the recessive RB tumor suppressor gene in the development of this malignancy has been mentioned earlier and is discussed in chapter 13. The hereditary form of this childhood tumor has also been the primary model for Knudson's two-hit carcinogenesis hypothesis [247]. Although there are no reports implicating dominant acting oncogenes in the development of either hereditary or sporadic forms of retinoblastoma, many genetic abnormalities other than del (13q) have been found in this malignancy [248], and the role of oncogenes in retinoblastomas has not been excluded.

Wilms' tumors

Along with retinoblastomas, Wilms' tumors also contain a putative tumor suppressor gene located at chromosome 11p13 which has been implicated in this malignancy [39] as well as two related syndromes, the Beckwith–Wiedemann syndrome (rhabdomyosarcoma, hepatoblastoma, and Wilms' tumor) and WAGR (Wilms' tumor, Aniridia, Genitourinary abnormalities, Retardation), each of which have a similar deletion affecting the short arm of chromosome 11 [39,249]. In one report [250], the loss of sequences on 11p13 were found isolated to maternal chromosomes in 5 of 5 tumors, suggesting that the original gene defect occurred in the paternal chromosome during spermatogenesis. According to this hypothesis, when the loss of the maternal allele occurred during childhood, the recessive and tumorgenic defect was unmasked [250].

There are two reports demonstrating N-*myc* mRNA overexpression in Wilms' tumor samples [251,252]; in both these reports an inverse correlation existed between the levels of N-*myc* and c-*myc* expression. Although the role of these related oncogenes in Wilms' tumor is not understood, Nisen et al. [252] has speculated that N-*myc* expression might be up-regulated in response to the allelic loss of a chromosome 11p13 gene.

Neuroblastomas

There are single case reports of N-*ras* gene amplification [253] and the finding of a new transforming oncogene, c-*neu* [254], in established neuroblastoma cell lines. In another study [255], a positive correlation was reported between p21^{ras} tumor expression and favorable prognosis in patients with neuroblastoma. With the exception of these few studies, however, the greatest interest in neuroblastomas has focused on N-*myc* amplification and its clinical correlations.

There is probably no other human malignancy where the association between oncogene activation and clinical tumor behavior is so well established as with N-*myc* amplification in neuroblastoma. In 1983, Schwab et al. [18] detected amplified N-*myc* copies in a single neuroblastoma cell line; subsequent studies by this same group [19,20] demonstrated that 14 of 18 neuroblastoma cell lines and 24 of 63 (38%) primary tumor samples carried this same amplification. No amplifications were found in 15 stage I–II tumors, but 24 of 48 (50%) stage III–IV tumors possessed N-*myc* amplifications. The amplifications were found to range from 20-fold to 100-fold excess gene copies, and the levels of the corresponding mRNA were approximately 80-fold higher than that measured in control tissues. The close association between undifferentiated tumor grade and N-*myc* amplification/overexpression has been verified by Amatruda et al. [256], who also showed that N-*myc* expression decreased in concert with both morphological differentiation and with inhibition of cellular proliferation in vitro when neuroblastoma cells were treated with the differentiating agent, retinoic acid.

The largest clinical analysis to date was reported by Seeger et al. [21], who confirmed the earlier results [18,19,20] and also showed that tumor-free survival correlated inversely with N-*myc* gene copy number. This prognostic correlation was invariant of tumor stage, suggesting that N-*myc* amplification plays an independent role in determining the clinical aggressiveness of neuroblastomas. The N-*myc* oncogene is located on chromosome 2, and another genetic abnormality, deletion of the short arm of chromosome 1, is also highly correlated with advanced stages of this disease [257]. These deletions are present in more than 90% of stage III–IV tumors, but never present in stage I–II tumors, and their relationship to N-*myc* activation in this disease remains unknown [258].

Recent results by Brodeur et al. [75] show that N-*myc* copy numbers are stable within given tumor masses, at different metastatic sites in individual patients, and at different time points during the course of disease. However, it is alarming that chemotherapy can apparently induce or accelerate the process of N-*myc* amplification, especially in poor-prognosis patients [259]. Thus, the determination of N-*myc* amplification has become almost a routine procedure in large centers treating neuroblastoma patients, and the decision to give more or less aggressive therapy is now dependent on the analysis of this oncogene abnormality. Because of the obvious pathogenetic role that N-*myc* amplification plays in neuroblastoma, similar oncogene abnormalities are being sought in other solid tumors in the hope that they too will contribute to our understanding and management of more common forms of adult malignancies.

Conclusions

Oncogenes activated by DNA amplification, gene rearrangement, mutation, or deletion have been identified in isolated cases of virtually every type of human malignancy. With few exceptions, however, there is insufficient evidence implicating individual oncogenes in the development or progression of specific types of solid tumors. Unfortunately, DNA, RNA, and protein studies on original tumor tissue looking for evidence of oncogene activation have been few in number and limited in scope. These studies have focused on only a few of the 40 or more known oncogenes, or have been technically restricted in their search for unknown and dominant acting transforming genes.

This review has summarized the reported findings about oncogenes involved in human solid tumors and gives attention to those tumor types in which the activation of specific oncogenes has apparent clinical significance. Some of the uncommon and familial childhood cancers possess localized chromosome abnormalities that appear to mark the loss or inactivation of recessive anti-oncogenes, or tumor suppressor genes, whose functional relationship to activated oncogenes remains unknown. There is some evidence to suggest that recessive gene defects such as those found in retinoblastomas may also occur in more common types of adult tumors including colon, breast, lung, bladder, and kidney cancers, as well as in meningiomas and the specific syndromes of Multiple Endocrine Neoplasia (MEN).

The best studied example of a clinically significant activation of a tumor-bearing oncogene is the amplification of N-*myc* found in the aggressive childhood malignancy, neuroblastoma. When identified by extraction of tumor DNA or by in situ cytologic analysis of individual tumor cells, the finding of N-*myc* amplification and overexpression not only implicates this oncogene in the process of tumor progression but also provides the clinician with a biological marker that is helpful in determining patient management and prognosis. Members of this same oncogene family (N-,c-,L-*myc*) have also been found amplified and overexpressed in a proportion of adult tumors, especially breast and cervix cancers and small cell lung cancers. For unknown reasons, some tumors (e.g., breast, prostate, and thyroid cancers) appear to produce excess oncogene RNA and protein products (e.g., c-*myc*, c-*erb*B-2, Ha-*ras*) in the absence of gene amplification, suggesting that the constitutive overexpression of some oncogenes may be more common than formerly suspected and may occur by deregulating mechanisms other than gene amplification. Oncogenes commonly activated by DNA amplification and found to be associated with specific tumor types are c-*erb*B-1 in non-small cell lung and gastric cancers, and the related tyrosine kinase receptor gene, c-*erb*B-2, in breast cancer.

Amplification of *ras* oncogenes, occasionally found in established tumor cell lines, is not commonly associated with any specific type of solid tumor. These transforming oncogenes (Ki-, Ha-, N-*ras*), however, are most sensitive to mutagenic activation involving codons 12, 13, and 61; and point mutations in *ras* have been found in 30%–50% of colorectal, pancreatic, thyroid, and non-small cell lung cancer specimens. While this evidence implicates mutational activation of *ras* in the development of some types of human tumors, studies using monoclonal antibodies to detect cellular expression of the $p21^{ras}$ oncoprotein product indicate that *ras* overexpression is clinically associated with aggressive forms of other types of human malignancies, including head and neck cancers, non-small cell lung cancers, prostate and bladder cancers.

In summary, there is evidence to suggest that oncogene activation occurs during the development and progression of most human malignancies. However, additional basic and clinical research is necessary to define the mechanistic relationships of known and yet-to-be-discovered oncogenes in the entire pathogenic process of malignant diseases, and to determine how we can best utilize this knowledge to improve our clinical detection and management of patients with life-threatening tumors.

Acknowledgements

This work was supported in part by grants CA-44768 and CA-36773 from the National Cancer Institute and CH-235 from the American Cancer Society. C.F.R. was supported by a grant from the German Volkswagon Stiftung, Hanover, West Germany. We thank Constance Benz for assisting in the preparation of this manuscript.

References

1. Varmus H: The molecular genetics of cellular oncogenes. Annu Rev Genet 18:553–612, 1984.
2. Land H, Parada L, Weinberg R: Cellular oncogenes and multistep carcinogenesis. Science 222:771–778, 1983.
3. Weinberg R: Ras oncogenes and their molecular mechanisms of carcinogenesis. Blood 64:1143–1145, 1984.
4. Varmus H: Viruses, genes, and cancer. Cancer 55: 2324–2328, 1985.
5. Bishop M: Viruses, genes, and cancer. Cancer 55: 2329–2333, 1985.
6. Weinberg R: The action of oncogenes in the cytoplasm and nucleus. Science 230:770–776, 1985.
7. Bishop M: Viral oncogenes. Cell 42:23–28, 1985.
8. Marshall C: Human oncogenes. In: Weiss R (ed): RNA Tumor Viruses, 2nd edition. New York, Cold Spring Harbor Laboratories, 1985, pp 487–558.
9. Sager R: Genetic suppression of tumor formation: a new frontier in cancer research. Cancer Res 46:1573–1580, 1986.
10. Barbacid M: Mutagens, oncogenes and cancer. Trends in Genetics 2:188–192, 1986.
11. Rosen N, Israel M: Genetic abnormalities as biological tumor markers. Sem Oncol 14: 213–231, 1987.
12. Marshall C: Oncogenes and growth control. Cell 49:723–725, 1987.
13. Moore J, Evan G: Immunoassays for oncoproteins. Nature 327:733–734, 1987.
14. Barbacid M: Ras genes. Annu Rev Biochem 56:779–827, 1987.
15. Bishop M: The molecular genetics of cancer. Science 235:305–311, 1987.
16. Friend S, Dryja T, Weinberg R: Oncogenes and tumor suppressing genes. N Engl J Med 318:618–622, 1988.
17. Durst M, Croce C, Gissmann L, Schwarz E, Huebner K: Papillomavirus sequences integrate near cellular oncogenes in some cervical carcinomas. Proc Natl Acad Sci USA 84:1070–1074, 1987.
18. Schwab M, Alitalo K, et al: Amplified DNA with limited homology to *myc* cellular oncogene is shared by human neuroblastoma cell lines and a neuroblastoma tumor. Nature 305:245–248, 1983.
19. Schwab M, Ellison J, et al.: Enhanced expression of the human gene N-*myc* consequent to amplification of DNA may contribute to malignant progression of neuroblastoma. Proc Natl Acad Sci USA 81:4940–4944, 1984.

20. Brodeur G, Seeger R, Schwab M, Varmus H, Bishop M: Amplification of N-*myc* in untreated human neuroblastomas correlates with advanced disease stage. Science 224: 1121–1124, 1984.
21. Seeger R, Brodeur G et al.: Association of multiple copies of the N-*myc* oncogene with rapid progression of neuroblastomas. N Engl J Med 313:1111–1116, 1985.
22. King R, Kraus M, Aaronson S: Amplification of a novel v-*erb*B-related gene in a human mammary carcinoma. Science 229:974–978, 1985.
23. Slamon D, Clark G, et al.: Human breast cancer: correlation of relapse and survival with amplification of the HER-2/*neu* oncogene. Science 235:177–182, 1987.
24. vd Vijver M, vd Bersselaar R, et al.: Amplification of the neu (c-*erb*B-2) oncogene in human mammary tumors is relatively frequent and is often accompanied by amplification of the linked c-*erb*A oncogene. Mol Cel Biol 7:2019–2023, 1987.
25. Little C, Nau M, Carney D, Gazdar A, Minna J: Amplification and expression of the c-*myc* oncogene in human lung cancer cell lines. Nature 306:194–196, 1983.
26. Saksela K, Bergh J, Lehto V–P, Nilsson K, Alitalo K: Amplification of the c-*myc* oncogene in a subpopulation of human small cell lung cancer. Cancer Res 45:1823–1927, 1985.
27. Nau M, Brooks B, et al.: A new *myc*-related gene amplified and expressed in human small cell lung cancer. Nature 318:69–73, 1985.
28. Nau M, Brooks B, et al.: Human small-cell lung cancers show amplification and expression of N-*myc* gene. Proc Natl Acad Sci USA 83:1092–1096, 1986.
29. Wong A, Ruppert J, et al.: Gene amplification of c-*myc* and N-*myc* in small cell carcinoma of the lung. Science 233:461–464, 1986.
30. Heighway J, Hasleton P: c-Ki-*ras* amplification in human lung cancer. Br J Cancer 53: 285–287, 1986.
31. Slamon D, deKernion J, Verma I, Cline M: Expression of cellular oncogenes in human malignancies. Science 224:256–262, 1984.
32. Aurias A, Rimbaut C, et al.: Chromosomal translocations in Ewings sarcoma. N Engl J Med 309(8):496–497, 1983.
33. Turc-Carel C, Phiklip I, et al.: Chromosomal translocations in Ewings sarcoma. N Engl J Med 309:497–498, 1983.
34. Bechet J–M, Bornkamp G, Lenoir G: The c-*sis* oncogene is not activated in Ewings sarcoma. N Engl J Med 310:393, 1984.
35. Kessel AGV, Turc-Carel C, et al. Translocation of oncogene c-*sis* from chromosome 22 to chromosome 11 in a Ewing sarcoma-derived cell line. Mol Cell Biol 5:427–429, 1985.
36. Drabkin H, Bradley C, Patterson D: Translocation of c-*myc* in the hereditary renal cell carcinoma associated with a t(3;8) (p14.2;q24;13) chromosomal translocation. Proc Natl Acad Sci USA 82:6980–6984, 1985.
37. Rodenhuis S, vd Wetering M, et al.: Mutational activation of the K-*ras* oncogene: a possible pathogenetic factor in adenocarcinoma of the lung. N Engl J Med 317:929–935, 1987.
38. Bos J, Fearon E, et al.: Prevalence of ras gene mutations in human colorectal cancers. Nature 327:293–297, 1987.
39. Forrester K, Almoguera C, et al.: Detection of high incidence of K-*ras* oncogenes during human colon tumorigenesis. Nature 327:298–303, 1987.
40. Cavenee W, Hansen M, et al.: Genetic origin of mutations predisposing to retinoblastoma. Science 228:501–503, 1985.
41. Koufos A, Hansen M, et al.: Loss of heterozygosity in three embryonal tumors suggests a common pathogenetic mechanism. Nature 316:330–334, 1985.
42. Brodeur G, Green A, et al.: Cytogenetic features of human neuroblastoma and cell lines. Cancer Res 41:4678–4686, 1981.
43. Solomon E, Voss R, et al.: Chromosome 5 loss in human colorectal carcinomas. Nature 328:616–619, 1987.
44. Okamoto M, Sasaki M, et al.: Loss of constitutional heterozygosity in colon carcinoma from patients with familial polyposis coli. Nature 331:273–277, 1988.
45. Atkin N, Baker M: Chromosome 10 deletion in carinoma of the prostate. N Engl J Med

312:315, 1985.
46. Teyssier J, Henry I, et al.: Recurrent deletion of the short arm of chromosome 3 in human renal cell carcinomas: shift of the c-*raf* locus. J Natl Cancer Inst 77:1187–1191, 1986.
47. Zbar B, Brauch H, Talmadge C, Linehan M: Loss of alleles on the short arm of chromosome 3 in renal cell carcinoma Nature 327:721–724, 1987.
48. Kok K, Osinga J, et al.: Deletion of a DNA sequence at the chromosomal region 3p21 in all major types of lung cancer. Nature 330:578–581, 1987.
49. Fearon E, Feinberg A, Hamilton S, Vogelstein B: Loss of genes on the short arm of chromosome 11 in bladder cancer. Nature 318:377–380, 1985.
50. Seizinger B, dl Monte S, et al.: Molecular genetic approach to human meningioma: loss of genes on chromosome 22. Proc Nat Acad Sci USA 84:5419–5423, 1987.
51. Mathew C, Smith B, et al.: Deletion of genes on chromosome 1 in endocrine neoplasia. Nature 328:524–526, 1987.
52. Mathew C, Chin K, et al.: Linked genetic marker for multiple endocrine neoplasia type 2A on Chromosome 10. Nature 328:527–528, 1987.
53. Simpson N, Kidd K et al.: Assignment of multiple endocrine neoplasia type 2A to chromosome 10 by linkage. Nature 328:528–530, 1987.
54. Larsson C, Skogseid B, et al.: Multiple endocrine neoplasia type 1 gene maps to chromosome 11 and is lost in insulinoma. Nature 332:85–87, 1988.
55. Miyaki M, Sato C, et al.: Amplification and enhanced expression of cellular oncogene c-Ki-*ras*-2 in human epidermoid carcinoma of the lung. Jpn J Cancer Res 76:260–263, 1985.
56. Taya Y, Hosogai K, et al.: A novel combination of K-*ras* and *myc* amplification accompanied by point mutational activation of Ki-*ras* in a human lung cancer. EMBO J 3: 2943–2946, 1986.
57. Yokota J, T-Yokota Y, et al.: Alternations of *myc*, *myb* and H*ras* proto-oncogenes in cancers are frequent and show clinical correlation. Science 231:261–265, 1986.
58. Balmain A, Pragnell I: Mouse skin carcinoma induced in vivo by chemical carcinogens have a transforming Harvey-*ras* oncogene. Nature 303:72–74, 1983.
59. Balmain A, Ramsden M, Bowden G, Smith J: Activation of the mouse cellular Harvey-*ras* gene in chemically induced benign shin papillomas. Nature 307:658–660, 1984.
60. Quintanilla M, Brown K, Ramsden M, Balmain A: Carcinogen-specific mutation and amplification of Ha-*ras* during mouse skin carcinogenesis. Nature 322:78–80, 1986.
61. Reynolds S, Stowers et al.: Detection and identification of activated oncogenes in spontaneously occurring benign and malignant hepatocellular tumors of the B6C3F1 mouse. Proc Natl Acad Sci USA 83:33–37, 1986.
62. Sukumar S, Notario V, Martin-Zanca D, Barbacid M: Induction of mammary carcinomas in rats by nitroso-methylurea involves malignant activation of H-*ras*-1 locus by single point mutations. Nature 306:658–661, 1983.
63. Johnson B, Ihde D, et al. *Myc* family oncogene amplification in tumor cell lines established from small cell lung cancer patients and its relationship to clinical status and course. J Clin Invest 79:1629–1634, 1987.
64. Sikora K, Chan S, et al.: C-*myc* oncogene expression in colorectal cancer. Cancer 59: 1289–1295, 1987.
65. Thor A, Hand H, et al.: Monoclonal antibodies define differential ras gene expression in malignant and benign colonic disease. Nature 311:562–565, 1984.
66. Monnat M, Tardy S, et al.: Prognostic implications of the cellular genes *myc*, *fos*, Ha-*ras*, and Ki-*ras* in colon carcinoma. Int J Cancer 40:293–299, 1987.
67. Lundy J, Grimson R, et al.: Elevated ras oncogene expression correlates with lymph node metastases in breast cancer patients. J Clin Oncol 4:1321–1325, 1986.
68. Viola M, Formowitz F, et al.: Expression of ras oncogene p21 in prostate cancer. N Engl J Med 314:133–137, 1986.
69. Riou G, Le M, et al.: C-*myc* protooncogene expression and prognosis in early carcinoma of the uterine cervix. Lancet 1:761–763, 1987.
70. Ohuchi N, Thor A, et al.: Expression of the 21,000 molecular weight was protein in a

spectrum of benign and malignant human mammary tissues. Cancer Res 46:2511–2519, 1986.
71. Gallick G, Kurzrock R, et al.: Expression of p21^{ras} in fresh primary and metastatic human colorectal tumors. Proc Nat Acad Sci USA 82:1795–1799, 1985.
72. Hendy-Ibbs P, Cox H, Evan G, Watson J: Flow cytometric quantitation of DNA and c-*myc* oncoprotein in archival biopsies of uterine cervix neoplasia. Br J Cancer 55:275–282, 1987.
73. Liu E, Dollbaum C, et al.: Molecular lesions involved in the progression of a human breast cancer. Oncogene, 3:323–327, 1988.
74. Hand P, Vilasi V, et al.: Quantitation of Harvey *ras* p21 enhanced expression in human breast and colon carcinomas. J Natl Cancer Inst 79:59–65, 1987.
75. Brodeur G, Hayes A, et al.: Consistent copy number in simultaneous or consecutive neuroblastoma samples from sixty individual patients. Cancer Res 47:4248–4253, 1987.
76. Rochlitz C, Scott G, et al.: Incidence of activating *ras* oncogene mutations associated with primary and metastatic human breast cancer. Cancer Res 49:357–360, 1989.
77. Capon D, Chen E, Levinson A: Complete nucleotide sequence of the T24 human bladder carcinoma oncogene and its normal homologue. Nature 302:33–37, 1983.
78. Krontiris T, DiMartino N, Colb M, Parkinson D: Unique allelic restriction fragments of the human Ha-*ras* locus in leukocyte and tumor DNAs of cancer patients. Nature 313:369–374, 1985.
79. Lidereau R, Escot C, et al.: High frequency of rare alleles of the human c-Ha-*ras*-1 proto-oncogene in breast cancer patients. J Natl Cancer Inst 77:697–701, 1986.
80. Heighway Y, Thatcher N, Cerny N, Haselton P: Genetic predisposition to lung cancer. Br J Cancer 53:453–458, 1986.
81. Ceccherini-Nelli L, DeRe V, et al.: Ha-*ras*-1 restriction fragment length polymorphism and susceptibility to colon adenocarcinoma. Br J Cancer 56:1–5, 1987.
82. Land H, Parada L, Weinberg R: Tumorigenic conversion of primary embryo fibroblasts requires at least two cooperating oncogenes. Nature 304:596–602, 1983.
83. Dalla-Favera R, Wong-Staal F, Gallo R: Oncogene amplification in promyelocytic leukemia cell line HL 60 and primary leukemic cells of the same patient. Nature 299:61–63, 1982.
84. Taya Y, Hosagai K, et al.: A novel combination of Ki-*ras* and *myc* amplification accompanied by point mutational activation of Ki-*ras* in a human lung cancer. EMBO J 3:2943–2946, 1984.
85. Yamada H, Sakamoto H, et al.: Amplifications of both c-Ki-*ras* with a point mutation and c-*myc* in a primary pancreatic cancer and its metastatic tumors in lymph nodes. Jpn J Cancer Res 77:370–375, 1986.
86. Nomura N, Yamamoto T, et al.: DNA amplification of the c-*myc* and c-*erb*B-1 genes in a human stomach cancer. Gann 77:1188–1192, 1986.
87. Cardiff R, Young L: Mouse mammary tumor biology: a new synthesis. In: Essex M, Todaro G, Zurhausen H (eds): Viruses in Naturally Occurring Cancers. Cold Spring Harbor, NY, 1980, pp 1105–1114.
88. Dickson C, Smith R, Brookes S, Peters G: Tumorigenesis by mouse mammary tumor virus: proviral activation of a cellular gene in the common integration region int-2. Cell 37:529–536, 1984.
89. Lidereau R, Callahan R, et al.: Amplification of the int-2 gene in primary human breast tumors. Oncogene Res 2:285–291, 1988.
90. Zarbel H, Sukumar S, et al.: Direct mutagenesis of Ha-*ras*-1 oncogenes by N-nitroso-N-methylurea during initiation of mammary carcinogenesis in rats. Nature 315:382–385, 1985.
91. Kraus M, Yuasa Y, Aaronson S: A position 12-activated H-*ras* oncogene in all HS578T mammary carcinosarcoma cells but not normal mammary cells of the same patient. Proc Natl Acad Sci USA 81:5384–5388, 1984.
92. Kozma S, Bogaard M, et al.: The human c-Kirsten *ras* gene is activated by a novel mutation in coden 13 in the breast carcinoma cell line MDA-MB231. Nucleic Acid Res 15:5963–5971, 1987.
93. Prosperi M–T, Even J, et al.: Two adjacent mutations at position 12 activate the K-*ras*2

oncogene of a human mammary tumor cell line. Oncogene Res 1:121–128, 1987.
94. Birchmeier C, Birnbaum D, et al.: Characterization of an activated human *ras* gene. Mol Cell Biol 6:3109–3116, 1986.
95. Kozbor D, Croce C: Amplification of the *c-myc* oncogene in one of five human breast carcinoma cell lines. Cancer Res 44:438–441, 1984.
96. Lebeau J, Goubin G: Amplification of the epidermal growth factor receptor gene in the BT20 breast carcinoma cell line. Int J Cancer 40:189–191, 1987.
97. Kasid A, Lippman M, et al.: Transfection of v-*ras*H DNA into MCF-7 human breast cancer cells bypasses dependence on estrogen for tumorigenicity. Science 228:725–728, 1985.
98. Muller W, Sinn E, Puttengale P, Wallace R, Leder P: Single-step induction of mammary adenocarcinoma in transgenic mice bearing the activated *c-neu* oncogene. Cell 54:105–115, 1988.
99. Escot C, Theillet C, et al.: Genetic alternations of the *c-myc* protooncogene (*myc*) in human primary breast carcinomas. PNAS 83:4834–4838, 1986.
100. Cline M, Battifora H, Yokota Y: Proto-oncogene abnormalities in human breast cancer: Correlations with anatomic features and clinical course of the disease. J Clin Oncol 5:999–1006, 1987.
101. Theillet C, Lidereau R, et al.: Loss of c-H-*ras*-1 allele and aggressive human primary breast carcinomas. Cancer Res 46:4776–4781, 1986.
102. Lidereau R, Mathieu-Mahul D, et al.: Presence of an allelic EcoRI restriction fragment of the *c-mos* locus in leukocyte and tumor cell DNAs of breast cancer patients. Proc Natl Acad Sci USA 82:7068–7070, 1985.
103. Hand H, Thor A, et al.: Monoclonal antibodies of predefined specificity detect activated *ras* gene expression in human mammary and colon carcinomas. Proc Natl Acad Sci USA 81:5227–5231, 1984.
104. Spandidos D, Agnantis N: Human malignant tumors of the breast as compared to their respective normal tissue have elevated expression of the Harvey *ras* oncogene. Anticancer Res 4:269–272, 1984.
105. Agnantis N, Parissi P, Anagnostakis D, Spandidos D: Comparative study of Harvey-*ras* oncogene expression with conventional clinicopathologic parameters of breast cancer. Oncology 43:36–39, 1986.
106. Mariani-Costantini R, Escot C, et al.: In situ *c-myc* expression and genomic status of the *c-myc* locus in infiltrating ductal carcinomas of the breast. Cancer Res 48:199–205, 1988.
107. Fitzpatrick S, Brightwell J, et al.: Epidermal growth factor binding by breast tumor biopsies and relationship to estrogen receptor and progestin receptor levels. Cancer Res 44:3448, 1984.
108. Perez R, Pascual M, Macias M, Lage A: Epidermal growth factor receptors in human breast cancer. Breast Cancer Res Treat 4:189, 1984.
109. Kraus M, Popescu N, Amsbaugh S, King R: Overexpression of the EGF receptor-related proto-oncogene *erb*B-2 in human mammary tumor cell lines by different molecular mechanisms. EMBO J 6:605–610, 1987.
110. Whittaker S, Walker R, Varley J: Differential expression of cellular oncogenes in benign and malignant human breast tissue. Int J Cancer 38:651–655, 1986.
111. Cattoretti G, Rilke F, et al.: P53 expression in breast cancer. Int J Cancer 41:178–183, 1988.
112. Hand H, Vilasi V, et al.: Quantitation of Harvey *ras* p21 enhanced expression in human breast and colon carcinomas. J Natl Cancer Inst 79:59–65, 1987.
113. DeBertoli M, Abou-Issa H, Haley B, Sang Cho-Chung Y: Amplified expression of p21 *ras* protein in hormone-dependent mammary carcinomas of humans and rodents. Biochem Biophys Res Comm 127:699–706, 1985.
114. Der C, Krontiris T, Cooper G: Transforming genes of human bladder and lung carcinoma cell lines are homologous to the *ras* genes of Harvey and Kirsten sarcoma viruses. Proc Natl Acad Sci USA 79:3637–3640, 1982.
115. Capon D, Seeburg P, et al.: Activation of Ki-*ras* 2 in human colon and lung carcinomas by

two different point mutations. Nature 304:507–513, 1983.
116. Shimizu K, Birnbaum D, et al.: Structure of the Ki-*ras* gene of the human lung carcinoma cell line Calu-1. Nature 304:497–500, 1983.
117. Valenzuela D, Groffen J: Four human cell lines with novel mutations in position 12 of c-K-*ras* oncogene. Nucleic Acid Res 14:843–852, 1986.
118. Fukui M, Yamamoto T, et al.: Detection of raf-related and two other transforming DNA sequences in human tumors maintained in nude mice. Proc Natl Acad Sci USA 82: 5954–5958, 1985.
119. Kagimoto M, Miyoski J, et al.: Isolation and characterization of an activation c-H-*ras*-1 gene from a squamous-cell lung carcinoma cell line. Int J Cancer 35:809–812, 1985.
120. Yuasa Y, Srivastava S, et al.: Acquisition of transforming properties by alternative point mutations within c-*bas*/has human proto-oncogene. Nature 303:755–770, 1983.
121. Little C, Nau M, et al.: Amplification and expression of the c-*myc* oncogene in human lung cancer cell lines. Nature 306:194–196, 1983.
122. Seifter E, Sausville E, Battey J: Comparison of amplified and unamplified c-*myc* gene structure and expression in human small cell lung carcinoma cell lines. Cancer Res 46: 2050–2055, 1986.
123. Yoshimoto K, Hirohashi S, Sekiya T: Increased expression of the c-*myc* gene without gene amplification in human lung cancer and colon cancer cell lines. Jpn J Cancer Res 77: 540–545, 1986.
124. Yoshimoto K, Shiraishi M, Seliya T: Rearrangement of the c-*myc* gene in two giant cell carcinomas of the lung. Jpn J Cancer Res 77:731–745, 1986.
125. Sherwin S, Minna J, et al.: Expression of epidermal and nerve growth factor receptors and soft agar growth production by human lung cancer cells. Cancer Res 41:3538–3542, 1981.
126. Hunts J, Ueda M, et al.: Hyperproduction and gene amplification of the EGF receptor in squamous cell carcinomas. Gann 76:663–666, 1985.
127. Hendler F, Ozanne B: Human squamous cell lung cancers express increased epidermal growth factor receptors. J Clin Invest 74:647–651, 1984.
128. Gamou S, Hunts J, et al.: Molecular evidence for the lack of epidermal growth factor receptor gene expression in small cell lung carcinoma cells. Cancer Res 47:2668–2673, 1987.
129. Johnson B, Ihde D, et al.: *Myc* family oncogene amplification in tumor cell lines established from small cell lung cancer patients and its relationship to clinical status and course. J Clin Invest 79:1629–1634, 1987.
130. Clin M, Battifora H: Abnormalities of protooncogenes in non-small cell lung cancer. Cancer 60:2669–2674, 1987.
131. Santos E, Martin-Zanca D, et al.: Malignant activation of a K-*ras* oncogene in lung carcinoma but not in normal tissue of the same patient. Science 223:661–664, 1984.
132. Nakano H, Yamamoto F, et al.: Isolation of transforming sequences of two human lung carcinomas: Structural and functional analysis of the activated c-K-*ras* oncogenes. Proc Natl Acad Sci USA 81:71–75, 1984.
133. Griffin C, Baylin S: Expression of the c-*myc* oncogene in human small cell lung carcinoma. Cancer Res 45:272–275, 1985.
134. Nau M, Carney D, et al.: Amplification, expression and rearrangement of c-*myc* and N-*myc* oncogenes in human lung cancer. Current Topics Microbiol Immunol 113:172–177, 1984.
135. Funa K, Steinholtz L, Nou E, Bergh J: Increased expression of N-*myc* in human small cell lung cancer biopsies predicts lack of response to chemotherapy and poor prognosis. Am J Clin Pathol 88:216–220, 1987.
136. Sainsbury J, Farndon J, Sherbet G, Harris A: Epidermal growth factor receptors and estrogen receptors in human breast cancer. Lancet 1:364, 1984.
137. Veale D, Ashcroft T, Harris A: Epidermal growth factor receptors in non-small cell lung cancer. Br J Cancer 55:513–516, 1987.
138. Kurzrock R, Gallick G, Guttermann J: Differential expression of p21*ras* gene products among histological subtypes of fresh primary human lung tumors. Cancer Res 46:1530–1534, 1986.

139. Hollstein M, Montesano R, Yamasaki H: Presence of an EcoRI RFLP of the c-*mos* locus in normal and tumor tissue of esophageal cancer patients. Nucleic Acids Res 14:8695, 1986.
140. Tsuboi K, Hirayoshi K, et al.: (1987). Expression of the c-*myc* gene in human gastrointestinal malignancies. Biochem Biophys Res Comm 146:699–704.
141. Fukushige S-I, Matsubara K–I et al.: Localization of a novel v-*erb*B-related gene, c-*erb*B-2, on human chromosome 17 and its amplification in a gastric cancer cell line. Mol Cell Biol 6:955–958, 1986.
142. Deng G, Lu Y, et al.: Activated c-Ha-*ras* oncogene with guanine to thymine transversion at the twelfth codon in a human stomach cancer cell line. Cancer Res 47:3195–3198, 1987.
143. Nakasato F, Sakamoto H, et al.: Amplification of the c-*myc* oncogene in human stomach cancers. Gann 75:737–742, 1984.
144. Shibuya M, Yokota J, Ueyama Y: Amplification and expression of a cellular oncogene (c-*myc*) in human gastric adenocarcinoma cells. Mol Cell Biol 5:414–418, 1985.
145. Bos J, Verlaan-de Vries M, et al.: A human gastric carcinoma contains a single mutated and amplified normal allele of the Ki-*ras* oncogene. Nucleic Acids Res 14:1209–1217, 1986.
146. Staal S: Molecular cloning of the *act* oncogene and its human homologues AKT1 and AKT2: Amplification of AKT1 in a primary human gastric adenocarcinoma. Proc Natl Acad Sci USA 84:5034–5037, 1987.
147. Seki T, Fujii G, et al.: Amplification of c-*yes*-1 proto-oncogene in a primary human gastric cancer. Gann 76:907–910, 1985.
148. O'Hara B, Oskarsson M, Tainsky M, Blair D: Mechanism of activation of human *ras* genes cloned from a gastric adenocarcinoma and a pancreatic carcinoma cell line. Cancer Res 46:4695–4700, 1986.
149. Nishida J, Kobayashi Y, Hirai H, Takaku F: A point mutation at codon 13 of the N-*ras* oncogene in a human stomach cancer. Biochem Biophys Res Comm 146:247–252, 1987.
150. Shimizu K, Nakatsu Y, et al.: Molecular cloning of an activated human oncogene, homologous to v-*raf*, from primary stomach cancer. Proc Natl Acad Sci USA 82:5641–5645, 1985.
151. Sakamoto H, Mori M, et al.: Transforming gene from human stomach cancers and a noncancerous portion of stomach mucosa. Proc Natl Acad Sci USA 83:3997–4001, 1986.
152. Koda T, Sasaki A, Matsushima S, Kakinuma M: A transforming gene, *hst*, found in NIH 3T3 cells transformed with DNA from three stomach cancers and a colon cancer. Gann 78:325–328, 1987.
153. Koda T, Matsushima S, et al.: C-*myc* gene amplification in primary stomach cancer. Gann 76:551–554, 1985.
154. Czerniak B, Herz F, Koss L, Schlom J: *Ras* oncogene p21 as a tumor marker in the cytodiagnosis of gastric and colonic carcinomas. Cancer 60:2432–2436, 1987.
155. Tahara E, Yasui W, et al.: Ha-*ras* oncogene product in human gastric carcinoma: Correlation with invasiveness, metastasis or prognosis. Gann 77:517–522, 1986.
156. Yasui W, Sumiyoshi H, et al.: Expression of epidermal growth factor receptor in human gastric and colonic carcinomas. Cancer Res 48:137–141, 1988.
157. Allum W, Newbold K, et al.: Evaluation of p62c-^{myc} in benign and malignant gastric epithelia. Br J Cancer 56:785–786, 1987.
158. Yander G, Halsey H, Kenna M, Augenlicht L: Amplification and elevated expression of c-*myc* in a chemically induced mouse colon tumor. Cancer Res 45:4433–4438, 1985.
159. McCoy M, Toole J, et al.: Characterization of a human colon/lung carcinoma oncogene. Nature 302:79–81, 1983.
160. Der C, Cooper G: Altered gene products are associated with activation of cellular rask genes in human lung and colon carcinomas. Cell 302:201–208, 1983.
161. Alitalo K, Schwab M, et al.: Homogeneously staining chromosomal regions contain amplification copies of an abundantly expressed cellular oncogene (c-*myc*) in malignant neuroendocrine cells from a human colon carcinoma. Proc Natl Acad Sci USA 80:1707–1711, 1983.
162. Meltzer S, Ahnen D, et al.: Protooncogene abnormalities in colon cancers and adenomatous polyps. Gastroenterology 92:1174–1180, 1987.
163. Alexander R, Buxbaum J, Raicht R: Oncogene alternations in primary human colon

tumors. Gastroenterology 91:1503–1510, 1986.
164. Erisman M, Rothberg P, et al.: Deregulation of c-*myc* gene expression in human colon carcinomas is not accompanied by amplification or rearrangement of the gene. Mol Cell Biol 5:1969–1976, 1985.
165. Bodmer W, Bailey C, et al.: Localization of the gene for familial adenomatous polyposis on chromosome 5. Nature 328:614–616, 1987.
166. Calabretta B, Kaczmarek L, et al.: Expression of c-*myc* and other cell cycle-dependent genes in human colon neoplasia. Cancer Res 45:6000–6004, 1985.
167. Rothberg P, Spandorfer M, et al.: Evidence that c-*myc* expression defines two genetically distinct forms of colorectal adenocarcinoma. Br J Cancer 52:629–632, 1985.
168. Augenlicht L, Augeron C, Yander G, Laboisse C: Overexpression of *ras* in mucus-secreting colon carcinoma cells of low tumorigenicity. Cancer Res 47:3763–3765, 1987.
169. Garin Chesa P, Rettig W, et al.: Expression of p21^{ras} in normal and malignant tissues: lack of association with proliferation and malignancy. Proc Natl Acad Sci USA 84:3234–3238, 1987.
170. Spandidos D, Kerr I: Elevated expression of the human *ras* oncogene family in premalignant and malignant tumors of the colorectum. Br J Cancer 49:681–688, 1984.
171. Jones D, Ghosh A, Moore M, Schofield P: A critical appraisal of the immunohistochemical detection of the c-*myc* oncogene product in colorectal cancer. Br J Cancer 56:779–783, 1987.
172. Stewart J, Evan G, Watson J, Sikora K: Detection of the c-*myc* oncogene product in colonic polyps and carcinomas. Br J Cancer 53:1–6, 1986.
173. Chester J, Gaissert H, Ross J, Malt R: Pancreatic cancer in the syrian hamster induced by N-nitrosobis(2-oxopropyl)amine: co-carcinogenic effect of epidermal growth factor. Cancer Res 46:2954–2957, 1986.
174. Yamada H, Yoshida T, et al.: Establishment of a human pancreatic adenocarcinoma cell line (PSN-1) with amplifications of both c-*myc* and activated c-Ki-*ras* by a point mutation. Biochem Biophys Res Comm 140:167–173, 1986.
175. Cooper D, Blair D, et al.: Characterization of human transforming genes from chemically transformed, teratocarcinoma, and pancreatic carcinoma cell lines. Cancer Res 44:1–10, 1984.
176. Hirai H, Okabe T, et al.: Activation of the c-Ki-*ras* oncogene in a human pancreas carcinoma. Biochem Biophys Res Comm 127:168–174, 1985.
177. Prassolov V, Sakamoto H, et al.: Activation of c-Ki-*ras* gene in human pancreatic cancer. Gann 76:792–795, 1985.
178. Dragani T, Manenti G, et al.: Expression of retroviral sequences and oncogenes in murine hepatocellular tumors. Cancer Res 46:1915–1919, 1986.
179. Ishikawa F, Takaku F, et al.: Activated c-*raf* gene in a rat hepatocellular carcinoma induced by 2-amino-3methylimidazo(4,5-f)quinoline. Biochem Biophys Res Comm 132:186–192, 1985.
180. Ishikawa F, Takaku F, et al.: Activation of rat c-*raf* during transfection of hepatocellular carcinoma DNA. Proc Natl Acad Sci USA 83:3209–3212, 1986.
181. Tashiro F, Morimur S, et al.: Expression of the c-Ha-*ras* and c-*myc* genes in aflatoxin B1-induced hepatocellular carcinomas. Biochem Biophys Res Comm 138:858–862, 1986.
182. Wiseman R, Strowers S, et al.: Activating mutations of the c-Ha-*ras* protooncogene in chemically induced hepatomas of the male B6C3F1 mouse. Proc Natl Acad Sci USA 83:5825–5829, 1986.
183. Hsieh L, Hsiao W-L, et al.: Expression of retroviral sequences and oncogenes in rat liver tumors induced by diethylnitrosamine. Cancer Res 47:3421–3424, 1987.
184. Fox T, Wantanabe P: Detection of a cellular oncogene in spontaneous liver tumors of B6C3F1 mice. Science 228:596–597, 1984.
185. Reynolds S, Stowers S, et al.: Detection and identification of activated oncogenes in spontaneously occurring benign and malignant hepatocellular tumors of the B6C3F1 mouse. Proc Natl Acad Sci USA 83:33–37, 1986.

186. Huber B, Dearfield K, et al.: Tumorigenicity and transcriptional modulation of c-*myc* and N-*ras* oncogenes in a human hepatoma cell line. Cancer Res 45:4322–4329, 1985.
187. Su T, Lin L, et al.: Expression of c-*myc* gene in human hepatoma. Biochem Biophys Res Comm 132:264–268, 1985.
188. Ochiya T, Fujiyama A, et al.: Molecular cloning of an oncogene from a human hepatocellular carcinoma. Proc Natl Acad Sci USA 83:4993–4997, 1986.
189. Merlino G, Xu Y: Amplification and enhanced expression of the epidermal growth factor receptor gene in human carcinoma cells. Science 224:417–419, 1984.
190. Rettenmeier C, Sacca R, et al.: Expression of the human c-*fms* proto-oncogene product (colony-stimulating factor-1 receptor) on peripheral blood mononuclear cells and choriocarcinoma cell lines. J Clin Invest 77:1740–1746, 1986.
191. Wang L-C, Vass W, Gao C, Chang K: Amplification and enhanced expression of the c-Ki-*ras*2 protooncogene in human embryonal carcinomas. Cancer Res 47:4192–4198, 1987.
192. Feig L, Bast R, Knapp R, Cooper G: Somatic activation of *ras*-k gene in a human ovarian carcinoma. Science 223:698–701, 1984.
193. Filmus J, Buick R: Stability of c-Ki-*ras* amplification during progression in a patient with adenocarcinoma of the ovary. Cancer Res 45:4468–4472, 1985.
194. Filmus J, Trent J, Pullano R, Buick R: A cell line from ovarian carcinoma with amplification of the K-*ras* gene. Cancer Res 46:5179–5182, 1986.
195. Xu Y-H, Richert N, et al.: Characterization of epidermal growth factor receptor gene expression in malignant and normal human cell lines. Proc Natl Acad Sci USA 81:7308–7312, 1984.
196. Gullick W, Marsden J, et al.: Expression of epidermal growth factor receptors on human cervical, ovarian and vulval carcinomas. Cancer Res 46:285–292, 1986.
197. Covington M, Sikora K, et al.: C-*myc* expression in cervical cancer. Lancet 1:1260–1261, 1987.
198. Riou G, Barrois M, et al.: Presence de genomes de papillomvirus et amplification des oncogenes c-*myc* et Ha-*ras* dans des cancers envahissants du col de l'uterus. CR Aca Sci 299:575–580, 1984.
199. Ocadiz R, Sauceda R, et al.: High correlation between molecular alterations of the c-*myc* oncogene and carcinoma of the uterine cervix. Cancer Res 47:4173–4177, 1987.
200. Sikora K, Evan G, Stewart J, Watson J: Detection of the c-*myc* oncogene product in testicular cancer. Br J Cancer 52:171–176, 1985.
201. Watson J, Stewart J, et al.: The clinical significance of flow cytometric c-*myc* oncoprotein quantitation in testicular cancer. Br J Cancer 53:331–337, 1986.
202. Fleming W, Hamel A, et al.: Expression of the c-*myc* protooncogene in human prostatic carcinoma and benign prostatic hyperplasia. Cancer Res 46:1535–1538, 1986.
203. Fujita J, Yoshida O, et al.: Ha-*ras* oncogenes are activated by somatic alterations in human urinary tract tumors. Nature 309:464–466, 1984.
204. Swenson E, Kadlubar F: In: Felkner IC (ed): Microbial Testers Probing for Carcinogenesis. New York, M. Dekker, 1981, pp 3–33.
205. Parada L, Tabin C, Shih C, Weinberg R: Human EJ bladder carcinoma oncogene is homologue of Harvey sarcoma virus *ras* gene. Nature 297:474–478, 1982.
206. Santos E, Tronick S, et al.: T24 human bladder carcinoma oncogene is an activated form of the normal human homologue of BALB- and Harvey-MSV transforming genes. Nature 298:343–347, 1982.
207. Tabin C, Bradley S, et al.: Mechanism of activation of a human oncogene. Nature 300:143–149, 1982.
208. Reddy P, Reynolds R, Santos E, Barbacid M: A point mutation is responsible for the acquisition of transforming properties by the T24 human bladder carcinoma oncogene. Nature 300:149–152, 1982.
209. Fujita J, Srivastava S, et al.: Frequency of molecular alterations affecting *ras* protooncogenes in human urinary tract tumors. Proc Natl Acad Sci USA 82:3849–3853, 1985.

210. Feinberg A, Vogelstein B, et al.: Mutations affecting the 12th amino acid of c-*ras* oncogene product occur infrequently in bladder cancer. Science 220:1175–1179, 1983.
211. Malone P, Visvanathan K, et al.: Oncogenes and bladder cancer. Br J Urology 57:664–667, 1985.
212. Ishikawa J, Maeda S, et al.: Lack of correlation between rare Ha-*ras* alleles and urothelial cancer in Japan. Int J Cancer 40:474–478, 1987.
213. Neal D, Marsh C, Bennett M: Epidermal growth factor receptors in human bladder cancers: Comparison of invasive and superficial tumors. Lancet 1:366, 1985.
214. Viola M, Fromowitz F, et al.: *Ras* oncogene p21 expression is increased in premalignant lesions and high grade bladder carcinoma. J Exp Med 161:1213–1218, 1985.
215. Friedman W, Rosenblum B, et al.: Oncogenes in laryngeal cancer: Serial passage of transformed cellular DNA. Otolaryngol Head Neck Surg 93:346–350, 1985.
216. Kasid U, Pfeifer A, et al.: The *raf* oncogene is associated with a radiation-resistant human laryngeal cancer. Science 237:1039–1041, 1987.
217. Azuma M, Furumoto N, et al.: The relation of *ras* oncogene product p21 expression to clinicopathological status criteria and clinical outcome in squamous cell head and neck cancer. Cancer J 1:375–380, 1987.
218. Field J, Lamothe A, Spandidos D: Clinical relevance of oncogene expression in head and neck tumors. Anticancer Res 5:221–224, 1985.
219. Field J, Spandidos D: Expression of oncogenes in human tumors with special reference to the head and neck region. J Oral Path 16:97–107, 1986.
220. Eisbruch A, Blick M, et al.: Analysis of the epidermal growth factor receptor gene in fresh human head and neck tumors. Cancer Res 47:3603–3605, 1987.
221. Lemoine N, Mayall E, et al.: Activated *ras* oncogenes in human thyroid cancers. Cancer Res 48:4459–4463, 1988.
222. Fusco A, Grieco M, et al.: A new oncogene in human thyroid papillary carcinomas and their lymph node metastases. Nature 328:170–172, 1987.
223. Terrier P, Sheng Z-M, et al.: Structure and expression of c-*myc* and c-*fos* proto-oncogenes in thyroid carcinomas. Br J Cancer 57:43–47, 1987.
224. Lens P, Altena B, Nusse R: Expression of c-*sis* and platelet-derived growth factor in in vitro-transformed glioma cells from rat brain tissue transplacentally treated with ethylnitrosourea. Mol Cell Biol 6:3537–3540, 1986.
225. Garson J, McIntyre P, Kemshead J: N-*myc* amplification in malignant astrocytomas. Lancet 2:718–719, 1985.
226. Libermann T, Nusbaum H, et al.: Amplification, enhanced expression and possible rearrangement of EGF receptor gene in primary human brain tumors of glial origin. Nature 313:144–147, 1985.
227. Albino A, LeStrange R, et al.: Transforming *ras* genes from human melanoma: a manifestation of tumor heterogeneity? Nature 308:69–72, 1984.
228. Padua R, Barrass N, Currie G: A novel transforming gene in a human malignant melanoma cell line. Nature 311:671–673, 1984.
229. Padua R, Barrass N, Currie G: Activation of N-*ras* in a human melanoma cell line. Mol Cell Biol 5:582–585, 1985.
230. Sekiya T, Fushimi M, et al.: Molecular cloning and the total nucleotide sequence of the human c-Ha-*ras*-1 gene activated in a melanoma from a Japanese patient, Proc Natl Acad Sci USA 81:4771–4775, 1984.
231. Sekiya T, Fushimi M, Hirohashi S, Tokunaga A: Amplification of activated c-Ha-*ras*-1 in human melanoma. Gann 76:555–558, 1985.
232. Kuzumaki N, Oda A, et al.: Establishment of four mouse hybridoma cell lines producing monoclonal antibodies reactive with *ras* oncogene product p21. J Natl Cancer Inst 77:1273–1279, 1986.
233. Gerhard D, Dracopoli N, et al.: Evidence against Ha-*ras* involvement in sporadic and familial melanoma. Nature 325:73–75, 1987.
234. Sutherland C, Shaw H, et al.: Harvey-*ras* oncogene restriction fragment alleles in familial

melanoma kindreds. Br J Cancer 54:787–790, 1986.
235. Sawey M, Hood A, Burns F, Garte S: Activation of c-*myc* and c-K-*ras* oncogenes in primary rat tumors induced by ionizing radiation. Mol Cell Biol 7:932–935, 1987.
236. Guerrero I, Villasante A, Corces V, Pellicer A: Activation of a c-Ki-*ras* oncogene by somatic mutation in mouse lymphomas induced by gamma radiation. Science 225:1159–1162, 1984.
237. Bizub D, Wood A, Skalka A: Mutagenesis of the Ha-*ras* oncogene in mouse skin tumors induced by polycyclic aromatic hydrocarbons. Proc Natl Acad Sci USA 83:6048–6052, 1986.
238. Roop D, Lowy D, et al.: An activated Harvey *ras* oncogene produces benign tumors in mouse epidermal tissue. Nature 323:822–824, 1986.
239. Merregaert J, Michiels L, et al.: Oncogene involvement in radiation- and virus-induced mouse osteosarcomas. Leukemia Res 10:915–921, 1986.
240. Graves D, Owen A, et al.: Detection of c-*sis* transcripts and synthesis of PDGF-like proteins by human osteosarcoma cells. Science 226:972–974, 1984.
241. Cooper C, Park M, et al.: Molecular cloning of a new transforming gene from a chemically transformed human cell line. Nature 311:29–33, 1984.
242. Bogenmann E, Moghadam H, DeClerck Y, Mock A: C-*myc* amplification and expression in newly established human osteosarcoma cell lines. Cancer Res 47:3808–3814, 1987.
243. Schon A, Michiels L, et al.: Expression of protooncogenes in murine osteosarcomas. Int J Cancer 38:67–74, 1986.
244. Marshall C, Hall A, Weiss R: A transforming gene present in human sarcoma cell lines. Nature 299:171–173, 1982.
245. Hall A, Marshall C, Spurr N, Weiss R: Identification of transforming gene in two human sarcoma cell lines as a new member of the *ras* gene family located on chromosome 1. Nature 303:396–400, 1983.
246. Tahira T, Hayashi K, et al.: Structure of the c-Ki-*ras* gene in a rat fibrosarcoma induced by 1,8-dinitropyrene. Mol Cell Biol 6:1349–1351, 1986.
247. Knudson A: Mutation and cancer: Statistical study of retinoblastoma. Proc Natl Acad Sci USA 68:820–823, 1971.
248. Potluri V, Helson L, et al.: Chromosomal abnormalities in human retinoblastoma. Cancer 58:663–671, 1986.
249. Porteous E, Bichmore W, et al.: HRAS1-selected chromosome transfer generates markers that co-localize aniridia and genitourinary dysplasia-associated translocation breakpoints and the Wilms' tumor gene within band 11p13. Proc Natl Acad Sci USA 84:5355–5359, 1987.
250. Schroeder W, Chao L-Y, et al.: Nonrandom loss of maternal chromosome 11 alleles in Wilms' tumors. Am J Hum Genet 40:413–420, 1987.
251. Weissman B, Saxon P. et al.: Introduction of a normal human chromosome 11 into a Wilms' tumor cell line controls its tumorigenic expression. Science 236:175–180, 1987.
252. Nisen A, Zimmermann K, et al.: Enhanced expression of the N-*myc* gene in Wilms' tumors. Cancer Res 46:6217–6222, 1986.
253. Shimizu K, Goldfarb M, Perucho M, Wigler M: Isolation and preliminary characterization of the transforming gene of a human neuroblastoma cell line. Proc Natl Acad Sci USA 80:383–387, 1983.
254. Schechter A, Hung M, et al.: The neu gene: an *erb*B-homologous gene distinct from and unlinked to the gene encoding the EGF receptor. Science 229:976–978, 1985.
255. Tanaka T, Slamon D, et al.: Expression of Ha-*ras* oncogene products in human neuroblastomas and the significant correlation with a patient's prognosis. Cancer Res 48:1030–1034, 1988.
256. Amatruda Y, Sidell N, Ranyard J, Koeffler P: Retinoic acid treatment of human neuroblastoma cells is associated with decreased N-*myc* expression. Biochem Biophys Res Comm 126:1189–1195, 1985.
257. Christiansen H, Franke F, et al.: Evolution of tumor cytogenetic aberrations and N-*myc*

oncogene amplification in a case of disseminated neuroblastoma. Cancer Genet Cytogenet 26:235–244, 1987.
258. Christiansen H, Franke F, et al.: (1987). Evolution of tumor cytogenetic aberrations and N-*myc* oncogene amplification in a case of disseminated neuroblastoma. Cancer Genet Cytogenet 26:235–244, 1987.
259. Tsuda T, Obara M, et al.: Analysis of N-*myc* amplification in relation to disease stage and histologic types in human neuroblastomas. Cancer 60:820–826, 1987.

10. Oncogenes in human leukemias and lymphomas

Edison Liu

Hematologic malignancies frequently have been used as model systems in the study of tumorigenesis owing to the ease of isolating neoplastic tissue and to the wealth of knowledge on the growth and differentiation of the hematopoietic elements. Since malignancy is due to perturbations in the control of growth and differentiation, it is hoped that identifying genetic elements that induce leukemias may also point to those factors that control normal cellular functions. Proto-oncogenes represent such genetic elements; they have important functions in normal cells but can be perturbed to become cancer-causing genes. In this chapter, we will examine the role of various oncogenes in the development of human hematopoietic malignancies, and will discuss them in two groups (see table 1): oncogenes with strong associations with the human leukemias and lymphomas (seen frequently and consistently in the human disease), and those with limited associations with the human disorders (seen occasionally in humans, but whose role in leukemogenesis and lymphomagenesis is suggested by association or is certain in animal systems). Tumor-suppressor genes also appear to be important participants in the malignant progression of these hematopoietic neoplasms. However, since specific leukemia/lymphoma-suppressor genes have not been isolated, they will be discussed in a separate section.

Though there is frequently clinical overlap between the lymphomas and the leukemias, we will center on oncogene aberrations mainly in human leukemias both in the preleukemic and leukemic states. Only the major genetic abnormalities associated with the lymphomas (*bcl*-1, *bcl*-2, and *myc*) will be discussed. Our review will confirm the observation that human hematopoietic malignancies can be initiated by different genetic events and can require multiple lesions for progression to the full malignant phenotype.

Oncogenes strongly associated with human leukemias

Four proto-oncogenes are frequently involved in human hematopoietic malignancies: *abl, ras, myc*, and *bcl*-2.

Benz, C. and Liu, E., (eds.), Oncogenes. © *1989 Kluwer Academic Publishers.*
ISBN 0-7923-0237-0. All rights reserved.

Table 1. Oncogenes associated with human leukemias and lymphomas

Strong associations
bcr-abl	ras
myc	bcl-2

Occasional associations
ets	myb	EGF receptor
fos	fes	p53
CSF-1/c-*fms*	bcl-1	

Chromosomal location of putative tumor suppressor genes
5q23–32	7q22–32
20q11	9p22

c-abl *and chronic myelogenous leukemia*

Chronic myelogenous leukemia (CML) is a disease characterized by a surfeit of granulocytes and their precursors whose morphology is otherwise normal. This expansion of the granulocyte pool leads to enlargement of the liver and spleen, and a lowering of other normal marrow elements including platelets and erythrocytes. All patients with CML will ultimately progress to a blast phase that is morphologically indistinguishable from acute leukemia. In 85%–90% of these cases, a reciprocal translocation involving the long arms chromosomes 9 and 22, t(9q;22q) (q34;q11), is present in the affected blood cells [1–3]. This translocation moves the c-*abl* gene from its normal position on chromosome 9q to chromosome 22q [4,5] resulting in the karyotypic abnormality known as the Philadelphia chromosome (Ph^1). Molecular cloning of the chromosomal breakpoints in CML revealed no consistent breakpoint on chromosome 9 [6]. However, breakpoints on chromosome 22 were located within a 5.8-kb segment in the first 17 Ph^1-positive or Ph^1-indeterminant CML patients studied [7]. In subsequent series, 214 of 215 Ph^1-positive cases exhibited breakpoints within the same segment on chromosome 22q, referred to as the breakpoint cluster region (*bcr*) [8,9]. Moreover, approximately half of the patients who are cytogenetically Ph^1-negative exhibit the *bcr-abl* rearrangement by Southern hybridization analysis [9–16]; thus, the molecular analysis is more sensitive than the karyotype analysis. The translocation of the c-*abl* locus to a segment of DNA representing 0.0002% of the human genome in 95% of CML patients is compelling evidence that this proto-oncogene in its new chromosomal location is a critical factor in the genesis of CML.

Further investigation revealed that this translocation produced a novel 8.5-kb *abl* transcript compared to the 6- and 7-kb mRNAs of the normal c-*abl* gene [17–19]. This abnormal transcript was due to a fusion of the 5' portion of a gene on chromosome 22q called *bcr* (also called *phl*) with the 3' end of a truncated c-*abl* translocated from chromsome 9q. Mapping of the exons involved in the translocation showed that the first 8 to 12 identifiable 5' *bcr* exons were spliced onto the second exon of the c-*abl* gene [20–22,58]. This fusion transcript thus predicts for a *bcr-abl* fusion protein and, indeed, while the normal c-*abl* protein has a molecular weight of 150 kDa the *bcr-abl* fusion product detected in CML cell lines and patient samples is 210 kDa [23].

Functional changes in the bcr-abl *fusion protein.* Structural changes in a protein product often are associated with functional alterations, and the search for functional differences between the normal and the fusion *abl* proteins yielded an interesting observation: the normal cellular protein, $p150^{abl}$, had no detectable tyrosine kinase activity in vivo; the $p210^{bcr-abl}$ hybrid protein, however, exhibited significant tyrosine kinase activity. Tyrosine kinases are enzymes that catalyze the transfer of phosphate from ATP to tyrosine residues in certain proteins. Such phosphorylation appears to alter the enzyme activity of target proteins. These findings were astonishing in that they recapitulated the genetic events leading to the generation of the v-*abl* oncogene in the Abelson-murine leukemia virus described years previously [24]. Here, conversion of the c-*abl* proto-oncogene to the v-*abl* oncogene during transduction is associated with truncation in the 5' and 3' portions of the *abl* gene, thus generating a fusion 5'-*gag-abl*-3'protein (*gag* is a retroviral-specific gene) [24,25]. Like *bcr-abl*, v-*abl* has significant in vivo tyrosine kinase activity compared to the undetectable enzyme activity of the normal murine c-*abl* homologue. Furthermore, mutational analysis of the v-*abl* gene linked the transforming activity of this retrovirus with its tyrosine kinase activity [26,27]. It is therefore assumed that the tyrosine kinase activity is important for the transforming potential of the *bcr-abl* fusion gene as well.

From this association, it might be anticipated that the study of phosphorylation substrates might uncover likely biochemical pathways leading to transformation by an activated *abl* oncogene. In this respect, Huhn and coworkers used antibodies against phosphotyrosyl proteins and identified several prominent phosophorylated proteins at 210, 185, 150, 120, 105, 63, 56, 36, and 32 kDa in a variety of CML cell lines and also in patient blood leukocytes [28]. The constancy with which these protein substrates are phosphorylated suggests that a common biochemical cascade is associated with transformation of hematopoietic cells by the *bcr-abl* protein. Moreover, these substrates are dissimilar to the phosphotyrosyl proteins seen in leukemic cell lines not harboring the *bcr-abl* rearrangement. Of these phosphoproteins, only pp210 has been identified; it was found to be the autophosphorylated *bcr-abl* fusion protein.

Experience with v-*abl* suggests that different sets of protein substrates are phosphorylated in different cell types transformed by the same activated *abl* oncogene. Pre-T-cells and pre-B-cells transformed by v-*abl* share only three of eight phosphotyrosyl proteins [29]. Furthermore, pre-B-cells and fibroblasts transformed by v-*abl* exhibit many more unshared phosphoproteins than shared ones [30]. These comparisons suggest that an activated *abl* oncogene may induce different transformation pathways in different cell types.

The nature of some of these phosophotyrosyl proteins induced by transforming *abl* alleles are beginning to be uncovered. Transformation of murine fibroblasts by v-*abl* results in the phosphorylation of a series of nuclear DNA-binding proteins, indicating a transformation pathway that is related to the regulation of gene expression [31]. Furthermore, in human CML samples and cell lines, a 53 kDa phosphoprotein appears complexed to the p210$^{bcr-abl}$ fusion protein. This protein is different from the p53, which is the cellular protein associated with the SV40 large T-antigen and which has an unknown function [32].

When the standard protein kinase assay was made more sensitive by a variety of modifications, in vitro protein kinase activity of the c-*abl* protein was detected, even though quantitatively lower than that of v-*abl* or *bcr-abl* [33]. Furthermore, two-dimensional electrophoretic gel profiles of the c-*abl* and *bcr-abl* proteins reveal autophosphorylation of c-*abl* occurring in one major fragment, whereas *bcr-abl* exhibited three different areas of autophosphorylation. Thus, different patterns of autophosphorylation may be involved in the oncogenic activation of the *abl* gene.

Transforming activity of the bcr-abl *fusion gene.* The biological effects of *bcr-abl* are subtle and dependent on the target cell type. Whereas v-*abl* efficiently transforms NIH3T3 cells in culture, *bcr-abl* does not [34]. However, in long-term bone marrow culture systems, *bcr-abl* induces an increased capacity for self-renewal, resulting in the clonal outgrowth of immature B-lymphoid cells. These cells all express the introduced *bcr-abl* hybrid gene, but differ in their ability to induce tumors in athymic nude mice [35]. The role of *bcr-abl* in the genesis of CML may therefore be to allow uncontrolled self-renewal of the affected stem cells, while the acute leukemic phenotype (i.e., blast crisis) requires subsequent genetic aberrations.

A different bcr-abl *fusion gene is seen in acute lymphocytic leukemia.* Deletion analysis of the Abelson-murine leukemia virus showed that the presence of *gag* sequences was essential for lymphoid transformation but not for fibroblast transformation [27]. This would imply that for the *bcr-abl* fusion gene, perturbations of the *bcr* portion might affect the range of target tissues that this oncogene can transform. In fact, data exist to support this notion. Approximately 10–20% of patients with de novo acute lymphocytic leukemia (ALL) exhibit the t(9q;22q) translocation seen in CML [36,37]; however, they often do not have their chromosome 22q breakpoints in the breakpoint cluster region (*bcr*) seen in common CML. Instead, the breakpoint in ALL is in the first intron of the *bcr* gene, leading to a fusion gene that contains only the first *bcr* exon linked to the second c-*abl* exon. Though the size of the first *bcr* intron is estimated as greater than 60 kb, the breakpoints in 6 of 7 Ph^1-positive ALL cases were mapped to a restricted 10.8-kb fragment at the 3' end of the first intron [38,39]. Thus when data from four studies are pooled, 22 of 35 patients (62%) with Ph^1-positive ALL showed this abnormal rearrangement occurring in the first *bcr* intron [33,40–42]. This fusion gene results in a novel *bcr-abl* protein of 180–190 kDa that also exhibits increased autophosphorylating activity [43–46]. One third of patients with common CML develop a lymphoid blast crisis morphologically undistinguishable from ALL. In the past, it was thought that such cases of Ph[1]-positive ALL were CML patients whose chronic phase eluded clinical detection. However, these recent studies have shown that while this may be true for many patients, others have a different disease as defined by molecular parameters. In childhood ALL, the presence of a Philadelphia chromosome is associated with a significantly shorter survival, despite treatment with aggressive chemotherapy [47]. Whether there is any difference in the clinical course of adult ALL patients bearing either the common or the variant *bcr-abl* rearrangement remains to be determined.

Genes involved in the progression of chronic to blast-phase CML. At the time of blast crisis, additional chromosomal abnormalities frequently are seen: +8, i(17q), +Ph[1], and +19. Except for +Ph[1], these cytogenetic aberrations do not identify the exact genes that are involved. Recently, mutations in the *ras* family of proto-oncogenes have been detected in both the chronic and blast phases of CML [48,49] with a suggestion that such mutations may be more prevalent in the blast phase of the disease [48,50]. One study detected mutant *ras* genes in 0 of 39 cases of Ph[1]-positive chronic-phase CML and in 1 of 18 (17%) blast-crisis samples. This difference was not statistically significant [50]. In view of the growing evidence of an important role for mutant *ras* alleles in the initiation and progression of human leukemias [51–55], it is surprising that *ras* mutations do not participate at least to a limited extent in the progression of CML cells to blast crisis. Thus, the low overall incidence of such mutations speaks against the importance of the *ras* genes in the chronic phase of CML [32,51].

As discussed previously, the *bcr* exons used to make up the *bcr-abl* fusion gene may determine, in part, the leukemic phenotype (i.e., ALL vs. CML). Recently, evidence has emerged that CML patients with breakpoints in the 3' portion of the 5.8-kb breakpoint cluster region progress to blast crisis more quickly than those patients with breakpoints in the 5' portion [56–59]. Although corresponding differences at the RNA and protein level have not been determined, DNA sequence analysis suggests that the 5' breakpoint results in the loss of one *bcr* exon as compared with the 3' breakpoint.

The level of *bcr-abl* expression may also play a role in the progression from chronic phase to blast crisis. Duplication of the Philadelphia chromosome (+Ph[1]) is a relatively common cytogenetic event in CML blast crisis, although gene amplification (>5 copies) has been described rarely in primary CML blood cells [60,61]. Nevertheless, increased expression of the fusion *bcr-abl* mRNA in blast crisis, as compared to chronic-phase CML, has been reported [62,63], and the level of $p210^{bcr-abl}$ also appears to be higher in Epstein–Barr virus (EBV) immortalized B-cell lines derived from patients in blast crisis [64]. These studies, however, were complicated by questions of sampling variation (EBV cell lines) and by tissue heterogeneity (RNA levels from mixed populations of granulocytes, lymphocytes, and blasts).

The involvement of other oncogenes in the progression of chronic myeloid leukemia to blast crisis has not been well documented. Amplification of c-*myc* appeared to be involved in the disease evolution in one of three episodes of blast crisis in one CML patient [65].

CML is an attractive model system to study multistep pathogenesis. Therefore, further investigations into the conversion from chronic to blast phase can be expected to uncover important principles in leukemic progression.

The importance of the bcr-abl *fusion gene in the maintenance of the CML phenotype*. Previous observations have suggested that the Philadelphia chromosome may not be the sole initiating event in CML. Patients have been described who initially are Ph^1-negative but who later acquire a Philadelphia chromosome [66,67]. Furthermore, in isolated cases, the nonmalignant B- or T-lymphocytes of Ph^1-bearing CML patients lacked the Philadelphia chromosome but were derived from the same clone as the Ph^1-positive leukemic myeloid cells [68,69]. This suggests that, in some cases, another transforming event may precede the emergence of the Philadelphia chromosome.

Additional evidence points to the fact that while the *bcr-abl* gene may be necessary to induce the chronic-phase phenotype, it may not be necessary to maintain the leukemic state. In this regard, several reports describe the presence of the *bcr-abl* rearrangement in chronic-phase CML and its loss in the blast crisis of individual patients [41,70,71].

Mutant ras *genes and preleukemia*

Preleukemia or the myelodysplastic syndrome (MDS) is a hematologic disorder characterized by abnormal-appearing blood elements (dysplastic morphology), low blood counts (anemia, thrombocytopenia, and neutropenia), and a 30% risk of progression to acute leukemia [72–74]. Because of its malignant potential, several investigators have examined tissue from MDS patients in order to define genetic lesions that may occur early in the course of leukemogenesis. Using a sensitive transfection/tumorigenicity assay, Hirai et al. [52] detected mutant N-*ras* genes in 3 of 8 MDS patients; and Liu et al. [53] found mutant K-*ras* alleles in 2 of 4 MDS patients and in one patient with acute leukemia arising from MDS. Significantly, in both studies the presence of a mutant *ras* allele appeared to predict for progression to acute leukemia within a two-year follow-up period. The importance of the *ras* mutation in the transformation process was exemplified by the finding that a K-*ras* codon 13 mutation was detected in a patient with RAEB (refractory anemia with excess blasts, one category of MDS) and in successive blood samples over a 1.5-year course, including a sample at the time of leukemic conversion [53].

Some studies point to mutations in the *ras* genes as among the earliest of genetic lesions in MDS. This is supported by the detection of an N-*ras* mutation in the lymphocytes, granulocytes, and monocytes of a patient with MDS [73], indicating the presence of the *ras* abnormality in a very primitive stem cell. However, there is also evidence that aberrations in *ras* are later events in the course of MDS. Two patients with chromosome 5 abnormalities and MDS showed no *ras* mutations at presentation but exhibited a clonal expansion of blast cells harboring aberrant N-*ras* alleles as the diseases progressed to acute leukemia [54].

The importance of *ras* mutations in predicting subsequent leukemic transformation has recently been questioned. In one study, only 3 of 31 cases of MDS harbored abnormal *ras* alleles, and with an observation period of less than one year, none of these cases progressed to acute leukemia. Within the same observation period, four other patients, having no detectable *ras* mutations, developed acute leukemia [75]. In another analysis, 20 of 50 MDS patients (40%) carried mutant *ras* genes, but no significant association between the genetic mutation and leukemic progression emerged [76]. Careful comparison of these different studies is hindered by the differences in the detection techniques (polymerase chain reaction, or transfection) and the clinical classification employed. Thus an elucidation of the role of *ras* in MDS awaits larger and more comprehensive studies.

The role of molecular analyses in redefining human preleukemic conditions.
Until recently, the nosology of the myeloproliferative syndromes has been based on morphologic distinctions made by light microscopy. The advent of cytogenetics allowed the distinction between Ph^1-positive (common) and Ph^1-negative (atypical) CML, a classification scheme that shows a shortened survival for those who are Ph^1-negative [77]. Further improvements in the detection of the *bcr-abl* rearrangement using molecular techniques have made even more stark the difference between the clinical course of CML with or without this genetic abnormality [14]. The molecular findings are sufficiently dramatic that in recent years several investigators have raised the question of whether there is any such entity as Ph^1-negative/*bcr-abl*-rearrangement-negative CML. Morphologically and clinically, Ph^1-negative CML is frequently similar to myelodysplasia [78,79]. Recently, it was found that 47% of patients with Ph^1-negative and *bcr-abl*-rearrangement-negative CML harbor a *ras* mutation [50]. The absence of the *bcr-abl* rearrangement and the high prevalence of *ras* mutations provides some evidence that atypical CML is also a molecularly distinct entity from common CML. It now appears that Ph^1-negative CML should be reclassified and placed alongside the myelodysplastic syndromes.

ras *mutations in acute leukemia*

Mutations in the *ras* gene family (N-*ras*, H-*ras*, K-*ras*) have been detected in 30% of acute leukemia samples [43,55,80–84]. There is no correlation between the presence of an aberrant allele and the cell of origin (lymphoid or myeloid) or the morphologic phenotype of the leukemic cells (as determined by the French–American–British classification system). To date, however, no study has examined the effect of mutant *ras* genes on the clinical response to therapy.

Analyses of acute leukemia blast cells have revealed several general points. First, lesions in N-*ras* predominate over those occurring in K-*ras* or H-*ras*. Second, a large number of *ras* codon 13 mutations have been detected in acute leukemic samples. These two observations are noteworthy since K-*ras* mutations are more frequently seen in epithelial tumors [85,86], and codon 13 mutations have been only rarely detected in nonleukemic neoplasia [87,88]. The reasons for this difference in the distribution of *ras* mutations remain unclear, but may relate to time of carcinogen exposure and type of carcinogen involved [88]. Third, mutant *ras* genes are not necessary to maintain the leukemic phenotype. This last point was demonstrated in one study where four leukemic patients harbored *ras* mutations prior to treatment, achieved remissions with chemotherapy, but lost their abnormal *ras* alleles in the leukemic cells at the time of relapse [55]. These examples may be interpreted either as *ras* mutations occurring late in leukemogenesis, or as *ras* mutations activating other more powerful transforming genes that can perpetuate the leukemic phenotype in the absence of the initiating *ras* abnormalities. Further studies will be needed to discern the two possibilities.

As was the case for the *abl* gene in CML, much can be learned of the biological function of *ras* in human leukemias by the study of v-*ras* in animal systems. Retroviruses containing mutant *ras* genes induce erythroleukemias and sarcomas when injected into newborn rodents [89]. In vitro infection efficiently transforms rodent hematopoietic cells of erythroid, myeloid, and lymphoid lineages [90–92]. Furthermore, Harvey murine sarcoma virus-transformed erythroid cells retain their capacity to differentiate as determined by the synthesis of hemaglobin after induction [91]. Similarly, *ras*-transformed myeloid cells can also differentiate when exposed to various inducing agents [93]. Thus mutant *ras* genes can transform hematopoeitic cells without severely perturbing differentiation pathways. These observations predicted what would be seen in human leukemias. As noted above, differentiated myeloid cells in MDS and CML have been found to contain the same mutant *ras* genes that have been detected in leukemic blast cells.

Oncogenes strongly associated with human lymphomas: myc

The importance of *myc* in malignancy first emerged in the analysis of avian, murine, and feline tumors where the c-*myc* locus was activated by retroviral insertion or transduction [94]. The biochemistry and activity of this oncogene have been discussed in chapter 3 and therefore will not be discussed in detail here. Of human hematopoietic malignancies, Burkitt's lymphomas are most frequently associated with perturbations of the c-*myc* gene. The first suggestion that this proto-oncogene was involved in Burkitt's lymphoma came from the observation that 80% of Burkitt's cases carry a t(8;14) (q24;32) translocation and that the c-*myc* locus was localized to precisely the breakpoint on chromosome 8q24 [95]. Further characterization of the genetic perturbations revealed that the c-*myc* gene was rearranged in approximately 50% of Burkitt's lymphomas, juxtaposing *myc* against different portions of the immunoglobulin IgH locus [18,95,96]. On chromosome 8, the c-*myc* gene is altered either in the 5' or 3' nontranscribed regions of the gene, by the removal of the noncoding exon 1, or by point mutations in noncoding or coding regions of the gene [19,97–99]. The consistent effect is dysregulation of *myc* expression, such that the normal fluctuations of *myc* in response to a variety of stimuli are perturbed [19,95]. Furthermore, the expression of the rearranged *myc* allele appears to suppress the expression of the untranslocated allele [100].

The theory that dysregulation of *myc* expression is necessary for the induction of lymphomas/leukemias is supported by the observation that transgenic mice bearing a normal c-*myc* coupled to the heavy chain enhancer (Eµ) develop lymphomas, whereas no lymphomas arise in transgenic mice bearing the normal *myc* gene alone [101]. All tumors express the Eµ-*myc* transgene well, but no endogenous normal *myc* transcript can be detected, a finding similar to that in Burkitt's lymphoma cells. The Eµ-*myc* transgene appears to be expressed exclusively in B-lymphoid cells [102] and induces a significant change in the differentiation characteristics of these cells [103]. Cell surface marker analysis of lymphoid tissues in young transgenic mice reveal a dramatic expansion of early B-lineage cells with a reduction in the fraction of mature B-cells. In older animals, the later pre-B-cell population also increases in numbers, resulting in a 4- to 5-fold increase in pre-B-cells and a 30% reduction in mature B-cells [103,104]. Bone marrow DNA in the Eµ-*myc*-bearing mice prior to development of leukemia/lymphoma show that the B-cell expansion is polyclonal. Of note is that the B-cells in these mice are devoid of small B220+ ThB+ pre-B-cells, and the analysis of cellular DNA content shows that one third of the B-cells are in cycle. Taken together, these data suggest that constitutive *myc* expression induces a proliferative state in lymphocytes. Almost all mice bearing the Eµ-*myc* transgene develop B-cell lymphomas or leukemias within a six-month period of observation. Some Eµ-*myc* transgenic strains appear to have slower rates of tumor formation, and experiments reveal a genetic basis for this resistance to transformation [105].

Burkitt's lymphomas are derived from a single malignant clone, as are the leukemia/lymphomas arising in the Eµ-*myc* transgenic mice [101]. This observation indicates that although an activated *myc* may be necessary for transformation, it alone is insufficient to induce the full lymphoma phenotype. Activation of other genes, therefore, is vital for complete transformation to occur. In Burkitt's lymphoma, an important genetic event, infection by the Epstein–Barr virus (EBV) appears to be one such cooperating factor. Endemic Burkitt's lymphomas uniformly carry the EBV genome in their cancer cells [95], suggesting an important role for this virus in the genesis of this disease. The introduction of an activated *myc* gene into EBV-infected primary lymphocytes efficiently renders these cells tumorigenic in athymic nude mice [106]. These data highlight the importance of the cooperation between EBV and an activated *myc* gene in the genesis of Burkitt's lymphoma. However, in nonendemic or sporadic Burkitt's lymphomas, only 15%–20% of cases are associated with EBV infection [95], and thus the same lymphomatous phenotype may arise using different combinations of genetic factors. This concept is further supported by the observation that in two patients, rearrangements of the c-*myc* allele occurred in blast cells that emerged during the progression of their t(14;18)-associated follicular lymphomas [107,108].

Oncogenes strongly associated with lymphomas: bcl-2

Approximately 80% of follicular lymphomas carry a t(14;18) (q24;q32) translocation [109] that on detailed molecular analysis juxtaposes segments of the IgH locus (normally residing on chromosome 14) next to a gene on chromosome 18 subsequently named *bcl-2* [110]. The translocation breakpoints involving *bcl-2* are remarkably precise. In 60%–70% of cases, the rearrangement interrupts a 100-base-pair region of this gene at the 3' end [110,111]; however, a second breakpoint cluster region involving *bcl-2* has recently been uncovered [112]. Using probes to both cluster regions, the precise molecular location of the *bcl-2* translocation can be determined in greater than 90% of follicular lymphomas bearing t(14;18) [112]. The *bcl-2* gene has two exons and produces three transcripts of 8.5, 5.5, and 3.5 kb as a result of differential splicing and polyadenylation [113]. The coding region of *bcl-2* is not perturbed in the translocation process. Two proteins are encoded, *bcl-2* alpha (239 amino acids long) and *bcl-2* beta (205 amino acids long), which are identical except at the carboxy terminus [114] and which share no homology with known proteins. Subcellular fractionation studies on *bcl-2* alpha localize this protein to the cell membrane [115]. Expression of the *bcl-2* protein may be important in B-lymphocyte development, since it is high during the early developmental stages of B-cells but progressively decreases with lymphocyte maturation [116]. When polyclonal antibodies against the *bcl-2* protein are applied to non-Hodgkin's lymphoma tissues, 37 of 41 follicular lymphomas showed expression of the *bcl-2* protein, whereas none of 30 non-malignant lymph nodes exhibited *bcl-2* expression [117]. When the *bcl-2* gene is cloned into an expression vector and transfected into NIH3T3 cells, no focus formation activity is seen; however, these transfected cells efficiently form tumors in athymic nude mice with short latency times, indicating an oncogenic potential for this gene [118].

The presence of *bcl-2* rearrangements and *bcl-2* protein expression is not limited to lymphomas of the follicular histology. Diffuse large-cell lymphomas represent a different class of lymphomas with a different natural history. Twenty-nine 114 (25%) patients with diffuse large-cell lymphomas show a rearrangement of *bcl-2* [119–121]. On the protein level, 13 of 38 patients with diffuse large-cell lymphoma express *bcl*-2 [117]. Although the exact clinical significance of *bcl*-2 rearrangement and expression in diffuse large cell lymphomas is presently unknown, these findings illustrate the molecular heterogeneity present in this class of lymphomas. Such molecular differences may later prove to be important prognostic variables.

Oncogenes occasionally associated with hematopoietic malignancies

Perturbations of several other oncogenes have been occasionally reported in human leukemias and therefore are implicated in some aspect of hematological malignancies. However, because they are infrequently found, it is unlikely that they have a major role in the initiation of leukemia, but may represent factors in the progression to the acute leukemic phenotype. The possibility still exists that when more refined molecular techniques and biological assays for transformation are developed, the function of these oncogenes in leukemic progression will become more clear. Oncogenes to be discussed in this section include *ets*, *myb*, c-*erb*B-1 (EGFR), *fes*, *myc*, *fos*, the growth factor and the growth factor receptor genes (CSF-1, c-*fms*), and p53.

The possibility that some of these oncogenes might be involved in human leukemogenesis comes from data showing retroviral activation of these genes in experimental leukemias. The avian myeloblastosis virus carried v-*myb* and induces myeloblastosis in chickens [123,124]; the E26 virus transforms both myeloblasts and erythroblasts and contains both v-*myb* and v-*ets* [125]; and retroviruses carrying the v-*erb*B oncogene cause erythroleukemias in chickens [126]. In human leukemias, these various oncogenes may be implicated in tumorigenesis by their overexpression, or by genetic aberrations such as amplification or rearrangements.

Oncogene overexpression

The evidence that *myb* may be involved in human leukemogenesis came with the observation that leukemic blasts showed greater expression of *myb* mRNA than normal bone marrow [127,128] and that *myb* overexpression was seen almost exclusively in primary hematopoietic malignancies [129,130]. More extensive surveys of leukemic samples revealed higher *myb*-specific expression in more immature forms of ALL and AML (pre-B ALL, and M1/M2 phenotypes of AML) [131]. The size of the transcripts, however, were normal, suggesting no obvious truncation of the c-*myb* proto-oncogene as had been documented with retroviral-induced activation of c-*myb* [132]. The importance of the c-*myb* proto-oncogene in normal marrow development was highlighted by experiments where antisense oligonucleotides directed against *myb* transcripts inhibited the growth of bone marrow cells in culture [133]. Furthermore, the inhibition was apparent only when the antisense oligonucleotides were applied soon after the plating of the cells, suggesting a role for the *myb* protein in the early stages of colony formation. Despite these associations, the possibility exists that the augmented expression of c-*myb* is a reflection of the undifferentiated nature of leukemic blast cells or an indicator of sustained proliferative potential, and that elevated levels of a normal *myb* protein do not induce the leukemic state.

Studies on the patterns of expression of other proto-oncogenes also revealed elevated *myb* expression occurring without gene amplification in 70%–85% of leukemias [134–137] and increased levels of *fes*, *fos*, and p53 mRNA in a large proportion of these patients [129,131,135]. High constitutive *fos* expression was detected mainly in AML patients with monocyte phenotype [138], suggesting a role for this proto-oncogene in determining the differentiation state of leukemic cells. Leukemic blasts with elevated p53 mRNA levels were associated with a greater in vitro self-renewal capacity [139], which is a parameter correlated with lower remission rates. When *ras*-specific antibodies were applied to human leukemic samples, all three *ras* proteins were detected; however, N-*ras* and K-*ras* were expressed to a greater degree than H-*ras* [140]. Other proto-oncogenes such as c-*sis*, c-*erb* B, and c-*src* were not expressed to any degree [131,137].

The expression of the hematopoietic growth factors and growth factor receptors in leukemic samples are of particular interest, since unregulated autocrine stimulation may be a mode of tumorigenesis [141]. Evidence of a role for this mechanism in leukemic progression comes in the insertion of the GM-CSF cDNA in the nonleukemic FD-CP1 hematopoietic cell line [142]. The secretion of GM-CSF by these cells caused them to attain a leukemic phenotype. In human leukemia, 10 of 17 cases studied exhibited CSF-1 transcripts, while 7 of 15 expressed c-*fms* (CSF-1 receptor). Co-expression of the two genes were detected in five of these cases, raising the possibility of autocrine stimulation in these leukemic cells [143].

Despite the association of oncogene overexpression with human leukemias, a causal relationship cannot be established from the available data. The difficulty lies in the heterogeneity of hematopoietic cells in a sample of blood or bone marrow. Normal blood cells are a mixture of lymphocytes, granulocytes, early blasts, and differentiated, mature hematopoietic elements, each with a set of expressed genes specific to a lineage and a differentiation pathway. The mRNA isolated from such samples represent at best the average output of many different cell types. Leukemic cells, by contrast, are enriched for a specific cell type, e.g., blasts, which otherwise comprise less than 5% of normal bone marrow cells. Thus a proto-oncogene that is expressed only in myeloblasts will seem overexpressed in M1 AML, but not expressed in normal bone marrow.

Oncogene rearrangements or amplification

Genetic rearrangements that occur in high frequency in hematopoietic malignancies, namely *myc*, *bcl*-2, and *bcr-abl*, have already been discussed. In human acute leukemias, other translocations or amplification of specific proto-oncogenes are not common [84,137,144,145]. Amplification of c-*myc* was detected in the HL-60 myeloid cell line and in the original primary leukemic cells [146] in one case of AML arising from a myelodysplastic syndrome [147] and in one case of CML progressing to blast crisis [65]. In general, however, larger screening efforts have uncovered further cases of *myc* amplification in acute leukemic samples [144,145,148].

The viral oncogene, v-*ets*, is found in the avian retrovirus E26, which is capable of inducing erythroblastosis [125,149]. Molecular dissection of this oncogene revealed its origin to be from two separate loci termed *ets*-1 and *ets*-2. In humans, *ets*-1 is a cytoplasmic proto-oncogene localized to chromosome 11q23, and the *ets*-2 gene is a nuclear proto-oncogene localized to chromosome 21q22. Of considerable interest is the fact that several chromosomal translocations frequently found in acute nonlymphocytic leukemias (ANLL) occur in precisely those locations: infant acute lymphocytic leukemias exhibit the translocation t(4;11) (q21;q23) [150,151]; other ANLLs show translocations involving chromosomes 6,9,10,17, and 19 and chromosome 11q23 [149]; and many M2 AMLs carry the translocation t(8;21) (q22;q22) [93]. The *ets*-1 locus is moved from chromosome 11 to other chromosomes in the translocations t(4;11) and t(9;11) [149,152], and the *ets*-2 gene is moved from chromosome 21 to 8 and t(8;21) [93]. Southern blot hybridization revealed a rearrangement of the *ets*-1 proto-oncogene in 3 of 13 cases of primary acute leukemia [153–155] with t(4;11), t(9;11), or indeterminate karyotype. However, none of eight cases with t(8;21) AML showed *ets*-2 rearrangements on Southern hybridization [154]. Though gene amplification of *ets*-1 was seen in an ANLL patient with a homogenous staining region in 11q23 [153], one case of t(4;11) ALL and two cases of t(8;21) AML exhibited reduced expression of the specific *ets* transcripts or loss of an *ets* hybridizing RNA band. This suggests that the activation of the *ets* proto-oncogenes is not due simply to augmentation of expression [153,154].

The t(11;14) (q13;32) translocation that occurs in chronic lymphocytic leukemias involved J_H segments on chromosome 14, and a putative oncogene on chromosome 11q13, *bcl*-1 [122]. The nature of *bcl*-1 has not been fully elucidated [95], but its role in common chronic lymphocytic leukemia (CLL) may be less than initially anticipated: rearrangements of *bcl*-1 could not be detected in 38 unselected cases of CLL [185]. It may be possible that *bcl*-1 is involved only in the subset of CLL cases with the t(11;14) translocation.

The epidermal growth factor receptor (EGFR) gene is the cellular homologue of the v-*erb*B oncogene and is localized to human chromosome 7p11 (see chapter 6). The EGFR transcript is expressed at very low levels in normal bone marrow and in the great majority of leukemia samples [128,131]. However, in three myelodysplasia patients with the translocation +der(1), t(1;7) (p11;p11), overexpression of the EGFR transcript was associated with a 20-fold gene amplification of this locus [156]. Thus despite the rarity of perturbations in the EGFR gene in human leukemic conditions, amplification and overexpression of this gene may have a role in the initiation or maintenance of the preleukemic state.

Recently a new class of oncogene has been identified that may have some importance to human leukemias. Myeloid leukemias can be induced by retroviral insertional activation. Several resultant transformed cell lines exhibited retroviral insertions in a common integration site called Evi-1 [157]. Subsequently a transcriptional unit activated by retroviral insertion was isolated from one cell line and was found to be a zinc finger protein homologous to a Xenopus RNA polymerase III transcription factor, TFIIIA [158]. The human homologue to this murine Evi-1 gene resides and inversions found in myelodysplastic syndromes and acute leukemias [158–160]. A peculiar characteristic of these leukemias is their association with high platelet counts [159].

Tumor-suppressor genes in hematopoietic malignancies

The location of genes that suppress the tumorigenic phenotype is frequently first suggested by cytogenetic studies showing loss of specific chromosomal material. Detailed molecular genetic analyses that follow may then lead to the identification and isolation of a putative suppressor gene. It was in this manner that the retinoblastoma suppressor gene was ultimately cloned. In human leukemias, cytogenetic data point to regions of 5q, 7q, 20q, and 9p as potential locations of leukemic suppressor genes, since deletion of genetic material in these regions occurs with some frequency in hematologic neoplasia [36,161].

Deletions in either chromosomes 5 or 7 are frequently associated with therapy-induced acute nonlymphocytic leukemias: 50 of 119 patients showed either a −5 or 5q-karyotype, and 79 of 119 patients exhibited either a −7 or 7q- configuration [162–164]. The critical region in chromosome 5 appears to be 5q23–5q32 where the genes for the growth factors, GM-CSF [165], CSF-1 [166], interleukin 3 [167], and the growth factor receptor, c-*fms* [168], have been localized. In many patients with the 5q- syndrome, these genes are deleted in the abnormal chromosome, resulting in hemizygosity [167,169]. Whether the loss of any number of these genes or of a yet unidentified linked gene is necessary for the myelodysplastic phenotype is unclear; however, one case of congenital hypothyroidism and ALL exhibited a homozygous deletion at the c-*fms* locus in the germ line, despite a normal-appearing chromosome 5 [170]. Although insufficient material remained to assess the expression of this abnormal c-*fms* gene, the possibility exists that a 'crippled" c-*fms* protein at least contributed to this clinical syndrome.

Deletions in chromosome 7q are also common in patients with myelodysplastic syndrome arising from prior mutagen exposure [163]. Minimal deletions have been detected at 7q22-32 where the *met* proto-oncogene resides, making this the likely critical chromosomal region (171,172). The prediction for the existence of a putative leukemia-suppressor locus in 7q22-32 is strengthened by the presence of familial cases of bone marrow monosomy 7 associated with a myeloproliferative disorder and childhood AML [173,174].

Deletions involving 20q are not uncommon in myeloproliferative disorders including MDS and AML, and have been localized to 20q11 [175]. The human *src* locus is not deleted in this disorder [176]; however, a new protein-tyrosine kinase expressed exclusively in hematopoietic cells, *hck*, has been localized to 20q11-12 [177]. This gene belongs to a family of tyrosine kinase genes that may have important functions in the differentiation of blood elements. It is conceivable therefore that deletion of *hck* may contribute to the pathogenesis of certain leukemic conditions by the removal of a differentiation factor for certain hematopoietic cells.

The loss of a band in chromosome 9p22 is frequently observed in ALL and in non-Hodgkin's lymphomas [178–180], where the alpha and beta1 interferon genes have been assigned [152,181]. Recently, 6 of 21 leukemic (ALL and AML) cell lines showed a homozygous deletion of the two interferon genes [182]. Furthermore, 7% of 42 ALL cases showed the same total loss of the interferon genes, and 19% of these patients exhibited hemizygosity at the interferon loci [182]. Since the interferons have antiproliferative effects mediated in part by various growth factors [183,184], their inactivation by genetic deletion may result in uncontrolled growth.

Conclusions

Perturbations in the cellular proto-oncogenes are frequently found in human leukemias and lymphomas, and the current evidence is that they play an important role in the genesis and progression of these disorders. At what point in the progression pathway they act and to what extent they contribute to the final phenotype are questions that remain uncertain, though there are now very intriguing clues. Different *bcr-abl* recombinations tend to induce different leukemic phenotypes: ALL versus chronic phase CML. Leukemic cells with high *fos* mRNA levels have monocytic features, and *myc* rearrangements are seen most frequently in high-grade lymphomas. Each individual oncogene may serve several functions in the varied pathways to malignancy: *myc* rearrangements may be the first steps in sporadic Burkitt's lymphomas but late steps in follicular lymphomas advancing to lymphoblastic lymphoma, and *ras* mutations may be early genetic events in myelodysplasia but late ones in de novo AML.

Despite their varied molecular origins, the final malignant phenotype may be indistinguishable: e.g., blast crisis CML, ANLL arising from myelodysplasia, and de novo AML. Yet knowledge of the molecular changes enables clinicians to predict clinical outcomes. Thus molecular diagnostics based on an understanding of oncogenes are becoming important aids to the clinician.

When the field is viewed as a whole, one is impressed with the complex genetic and epigenetic interactions necessary to achieve the malignant phenotype. Equally impressive is how many different ways there are to become a cancer cell, and how difficult it will be to fight such a versatile opponent.

Acknowledgments

The author wishes to thank Drs. Andreas and Beatrix Neubauer for their help in preparation of the manuscript.

References

1. Rowley JD: A new consistent chromosomal abnormality in chronic myelogenous leukaemia identified by quinacrine fluorescence and giemsa staining. Nature 243:290–293, 1973.
2. Whang-Peng J, Henderson RS, Knutsen T, Freireich EJ, Gart JJ: Cytogenetic studies in acute myelocytic leukemia with special emphasis on the occurrence of the Ph1 chromosome. Blood 36:448–457, 1970.
3. Rowley JD: Ph^1-positive leukaemia, including chronic myelogenous leukemia. Clin. Haematol 9(1):55–85, 1980.
4. Bartram CR, de Klein A, Hagemeijer A: Translocation of the c-*abl* oncogene correlates with the presence of a Philadelphia chromosome in chronic myelocytic leukemia. Nature 306:277–280, 1983.
5. de Klein A, Geurts van Kessel A, Grosveld GC, Bartram CR, Hagemeijer A, Bootsma D, Spurr NK, Heisterkamp N, Groffen J, Stephenson JR: A cellular oncogene (c-*abl*) is translocated to the Philadelphia chromosome in chronic myelogenous leukemia. Nature 300:765–767, 1982.
6. Heisterkamp N, Stephenson JR, Groffen J, Hansen PF, de Klein A, Bartram CR, Grosveld G: Localization of the c-*abl* oncogene adjacent to a translocation breakpoint in chronic myelogenous leukemia. Nature 306:239–242, 1983.
7. Groffen J, Stephenson JR, Heisterkamp N, de Klein A, Bartram CR, Grosveld G: Philadelphia chromosomal breakpoints are clustered within a limited region, *bcr*, on chromosome 22. Cell 36:93–99, 1984.
8. Hirosawa S, Aoki N, Matsushime H, Shibua M: Undetectable *bcr-abl* rearrangement in some CML patients are due to a deletion mutation in the *bcr* gene. Am J Hematol 28: 33–36, 1988.
9. Biennerhassett GT, Furth ME, Anderson A, Burns JP, Chaganti RSK, Blick M, Talpaz M, Dev VG, Chan LC, Wiedemann LM, Greaves MF, Hagemeijer A, van der Plas D, Skuse G, Wang N, Stam K: Clinical evaluation of a DNA probe assay for the Philadelphia translocation in chronic myelogenous leukemia. Leukemia 2(10):648–657, 1988.
10. Morris CM, Reeve AE, Fitzgerald PH, Hollings PE, Beard ME, Heaton DC: Genomic diversity correlates with clinical variation in Ph^1-negative chronic myelogenous leukemia. Nature 32:281–283, 1986.
11. Teyssier JR, Bartram CR, Deville J, Potion G, Pigeon F: C-*abl* oncogene and chromosome 22 '*bcr*' juxtaposition in chronic myelogenous leukemia. N Engl J Med 312(21):1393–1394, 1985.
12. de Klein A, Bartram CR, Hagemeijer A, Heisterkamp N, Stam K, Groffen J, Grosveld G: The c-*abl* oncogene in chronic myelogenous leukemia. Hematologica 72:19–22, 1987.
13. Ganesan S, Rassol F, Guo AP, Young BD, Galton DAG, Goldman JM: Rearrangement of the *bcr* gene in Philadelphia chromosome negative chronic myelogenous leukemia.

Haematology and Blood Transfusions 31:153–159, 1987.
14. Ezdinli EZ, Sokal JE, Crosswhite L, Sandberg AA: Philadelphia-chromosome-positive and -negative chronic myelocytic leukemia. Ann Intern Med 72:175–182, 1970.
15. Kurzrock R, Blick MB, Talpaz M et al.: Rearrangement in the breakpoint cluster region and the clinical course in Philadelphia-negative chronic myelogenous leukemia. Ann Intern Med 105:673–679, 1986.
16. Bartram CR, Kleihauer E, de Klein A, et al.: C-*abl* and *bcr* are rearranged in a Ph^1-negative CML patient. EMBO J 4:683–686, 1985.
17. Shtivelman E, Gale RP, Dreazen O, et al.: *Bcr-abl* RNA in patients with chronic myelogenous leukemia. Blood 69:971–973, 1987.
18. Haluska FG, Finver S, Tsujimoto Y, Croce CM: The t(8;14) chromosomal translocation occurring in B-cell malignancies results from mistakes in V-D-J joining. Nature 324:158–161, 1986.
19. Haluska FG, Tsujimoto Y, Croce CM: Mechanisms of chromosomal translocation in B- and T-cell neoplasia. Trends Genet 3:11–15, 1987.
20. Heisterkamp N, Stam K, Groffen J, de Klein A, Grosveld G: Structural organization of the *bcr* gene and its role in the Ph^1 translocation. Nature 315:758–761, 1985.
21. Shtivelman E, Lifshitz B, Gale RP, Canaani E: Fused transcript of *abl* and *bcr* genes in chronic myelogenous leukaemia. Nature 315:550–554, 1985.
22. Mes-Masson AM, McLaughlin J, Daley GQ, Paskind M, Witte ON: Overlapping cDNA clones define the complete coding region for the P210-*cabl* gene product associated with chronic myelogenous leukemia cells containing the Philadelphia chromosome. Proc Natl Acad Sci USA 83:9768–9772, 1986.
23. Konopka JB, Watanabe SM, Singer JW, Collins SJ, Witte ON: Cell lines and clinical isolates derived from Ph^1 positive chronic myelogenous leukemia patients express c-*abl* proteins with a common structural alteration. Proc Natl Acad Sci USA 82:1810–1814, 1985.
24. Baltimore D, Shields A, Otto G, Goff S, Besmer PR, Witte O, Rosenberg N: Structure and expression of the Abelson murine leukemia virus genome and its relationship to a normal cell gene. Cold Spring Harbor Symp Quant Biol 44:849–854, 1980.
25. Konopka JB, Witte ON: Activation of the *abl* oncogene in murine and human leukemias. Biochim Biophys Acta 823:1–17, 1985.
26. Prywes R, Foulkes JG, Baltimore D: The minimum transforming region of c-*abl* is the segment encoding protein-tyrosine kinase. J Virol 54:114–122, 1985.
27. Prywes R, Foulkes JG, Rosenberg N, Baltimore D: Sequences of the A-MuLV protein needed for fibroblast and lymphoid cell transformation. Cell 34:569–579, 1983.
28. Huhn RD, Marshall R, Posner MR, Rayter SI, Foulkes JG, Frackelton AR: Cell lines and peripheral blood meukocytes derived from individuals with chronic myelogenous leukemia display virtually identical proteins phosphorylated on tyrosine residues. Proc Natl Acad Sci USA 84:4408–4412, 1987.
29. Saggioro D, Ferracini R, DiRenzo MF, Naldini L, Chieco-Bianchi L, Comoglio PM: Protein phosphorylation at tyrosine residues in v-*abl* transformed mouse lymphocytes and fibroblasts. Int J Cancer 37:623–628, 1986.
30. Frackelton AR: Characterization of phosphotyrosyl proteins in cells transformed by Abelson murine leukemia virus: use of a monoclonal antibody to phosphotyrosine. In: Feramisco L, Ozanne B, Stiles C (ed): Growth Factors and Transformation. Cold Spring Harbor, NY: Cold Spring Harbor Laboratory, 1985, pp 339–345.
31. Bell JC, Mahadevan LC, Colledge WH, Frackelton AR Jr, Sargent MG, Foulkes JG: Abelson-transformed fibroblasts contain nuclear phosphotyrosyl-proteins which preferentially bind to murine DNA. Nature 325:552–554.
32. Wanjun L, Kloetzer WS, Arlinghaus RB: A novel 53kD protein complexed with p210$^{bcr-abl}$ in human chronic myelogenous leukemia cells. Oncogene 2:559–566, 1988.
33. Konopka JB, Witte ON: Detection of *abl* tyrosine kinase activity in vitro permits direct comparison of normal and altered *abl* gene products. Mol Cell Biol 5:3116–3123, 1985.
34. Daley GQ, McLaughlin J, Witte ON, Baltimore D: The CML specific p210 *bcr/abl* protein,

unlike v-*abl*, does not transform NIH/3T3 fibroblasts. Science 237:532–535, 1987.
35. Young JC, Witte ON: Selective transformations of primitive lymphoid cells by the *bcr/abl* oncogene expressed in long term lymphoid or myeloid cultures. Mol Cell Biol 8:4079–4087, 1988.
36. Rowley JD: Clinical significance of chromosomal abnormalities in acute lymphoblastic leukemia. Cancer Genet Cytogenet 4:111–37, 1981.
37. Hirosawa S, Aoki N, Shibuya M, Onozawa Y: Breakpoints in Philadelphia chromosome (Ph^1)-positive leukemias. Jpn J Cancer Res 78:590–595, 1987.
38. Erikson J, Griffin CA, ar-Rushdi A, et al.: Heterogeneity of chromosome 22 breakpoint in Philadelphia-positive acute lymphoblastic leukemia. Proc Natl Acad Sci USA 83:1807–1811, 1986.
39. Chen SJ, Chen Z, Grausz D, Hillion J, d'Auriol L, Flandrin G, Larsen CJ, Berger R: Molecular cloning of a 5′ segment of the genomic Ph^1 gene defines a new breakpoint cluster region (*bcr2*) in Philadelphia positive acute leukemia. Leukemia 2(10):634–641, 1988.
40. Erikson J, Griffin CA, ar-Rushdi A, Valitieri M, Hoxie J, Finon J, Emanuel BS, Rovera G, Nowell PC, Croce CM: Heterogeneity of chromosome 22 breakpoint in Philadelphia-positive (Ph$^+$) acute lymphocytic leukemia. Proc Natl Acad Sci USA 83:1807–1811, 1986.
41. de Klein A, Hagemeijer A, Bartram CT, et al.: *Bcr* rearrangement and translocation of the c-*abl* oncogene in Philadelphia positive acute lymphoblastic leukemia. Blood 68:1369–1375, 1986.
42. Hermans A, Gow J, Selleri L, von Lindern M, Hagemeijer A, Wiedeman LM, Grosveld G: *Bcr-abl* oncogene activation in Philadelphia chromosome positive acute lymphoblastic leukemia. Leukemia 2(10):628–633, 1988.
43. Kurzrock R, Shtalrid M, Romero R, et al.: A novel c-*abl* protein produce in Philadelphia-positive acute lymphoblastic leukemia. Nature 325:631–635, 1987.
44. Clark SS, McLaughlin J, Crist WM, Champlin TR, Witte ON: Unique forms of the *abl* tyrosine kinase distinguish Ph^1-positive CML from Ph^1 ALL. Science 235:85–88, 1987.
45. Chan LC, Karhi KK, Rayter SI, Heisterkamp N, Eridani S, Powles R, Lawler SD, Groffen J, Foulkes JG, Greaves MF, Wiedemann LM: A novel *abl* protein expressed in Philadelphia chromosome positive acute lymphoblastic leukaemia. Nature 325:635–637, 1987.
46. Kurzrock R, Shtalrid M, Romero P, Kloetzer WS, Talpas M, Trujillo JM, Blick M, Beran M, Gutterman JU: A novel c-*abl* protein produce in Philadelphia-positive acute lymphoblastic leukemia. Nature 325:631–635, 1987.
47. Ribeiro RC, Abromowitsch M, Raimondi SC, Murphy SB, Behm F, Williams DL: Clinical and biological hallmarks of the Philadelphia chromosome in childhood acute lymphoblastic leukemia. Blood 70:948–953, 1987.
48. Liu E, Hjelle B, Bishop JM: Transforming genes in chronic myelogenous leukemia. Proc Natl Acad Sci USA 85:1952–1956, 1988.
49. Hirai H, Tanaka S, Azuma M, Anrahn Y, Kobayashi Y, Fujisawa M, Okabe T, Urable A, Takaku F: Transforming genes in human leukemia cells. Blood 66:1371–1378, 1985.
50. Cogswell P, Liu E: Frequency of ras mutations in chronic myelogenous leukemia. Submitted.
51. Janssen JWG, Steenvoorden ACM, Lyons J, Anger B, Bohlke JU, Bos JL, Seliger H, Bartram CR: Ras gene mutations in acute and chronic myelocytic leukemias, chronic myeloproliferative disorders, and myelodysplastic syndromes. Proc Natl Acad Sci USA 84:9228–9232, 1987.
52. Hirai H, Kobayashi Y, Mano H, Hagiwara K, Maru Y, Omine M, Mizoguchi H, Nishida J, Takaku F: A point mutation at codon 13 of the N-*ras* oncogene in myelodysplastic syndrome. Nature 327:430–432, 1987.
53. Liu E, Hjelle B, Morgan R, Hecht F, Bishop JM: Mutations of the Kirsten *Ras* proto-oncogene in myelodysplastic syndrome. Nature 327:430–432, 1987.
54. Hirai H, Okada M, Mizoguchi H, Mano H, Kobayashi Y, Nishida J, Takaku F: Relationship between an activated N-*ras* oncogene and chromosomal abnormality during leukemic progression from myelodysplastic syndrome. Blood 71:256–258, 1988.

55. Farr CJ, Saiki RK, Erlich HA, McCormick F: Analysis of *ras* gene mutations in acute myeloid leukemia by polymerase chain reaction and oligonucleotide probes. Proc Natl Acad Sci USA 85:1629–1633, 1988.
56. Mills KI, Mackenzie ED, Birnie GD: The site of the breakpoint within the *bcr* is a prognostic factor in Philadelphia-positive CML patients. Blood 72(4):1237–1241, 1988.
57. Schaefer-Rego K, Dudek H, Popenoe D, Arlin Z, Mears JG, Bank A, Leibowitz D: CML patients in blast crisis have breakpoints localized to a specific region of the *bcr*. Blood 70:448–455, 1987.
58. Kurzrock R, Gutterman JU, Talpaz M: The molecular genetics of Philadelphia chromosome-positive leukemias. N Engl J Med 319:990–998, 1988.
59. Shtalrid M, Talpaz M, Kurzrock R, Kantarjian H, Trujillo J, Gutterman J, Yoffe G, Blick M: Analysis of *bcr* gene and correlation with clinical course in Ph-positive chronic myelogenous leukemia. Blood 72:485–491, 1988.
60. Collins SJ: Breakpoints on chromosomes 9 and 22 in Philadelphia chromosome-positive chronic myelogenous leukemia (CML): amplification of rearranged *c-abl* oncogenes in CML blast crisis. J Clin Invest 78:1392–1396, 1986.
61. Collins SJ, Groudine MT: Chronic myelogenous leukemia: amplification of a rearranged *c-abl* oncogene in both chronic phase and blast crisis. Blood 69:893–898, 1987.
62. Collins SJ, Kubonishi I, Miyoshi I, Groudine M: Altered transcription of the *c-abl* oncogene in K-562 and other chronic myelogenous leukemia cells. Science 225:72–74, 1984.
63. Collins S, Colman H, Groudine M: Expression of *bcr* and *bcr/abl* fusion transcripts in normal and leukemic cells. Mol Cell Biol 7:2870–2876, 1987.
64. Konopka JB, Clark S, McLaughlin J, Nitta M, Kato Y, Strife A, Clarkson B, Witte ON: Variable expression of the translocated *c-abl* oncogene in Philadelphia-chromosome positive B-lymphoid cell lines from chronic myelogenous leukemia patients. Proc Natl Acad Sci USA 83:4049–4052, 1986.
65. McCarthy DM, Rassool FV, Goldman JM, Graham SV, Birnie GD: Genomic alterations involving the *c-myc* proto-oncogene locus during the evolution of a case of chronic granulocytic leukemia. Lancet 2:1362–1365, 1984.
66. Lisker R, Caras L, Mutdrinick O, Perez-Chavez F, Labardini J: Late-appearing Philadelphia chromosome in two patients with chronic myelogenous leukemia. Blood 56:812–814, 1980.
67. Hayata J, Sakurai M, Kakati S, Sandberg AA: Banding studies of chronic myelocytic leukemia, including five unusual Ph[1] translocations. Cancer 36:1177–1191, 1975.
68. Fialkow PJ, Martin PJ, Najfeld V, Penfold GK, Jacobsen RJ, Hansen JA: Evidence for a mutlistep pathogenesis of chronic myelogenous leukemia. Blood 58:158–163, 1981.
69. Najfeld V, Seremetis S, Sanders N, Jacobson R, Aledort L, Troy K, Arlin Z, Fialkow PJ: Origin of T-lymphocytes in Philadelphia chromosome positive chronic myelogenous leukemia (abstr). Blood 66 (Suppl 1):100a, 1985.
70. Bartram CR, Janssen JWG, Becher R: Persistance of CML despite deletion of rearranged *bcr/c-abl* sequences. Haematology and Blood Transfusions 31:145–147, 1987.
71. Bartram CR, Janssen JW, Becher R, de Klein A, Grosveld G: Persistence of chronic myelocytic leukemia despite delegation of rearranged *bcr-abl* sequences in blast crisis. J Exp Med 164:1389–1396, 1986.
72. Greenberg PL: The smoldering myeloid leukemic states: clinical and biological features. Blood 61:1035–1044, 1983.
73. Coiffier B, Adeleine P, Viala JJ, Bryon PA, Fiere D, Gentilhomme O, Vuuan H: Dysmyelopoietic syndromes. A search for prognostic factors in 193 patients. Cancer 52:83–90, 1983.
74. Mufti GJ, Stevens JR, Oscier DG, Hamlin TJ, Machin D: Myelodysplastic syndromes: a scoring system with prognostic significance. Br J Haematol 59:425–433, 1985.
75. Lyons J, Janssen JWG, Bartram C, Layton M, Mufti GJ: Mutation of Ki-*ras* and N-*ras* oncogenes in myelodysplastic syndromes. Blood 71:1707–1712, 1988.
76. Padua RA, Carter G, Hughes D, Gow J, Farr C, Oscier D, McCormick F, Jacobs A: *Ras*

mutations in myelodysplasia detected by amplification, oligonucleotide hybridization, and transformation. Leukemia 2(8):503–510, 1988.
77. Kantarjan HM, Smith TL, McCredie KB, et al.: Chronic myelogeneous leukemia: a multivariate analysis of the association of patients characteristics and survival. Blood 66:1326–35, 1985.
78. Pugh WC, Pearson M, Vardiman JW, Rowley JD: Philadelphia chromosome-negative chronic myelogenous leukemia: a morphological reassessment. Br J Haematol 60:457–467, 1985.
79. Travis LB, Pierre RV, DeWald GW: Ph^1 negative chronic granulocytic leukemia: a nonentity. Am J Clin Path 85(2):186–193, 1986.
80. Gambke CA, Hall A, Moroni C: Activation of an N-*ras* gene in acute myeloblastic leukemia through somatic mutation in the first exon. Proc Natl Acad Sci USA 82:879–882, 1985.
81. Needleman SW, Kraus MH, Srivastva SK, Levine PH, Aaronson SA: High frequency of N-*ras* activation in acute myelogenous leukemia. Blood 67:753–757, 1986.
82. Bos JL, Toksoz D, Marshall CJ, Verlaan-de Vries M, Veeneman GH, van der Eb AJ, van Boom JH, Janssen JWG, Steenvoorden ACM: Amino acid substitution at codon 13 of the N-*ras* oncogene in human acute myeloid leukemia. Nature 315:726–730, 1985.
83. Bos JL, Verlaan-de Vries M, van der Eb AJ, Janssen JWG, Delwel R, Lowenberg B, Colly LP: Mutations in N-*ras* predominate in acute myeloid leukemia. Blood 69:1237–1241, 1987.
84. Rodenhuis S, Bos JL, Slater RM, Behrendt H, van't Heer M, Smets SO: Absence of oncogene amplifications and occasional activation of N-*ras* in lymphoblastic leukemia of childhood. Blood 67:1698–1704, 1986.
85. Bos JL, Fearon ER, Hamilton SR, Verlaan-de Vries M, van Boom JH, van der Eb AJ, Vogelstein B: Prevalence of ras mutations in human colorectal cancers. Nature 327:293–297, 1987.
86. Rodenhuis S, van de Wetering ML, Mooi WJ, Evers SG, van Zanwijk N, Bos JL: Mutational activation of the K-*ras* oncogene; a possible pathogenic factor in adeoncarcinoma of the lung. N Engl J Med 317:929–935, 1987.
87. Rochlitz CF, Scott GK, Dodson JM, Liu E, Dollbaum C, Smith HS, Benz CC: Incidence of activating *ras* oncogene mutations associated with primary and metastatic human breast cancer. Cancer Res, in press.
88. Barbacid M: *Ras* genes. Annu Rev Biochem 56:779–827, 1987.
89. Tabin CJ, Weinberg RA: Analysis of viral and somatic activations of the cHa-*ras* gene. J Virol 53:260–265, 1985.
90. Rein A, Keller J, Schultz AM, Holmes KL, Medicus R, Ihle JN: Infection of immune mast cells by Harvey sarcoma virus:immortalization without loss of requirement for interleukin-3. Mol Cell Biol 5:2257–2264, 1985.
91. Hankins WD, Scolnick EM: Harvey and Kirsten sarcoma viruses promote the growth and differentiation fo erythroid precursor cells in vitro. Cell 26:91–97, 1981.
92. Pierce JH, Aaronson SA: Myeloid cell transformation by *ras*-containing murine sarcoma viruses. Mol Cell Biol 5(4):667–674, 1985.
93. LeBeau MM, Rowley JD, Sacchi N, Watson DK, Papas TS, Diaz MO: Hu-ets-2 is translocated to chromosome 8 in the t(8;21) in acute myelogenous leukemia. Cancer Genet Cytogenet 23:269–274, 1986.
94. Cole MD: The *myc* oncogene: its role in transformation and differantiation. Annu Rev Genet 20:361–384, 1986.
95. Haluska FG, Tsujimoto Y, Croce CM: Oncogene activation by chromosome translocation in human malignancy. Annu Rev Genet 21:321–345, 1987.
96. Bernard O, Cory S, Gerondakis S, Webb E, Adams JM: Sequence of the murine and human cellular *myc* oncogenes and two modes of *myc* transcription resulting from chromosomal translocation in B lymphoid tumors. EMBO J 2:2375–2383, 1983.
97. Murphy W, Sarid J, Taub R, Vasicek T, Battey J, Lenoir G, Leder P: A translocated human c-myc oncogene is altered in a conserved coding sequence. Proc Natl Acad Sci

USA 83:2939–2943, 1986.
98. Rabbitts TH, Forster A, Hamlyn P, Baer R: Effect of somatic mutation within translocated c-*myc* genes in Burkitt's lymphoma. Nature 309:592–597, 1984.
99. Pelicci PG, Knowles DM, Magrath I, Dalla-Favera R: Chromosomal breakpoints and structural alterations of the c-*myc* locus differ in endemic and sporadic forms of Burkitt lymphoma. Proc Natl Acad Sci USA 83:2984–2988, 1986.
100. ar-Rushdi A, Nishikura K, Erikson J, Watt R, Rovera G, et al.: Differential expression of the translocated and the untranslocated c-*myc* oncogene in Burkitt lymphoma. Science 222:390–393, 1983.
101. Adams JM, Harris AW, Pinkert CA, Corcoran LM, Alexander WS, Cory S, Palmiter RD, Brinster RL: The c-*myc* oncogene driven by immunoglobulin enhancers induces lymphoid malignancy in transgenic mice. Nature 318:533–538, 1985.
102. Alexander WS, Schrader JW, Adams JM: Expression of the c-*myc* oncogene under control of an immunglobulin enhancer in Eµ-*myc* transgenic mice. Mol Cell Biol 7:1436–1444, 1987.
103. Langdon WY, Harris AW, Cory S, Adams JM: The c-*myc* oncogene perturbs B lymphocyte development in Eµ-*myc* transgenic mice. Cell 47:11–18, 1986.
104. Cory S, Harris AW, Langdon WY, Alexander WS, Corcoran LM, Palmiter RD, Pinkert CA, Brinster RL, Adams JM: The *myc* oncogene and lymphoid neoplasia: from translocations to transgenic mice. Haematology and Blood Transfusions 31:248–251, 1987.
105. Harris HW, Pinkert CA, Crawford M, Langdon WY, Brinster RL, Adams JW: The Eu-*myc* transgenic mouse: a model for high-incidence spontaneous lymphoma and leukemia of early B cells. J Exp Med 167:353–371, 1988.
106. Lombardi L, Newcomb EW, Dalla-Favera R: Pathogenesis of Burkitt lymphoma: expression of an activated c-*myc* oncogene cases the tumorigenic conversion of EBV infected human B lymphocytes. Cell 49:161–170, 1987.
107. De Jong D, Voetdijk BMH, Beverstock GC, van Ommen GJB, Willemze R, Klium PM: Activation of the c-*myc* oncogene on a precursor B-cell blast crisis of follicular lymphoma, presenting as composite lymphoma. N Engl J Med 318:1373–1378, 1988.
108. Gauwerky CE, Hoxie J, Nowell PC, Croce CM: Pre-B cell leukemia with a t(8;14) and a t(14;18) translocation is preceded by follicular lymphoma. Oncogene 2:431–435, 1988.
109. Yunis JJ, Frizzera G, Oken MM, McKenna J, Theologides A, Arnesen M: Multiple recurrent genomic defects in follicular lymphoma. A possible model for cancer. N Engl J Med 316:79–84, 1987.
110. Tsujimoto Y, Cossman J, Jaffe E, Croce CM: Involvement of the *bcl*-2 gene in human follicular lymphoma. Science 228:1440–1443, 1985.
111. Tsujimoto Y, Bashir MM, Givol I, Cossman J, Jaffe E, Croce CM: DNA rearrangements in human follicular lymphoma can involve the 5' or the 3' region of the *bcl*-2 gene. Proc Natl Acad Sci USA 84:1329–1331, 1987.
112. Galili N, Cleary ML, Sklar J: Human follicular lymphomas: identification of a second t(14;18) breakpoint cluster region. Haematology and Blood Transfusions 31:167–171, 1987.
113. Tsujimoto Y, Croce CM: Analysis of the structure, transcripts, and protein products of *bcl*-2, the gene involved in human follicular lymphoma. Proc Natl Acad Sci USA 83:5214–5218, 1986.
114. Cleary ML, Smith SD, Sklar J: Cloning and structural analysis of cDNAs for *bcl*-2 and a hybrid *bcl*-2/immunoglobulin transcript resulting from the t(14;18) translocation. Cell 47:19–28, 1986.
115. Tsujimoto Y, Ikegaki N, Croce CM: Characterization of the protein product of *bcl*-2, the gene involved in human follicular lymphoma. Oncogene 2:3–7, 1987.
116. Graninger WB, Seto M, Boutain B, Goldman P, Korsmeyer SJ: Expression of *bcl*-2 and *bcl*-2-Ig fusion transcripts in normal and neoplastic cells. J Clin Invest 80:1512–1515, 1987.
117. Ngan BY, Chen-Levy Z, Weiss LM, Warnke RA, Cleary ML: Expression in non-Hodgkin's lymphoma of the *bcl*-2 protein associated with the t(14;18) chromosomal translocation. N

Engl J Med 318:1738–1644, 1988.
118. Reed JC, Cuddy M, Slabiak T, Croce CM, Nowell PC: Oncogenic potential of *bcl*-2 demonstrated by gene transfer. Nature 336:259–261, 1988.
119. Lee MS, Blick MB, Trujillo JM, Butler JJ, Katz RL, McLaughlin P, Hagemeister FB, Velasquez WS, Goodacre A, Cork A, Gutterman JU, Cabanillas F: The gene located at chromosome 18 band q21 is rearranged in uncultured diffuse lymphomas as well as follicular lymphomas. Blood 70:90–95, 1987.
120. Aisenberg AC, Wilkes BM, Jacobson JO: The *bcl*-2 gene is rearranged in many diffuse B-cell lymphomas. Blood 71:969–972, 1988.
121. Weiss LM, Warnke RA, Sklar J, Cleary ML: Molecular analysis of the t(14;18) chromosomal translocation in malignant lymphomas. N Engl J Med 317:1185–1189, 1987.
122. Erikson J, Finan J, Tsujimoto Y, Nowell PC, Croce CM: The chromosome 14 breakpoint in neoplastic B cells with the t(11;14) translocation involves the immunoglobulin heavy chain locus. Proc Natl Acad Sci USA 81:4144–4148, 1984.
123. Moscovici C, Samarut J, Gazzolo L, Moscovici MG: Myeloid and erythroid neoplastic response to avian defective leukemia viruses in chickens and in quail. Virology 68:1172–181, 1981.
124. Rosson D, Reddy EP: Mechanism of activation of the *myb* oncogene in myeloid leukemias. Ann NY Acad Sci 551:219–231, 1987.
125. Radke K, Beug H, Kornfeld S, Graf T: Transformation of botherythroid and myeloid cells by E26, an avian leukemia virus that contains the *myb* gene. Cell 31:643–653, 1982.
126. Frykberg L, Palmieri S, Beug H, Graft T, Hayman MJ, Vennstrom B: Transforming capacities of avian erythroblastosis virus mutants deleted in their *erb* A or *erb* B oncogenes. Cell 32:227–238, 1983.
127. Blick, M, Westin N, Gutterman J, Wong-staal F, Gallo R, McCredie K, Keating M, Murphy E: Oncogene expression in human leukemia. Blood 64:1234–1239, 1984.
128. Evinger-Hodges MJ, Dicke KA, Cutterman JU, Blick M: Proto-oncogene expression in human normal bone marrow. Leukemia: 1:597–602, 1987.
129. Slamon DJ, deKernion JB, Verma IM, Cline MJ: Expression of cellular oncogenes in human malignancies. Science 224:256–262, 1986.
130. Slamon DJ, Boone TFC, Murdock DC, Keith DE, Press MF, Larson RA, Souza LM: Studies of the human c-*myb* gene and its product in human acute leukemias. Science 233:347–351, 1986.
131. Mavilio F, Sposi NM, Petrini M, Bottero N, Marinucci M, De Rossi G, Amadori S, Mandelli F, Peschle C: Expression of cellular oncogenes in primary cells from human acute leukemias. Proc Natl Acad Sci USA 83:4394–4398, 1986.
132. Weinstein Y, Ihle JN, Lavu S, Reddy EP: Truncation of the c-*myb* gene by a retroviral integration in an interleukin 3-dependent myeloid leukemia cell line. Proc Natl Acad Sci USA 83:5010–5014, 1986.
133. Gewirtz AM, Calabretta B: A c-*myb* antisense oligodeoxynucleotide inhibits normal human hematopoiesis in vitro. Science 242:1303–1306, 1988.
134. Rothberg PG, Erisman MD, Diehl RE, Rovigatti UG, Astrin SM: Structure and expression of the oncogene c-*myc* in malignancies. Mol Cell Biol 4:1096–1103, 1984.
135. Birnie GD, Warnock AM, Burns JH, Clark P: Expression of the *myc* gene locus in populations of leukocytes from leukemia patients and normal individuals. Leukemia Res 10:515–526, 1986.
136. Ferrari S, Narni F, Mars W, Kaczmarek L, Venturelli D, Anderson B, Calabretta B: Expression of growth-regulated genes in human acute leukemias. Cancer Res 46:5162–5166, 1986.
137. Butturini A, Shtivelman E, Canaani E, Gale RP: Oncogenes in human leukemias. Acta Haemat 78(Suppl 1):2–10, 1987.
138. Pinto A, Colletta G, Del Vecchiol L, Rosati R, et al.: C-*fos* oncogene expression in human hematopoietic malignancies is restricted to acute leukemias with monocytic phenotype and to subsets of B cell leukemias. Blood 70:1450–1457, 1987.

139. Smith LJ, McCullough EA, Benchimol S: Expression of the p53 oncogene in acute myeloblastic leukemia. J Exp Med 164:751–761, 1986.
140. Shen WPV, Alfrich TH, Venta-Perez G, Franza BR, Furth ME: Expression of normal and mutant *ras* proteins in human acute leukemia. Oncogene 1:157–165, 1987.
141. Roussel MF, Dull TJ, Rettenmier CW, Ralph P, Ullrich A, Sherr CJ: Transforming potential of the c-*fms* proton-oncogene (CSF-1 Receptor). Nature 325:549–552, 1987.
142. Lang RA, Metcalf D, Gough NM, Dunn AR, Gonda TJ: Expression of a hematopoieitic growth factor cDNA in a factor-dependent cell line results in autonomous growth and tumorigenicity. Cell 41:677–683, 1985.
143. Rambaldi A, Wakamiya N, Vellenga E, Horiguchi J, Warren MK, Kufe D, Griffin JD: Expression of the macrophage colony stimulating factor and c-*fms* genes in human acute myeloblastic leukemia cells. J Clin Invest 81:1030–1035, 1988.
144. Boehm TLJ, Hirth HP, Kornhuber B, Drahovsky D: Oncogene amplification and clonal evolution in acute leukemia. Eur J Cancer Clin Oncol 23:871–873, 1987.
145. Yokota J, Tsumestugo-Yokota Y, Battiflora H, Slamon D, Cline M: Alteration of *myc*, *myb*, and *ras*Ha proto-oncogenes in cancer are frequent and show clinical correlation. Science 231:261–2650, 1986.
146. Dalla Favera R, Wong-staal F, Gallo RC: Oncogene amplification in promyelocytic leukemia cell line HL-60 and primary leukemia cells of the same patient. Nature 299:61–63, 1982.
147. Alitalo K, Saksela K, Wingvist R, Alitalo R, Keski-Oja J, Laiho M, Ilvonen M, Knuutila S, de la Chapelle A: Acute myelogenous leukemia with c-*myc* amplification and double minute chromosome. Lancet 11:1035–1038, 1985.
148. Diaz MO, LeBeau MM, Harden A, Rowley JD: Trisomy 8 in human haematologic neoplasia and the c-*myc* and c-*mos* oncogenes. Leukemia Res 9:1437–1442, 1985.
149. Papas TS, Watson DK, Sacchi N, O'Brien S, Ascione R: The cellular ets genes: molecular probes in human neoplasia. Hematologica 72(Suppl 6):6–18, 1987.
150. Van den Berghe H, David G, Broeckart-Van Orshoven A, Louwagie K, Verwilghen R, Casteels-Van Daele M, Eggermont E, Eeckels R: A new chromosome anomaly in acute lymphoblastic leukemia (ALL). Hum Genet 46:173–180, 1979.
151. Arthur DC, Bloomfield CD, Linquist LL, Nesbit ME: Translocation 4;11 in acute lymphoblastic leukemia: clinical characteristics and prognostic significance. Blood 59:96–99, 1982.
152. Diaz MO, LeBeau MM, Pitha P, Rowley JD: Interferon and c-*ets*-1 genes in the translocation (9;11) (p22;q23) in human acute monocytic leukemia. Science 231:265–2657, 1986.
153. Rovigatti U, Watson DK, Yunis JJ: Amplification and rearrangement of Hu-*ets*-1 in leukemia and lymphoma with involvement of 11q23. Science 232:398–400, 1986.
154. Papas TS, Watson DK, Sacchi N, O'Brien S, Ascione R: The cellular ets genes: molecular biology and clinical amplifications in human leukemias. Cancer Invest 4:555–574, 1986.
155. Goyns MH, Hann IM, Stewart J, Gegonne A, Birnie GD: The c-*ets*-1 proto-oncogene is rearranged in some cases of acute lymphoblastic leukemia. Br J Cancer 56:611–613, 1987.
156. Woloschak KE, DeWald GW, Bahn RS, Kyle RA, Greipp PR, Ash RC: Amplification of RNA and DNA specific for *erb* B in unbalanced 1;7 chromosomal translocation associated with myelodysplastic syndrome. J Cell Biochem 32:23–34, 1986.
157. Mucenski ML, Taylor BA, Ihle JN, Hartley JW, Morse HC, Jenkins NA, Copeland NG: Identification of a common ecotropic viral integration site Evi-1 in the DNA of AKXD murine myeloid tumors. Mol Cell Biol 8:301–308, 1988.
158. Morishita K, Parker DS, Mucenski DML, Jenkins NA, Copeland NG, Ihle JN: Retroviral activation of a novel gene encoding a zinc finger protein i IL-3 dependent myeloid leukemia cell lines. Cell 54:831–840, 1988.
159. Bitter MA, Neilly ME, LeBeau MM, Pearson MG, Rowley JD: Rearrangements of chromosome 3 involving bands 3q21 and 3q16 are associated with normal or elevated platelet counts in acute nonlymphocytic leukemia. Blood 66:1362–1370, 1985.
160. Akahoshi M, Oshimi K, Mizoguchi H, Okada M, Enomoto Y, Watanabe Y: Myelopro-

liferative disorders terminating in acute megakaryoblastic leukemia with chromosome 3q16 abnormality. Cancer 60:2654–2661, 1987.
161. Rowley JD: Chromosome abnormalities in human leukemia. Ann Intern Med 14:17–39, 1980.
162. Pederson-Bjergaard J, Philip P: Cytogenetic characteristics of therapy-related acute non-lymphocytic leukemia, preleukemia, and acute myeloproliferative syndrome: correlation with clinical data for 61 consecutive cases. Br J Haematol 66:199–207, 1987.
163. LeBeau MM, Albain KS, Larson KS, Vardiman JW, Davis EM, Blough RR, Golomb HM, Rowley JD: Clinical and cytogenetic correlations in 63 patients with therapy-related myelodysplastic syndromes and acute nonlymphoblastic abnormalities of chromosomes 5 and 7. J Clin Oncol 4:325–345, 1986.
164. Pedersen-Bjergaard J, Janssen JWG, Lyons J, Philip P, Bartram CR: Point mutations of the *ras* proto-oncogenes and chromsome aberrations on acute nonlymphoblastic leukemia and preleukemia related to therapy with alkylating agents. Cancer Res 48:1812–1817, 1988.
165. Huebner K, Isobe M, Croce CM, Golde DW, Kaufman SE, Gasson JC: The human gene encoding GM-CSF is at 5q21-q32, the chromosome region deleted in the 5q- abnormality. Science 230:1282–1285, 1985.
166. Pettenati MJ, LeBeau MM, Lemons RS, Shima EA, kawasaki ES, Larson RA, Sherr CJ, Diaz MO, Rowley JD: Assignment of CSF-1 to 5q33.1: evidence for clustering of genes regulating hematopoiesis and their involvement on the deletion of the long arm of chromosome 5 in myeloid disorders. Proc Natl Acad Sci USA 84:2970–2974, 1987.
167. LeBeau MM, Epstein ND, O'Brien SJ, Nienhuis AW, Yang YC, Clark SC, Rowley JD: The interleukin 3 gene is located on human chromosome 5 and is deleted in myeloid leukemias with a deletion of 5q. Proc Natl Acad Sci USA 84:5913–5917, 1987.
168. Groffen J, Heisterkamp N, Spurr N, Dana S, Wasmuth JJ, Stephenson JR: Chromsomal localization of the human c-*fms* oncogene. Nucleic Acids Res 11:6331–6339, 1983.
169. Nienhuis AW, Bunn HF, Turner P, Gopal TV, Nash WG, O'Brien SJ, Sherr CJ: Expression of the human c-*fms* proto-oncogene in hematopoietic cells and its deletion in the 5q- syndrome. Cell 42:421–428, 1985.
170. Verbeek JS, van Heerikhuizen J, de Pauw BE, Haanen C, Bloemers HPJ, Van de Ven WJM: A hereditary abnormal c-*fms* proto-oncogene in a patient with acute lymphocytic leukemia and congenital hypothyroidism. Br J Haematol 61:135–138, 1985.
171. Yunis JJ, Rydell RE, Oken MM, Arnesen MA, Mayer MG, Lobell M: Refined chromosome analysis as an independent prognostic indicator in de novo myelodysplastic syndromes. Blood 67:1721–1730, 1986.
172. Kere J, Ruutu T, Lahtinen R, de la Chapelle A: Molecular characterization of chromosome 7 long arm deletions in myeloid disorders. Blood 70:1349–1353, 1987.
173. Carroll WL, Morgan R, Glader BE: Childhood bone marrow monosomy 7 syndrome: a familial disorders?. J Pediatr 107:578–580, 1985.
174. Larsen WE, Schimke N: Familial acute myelogenous leukemia with associated c-monosomy in two affected members. Cancer 38:841–845, 1976.
175. Testa JR, Kinnealey A, Rowley JD, Golde DW, Pooter D: Deletion of the long arm of chromosome 20 (del (20) (q11)) in myeloid disorders. Blood 52:868–877, 1978.
176. LeBeau MM, Westbrook CA, Diaz MO, Rowley JD: C-*src* is consistently conserved in the chromosomal deletion 20q observed in myeloid disorders. Proc Natl Acad Sci USA 82:6692–6696, 1985.
177. Quintrell N, Lebo R, Varmus H, Bishop JM, Pettenati MJ, LeBeau MM, Diaz MO, Rowley JD: Identification of a human gene (HCK) that encodes a protein-tyrosine kinase and is expressed in hematopoeitic cells. Mol Cell Biol 7:2267–2275, 1987.
178. Chilcote RR, Brown E, Rowley JD: Lymphoblastic leukemia with lymphomatous features associated with abnormalities of the short arm of chromosome 9. N Engl J Med 313:286–291, 1985.
179. Pollak C, Hagemeijer A: Abnormalities of the short arm of chromosome 9 with partial loss of material in hematological disorders. Leukemia 1:541–548, 1987.

180. Carroll AJ, Castleberry RP, Crist WM: Lack of association between abnormalities of the chromosome 9 short arm and either 'lymphomatous' features or T cell phenotype in childhood acute lymphocytic leukemia. Blood 69:735–738, 1987.
181. Trent JM, Olson S, Lawn RM: Chromosomal localization of human leukocyte, fibroblast, and immune interferon genes by means of in situ hybridization. Proc Natl Acad Sci USA 79:7809–7813, 1982.
182. Diaz MO, Ziemin S, LeBeau MM, Pitha P, Smith SD, Chilcote RR, Rowley JD: Homozygenous deletion of the alpha and beta1 interferon genes in human leukemia and derived cell lines. Proc Natl Acad Sci USA 85:5259–5263, 1988.
183. Moore RN, Larsen HS, Horohov DW, Rouse BT: Endogenous regulation of macrophage proliferative expansion by colony-stimulating factor-induced interferon. Science 223:178–181, 1984.
184. Zullo JN, Cochran BH, Huang AS, Stiles CD: Platelet-derived growth factor and double-stranded ribonucleic acids stimulate expression of the same genes in 3T3 cells. Cell 43: 793–800, 1985.
185. Rechavi G, Katzir N, Brok-Simoni F, Holtzman F, Gurfinkel N, Givol D, Ben-Bassay I, Ramot B: A search for *bcl*1, *bcl*2, and c-*myc* oncogene rearrangements in chronic lymphocytic leukemia. Leukemia 3:57–60, 1988.

11. Human retrovirus-associated malignancy

Michael S. McGrath and Valerie L. Ng

This two-part review will focus on clinical and molecular characteristics of non-Hodgkins lymphomas (NHLs) that arise in individuals infected with human leukemia viruses compared with NHLs associated with the acquired immunodeficiency syndrome (AIDS). Both classes of NHL arise in individuals infected with a retrovirus, a class of RNA virus that carried the enzyme reverse transcriptase [1].

Retroviral infection has been implicated in the pathogenesis of sarcomas, leukemias, and lymphomas, as well as immunodeficiency states in many different animal model systems. However, the search for a human retrovirus associated with human disease was unsuccessful until the discovery of T-cell growth factor (interleukin 2, Il-2) [2]. Inclusion of this growth factor in culture medium permitted, for the first time, the long-term in vitro culture of human T-lymphocytes, from which the recently discovered human retroviruses were first isolated.

The human retroviruses can be classified into two of the retrovirus subfamilies, leukemia viruses and lentiviruses. The human T-cell leukemia viruses, types I, II and V (HTLV-I, HTLV-II, and HTLV-V, respectively), belong to the oncovirus subfamily [3]. HTLV-I is believed to be the etiologic agent of adult T-cell leukemia/lymphoma (ATLL), and will be discussed in detail in the first part of this review. The association of HTLV-II with disease is unclear at present. There have only been four isolates of HTLV-II to date [4–7]; two of these isolates have been associated with an atypical form of hairy cell leukemia [4,5]. One isolate of HTLV-V has been obtained from a patient with a malignant cutaneous lymphoma [8]; the role of this virus in causing disease awaits further study. HTLV-I and HTLV-II are highly related viruses and share 50% nucleotide homology. The human immunodeficiency viruses (HIV-1, HIV-2), the etiologic agents of the acquired immunodeficiency syndrome (AIDS), are lentiviruses [9–12], and to date have not been shown to transform lymphocytes, although the frequency of high-grade B-cell lymphoma in HIV-infected individuals is substantially higher than in uninfected individuals. The following two sections will summarize characteristics of HTLV-I and its associated T-cell lymphomas and will present a clinical description and summary of possible transformation mechanisms resulting in

Benz, C. and Liu, E., (eds.), Oncogenes. © 1989 Kluwer Academic Publishers.
ISBN 0-7923-0237-0. All rights reserved.

the high-grade B-cell lymphomas that occur in individuals infected with HIV-1.

Evidence for HTLV-I involvement in adult T-cell leukemia/lymphoma

Clinical aspects of HTLV-I infection

The first cases of an unusual form of adult T-cell lymphoma/leukemia (ATLL) in Japanese patients were reported in 1977 [13]. Similar cases were reported within the next few years from the United States and the West Indies [14,15].

ATLL patients often presented with hypercalcemia, skin lesions (often indistinguishable from mycosis fungoides or Sezary's syndrome), elevated white blood cell counts, peripheral and retroperitoneal lymphadenopathy (notably with the absence of mediastinal masses), hepatosplenomegaly, multiple metabolic abnormalities (i.e., hyperuricemia), and opportunistic infections [14–16]. The circulating malignant T-cells, always of the helper (OKT4, Leu3) T-cell phenotype, were markedly pleomorphic and contained highly lobulated nuclei (flower cells) [17]. The clinical course of patients presenting with such symptoms proved to be rapidly fatal (usually within one year of diagnosis regardless of chemotherapeutic intervention) [14].

The above constellation of symptoms coupled with the rapidly fatal clinical course has now been categorized as acute ATLL. A condition known as chronic ATLL has been described, and is characterized by cutaneous involvement, lymphadenopathy, and 1%–10% circulating leukemic flower cells [17,18]. Chronic ATLL may be present for many years and may run an indolent clinical course, although transformation into acute ATLL can occur.

In vitro characteristics of HTLV-I

In vitro culture of malignant T-cells from patients with ATLL in the presence of Il-2 yielded the first isolates of HTLV-I [19–21]. The in vitro transmission of HTLV-I to uninfected cord blood lymphocytes was only accomplished through cocultivation of irradiated HTLV-I-infected cells with Il-2-stimulated uninfected cells. Transformed HTLV-I-infected cells that emerged after cocultivation were primarily of the helper T-cell phenotype similar to the original ATLL cells. Further evidence for the role of HTLV-I in ATLL was the observation that long-term in vitro cultures of malignant T-lymphocytes expressed HTLV-I viral antigens [19–21], even though the freshly isolated tissue/cells failed to express detectable HTLV-I antigens [22]. Although HTLV-I virions produced in in vitro cell lines have a characteristic type C morphology, free virus is poorly infectious and free virions have not been observed in vivo. The constant presence of antibodies to HTLV-I in the blood of infected individuals is thought to down-regulate expression of HTLV-I antigens in infected cells in vivo [23]. HTLV-I genes, although virtually non-expressed in vivo are present in ATLL freshly isolated tumor tissue/cells as integrated proviral DNA [24,25].

Epidemiology of HTLV-I infection

The establishment of HTLV-I-producing cell lines allowed the development of serological assays capable of detecting human anti-HTLV-I antibodies. Individuals who had been exposed to the virus tested positive in these assays [26–28], and virtually all ATLL patients had antibodies to HTLV-I [29,30]. Other studies revealed a high seroprevalence of antibodies to HTLV-I in Southern Japan (an incidence ranging from 6%–26%), the Caribbean, parts of Africa, and the southeastern United States [31], all areas that corresponded to endemic areas of ATLL.

Seroepidemiology studies have identified many healthy HTLV-I seropositive individuals (carriers). In one Japanese study, HTLV-I seroprevalence was higher in women than in men; yet the prevalence of ATLL was highest in men [32]. The basis for this discrepancy is unclear. Current predictions estimate the highest risk of ATLL following HTLV-I infection at 2.04 patients annually per 1000 seropositive adults in men aged 60–69 years [32]. The morbidity risk for women in the same age group is only 0.74 per 1000 seropositive cases [32]. The overall lifetime risk of developing ATLL following HTLV-I infection is estimated to be 1 in 20 over 50 years [33]: This long latency period may explain why no cases of transfusion-associated ATLL have been observed to date.

There have been several cases of Japanese ATLL where patients presented with classical symptoms yet lacked serological evidence of infection with HTLV-I; cultivated tumor cells failed to express HTLV-I antigens, and molecular hybridization studies did not detect integrated provirus [16,34]. Furthermore, there was no serological evidence of HTLV-I infection in closely related family members. Similar findings of ATLL not associated with evidence of HTLV-I infection have been reported for some patients with non-Hodgkin's lymphoma in Jamaica [35]. With these few exceptions, the majority of ATLL cases described to date have been associated with HTLV-I infection. However, the description of these few cases of ATLL *not* associated with HTLV-I infection has led one group of authors to conclude that the role of HTLV-I in ATLL is similar to the role of Epstein–Barr virus in Burkitt's lymphoma—the virus may be present, but its exact role in pathogenesis is unclear [16,34].

Transmission of HTLV-I

HTLV-I is transmitted by blood transfusion, sexual intercourse (predominantly male-to-female transmission), and breast-feeding [36–38]. Because free viral particles have virtually never been seen in vivo [23], virus infection occurs by transmission of living infected cells, which can be present in blood products containing cellular material, in breast milk, and in semen. The observation that HTLV-I is primarily a cell-associated virus is supported by the lack of virus transmission following transfusion of cell-free blood products (i.e., fresh plasma) [36]. In contrast, transfusion of red cells or whole blood from seropositive donors resulted in a 65% seroconversion rate in the recipients.

The prevalence of HTLV-I seropositivity rises with age, suggesting that the primary mode of infection is by sexual intercourse [37]. Breast-feeding is believed to be the route by which infants and young children become infected [38]. These modes of virus transmission explain the high familial incidence of HTLV-I infection.

The molecular biology of HTLV-I

In attempting to define the mechanism(s) by which HTLV-I is capable of causing ATLL, a concentrated effort has been directed at understanding the molecular biology of HTLV-I. The genomic structure and virally encoded proteins of HTLV-I are depicted in figure 1. The virus consists of a 9-kilobase RNA genome that encodes the three structural genes necessary for virus replication. The *gag* gene specifies the information for the virion core proteins, p19, p24, and p15. The *pol* gene encodes the information for the virion reverse transcriptase, a magnesium-dependent RNA-dependent DNA polymerase. The *env* gene encodes the viral envelope proteins, gp46 and p20E.

As with all other animal retroviruses, HTLV-I proteins are synthesized first as precursor polyproteins, which are then cleaved to yield the mature viral proteins [39]. The protease responsible for cleaving the *gag* gene precursor polyprotein, Pr53, is a virally encoded protein (p27) that is translated

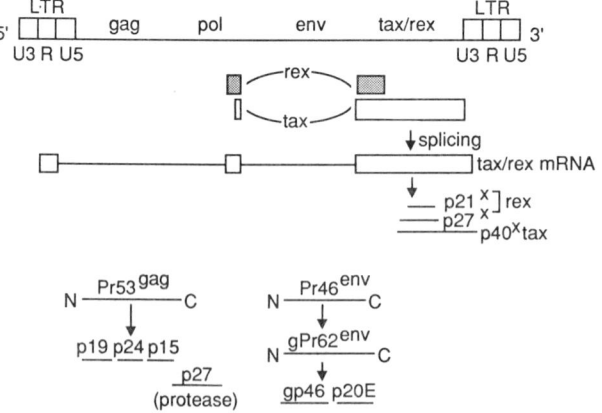

Figure 1. The genomic structure and viral proteins of HTLV-I. Abbreviations used: LTR: long terminal repeat; gag: group antigens; pol: polymerase; env: envelope; tax: transactivator; rex: regulator of expression of virion proteins; p: protein; Pr: precursor polyprotein; gp: glycoprotein; gPr: glycosylated precursor polyprotein; E: envelope; N: N-terminus; C: C-terminus.

from a different reading frame from a gene overlapping the 3' end of the *gag* gene [40,41]. The protease responsible for cleavage of the envelope precursor polyprotein, gp62, is believed to be of cellular origin. Processing of the *pol* gene product has not been studied.

Although HTLV-I is classified as an oncovirus because of its ability to cause cell transformation, it does not contain an oncogene derived from cellular sequences. Instead, it contains an extra gene (*tax*, formerly known as pX or *lor*), different forms of which are shared by all members of the HTLV family (i.e., HTLV-I, HTLV-II, bovine leukosis virus, and simian T-cell leukemia virus, type I), that influences virus replication and may be involved in transformation [42,43]. The *tax* gene is an additional coding region at the 3' end of the viral genome and encodes information for at least three different gene products. These proteins are encoded by mRNAs formed through double-splicing events involving regions of the LTR and *pol* genes as well as the *tax* gene. $p40^x$ is the *tax* gene product, and the *rex* (regulator of expression, virion proteins) gene encodes two forms of protein, $p27^x$ and $p21^x$.

What are the roles of the *tax/rex* gene products? The $p40^x$ protein has a relatively short half-life (12 minutes) [44] and functions as a transactivator by interacting with the LTR in a *trans* fashion to increase transcription of the integrated viral genome [42]. $p27^x$ and $p21^x$ differ only in their N-terminal amino acids, and are rich in proline (21%) and serine (15%) residues. In addition, $p27^x$ is a phosphoprotein, whose N-terminus contains 19 amino acids rich in basic residues derived from the extreme 3' region of the *pol* gene. It has been suggested that $p27^x$ may have an affinity for nucleic acids due to the contribution of *pol*-gene-derived sequences, as well as the high content of basic amino acide residues [45]. $p27^x$ is required for efficient expression of *gag* gene mRNA and synthesis of *gag* gene proteins [46], and may be necessary for optimal $p40^x$-mediated transactivation [47]. $p40^x$ and $p27^x$ have been localized to the nucleus of infected cells [44,48,49], a subcellular location consistent with the hypothesis that these proteins interact with nucleic acids and have a regulatory role in viral replication. $p21^x$ is found in the cytoplasm of infected cells; its function is unknown.

An HTLV-II protein ($p38^x$) with functions similar to those of the HTLV-I $p40^x$ has been described [43]. The *tax* genes of HTLV-I (tax_1) and HTLV-II (tax_2) are approximately 75% homologous (as compared to an overall 50% nucleotide homology between HTLV-I and HTLV-II) [43].

Mechanisms of transformation by HTLV-I

The exact mechanism(s) by which HTLV-I transforms cells is not known. However, many different mechanism have been proposed, and will be discussed here.

In many animal retrovirus systems, a preferred site of integration in the host genome next to a cellular gene (with resultant overproduction of the cellular gene product) is thought to be the mechanism by which cellular transformation occurs. For example, avian leukosis virus is thought to induce B-cell lymphomas in chickens by integrating near and activating the host cellular c-*myc* gene [50]. Overproduction of this cellular protein would then be instrumental in cell transformation. Molecular studies of fresh and cultured HTLV-I-infected tumor cells from ATLL patients demonstrated that tumor cells from an individual patient represented a clonal population of T-cells, in which the HTLV-I genome was integrated at only one location in the host genome. Comparison of integration sites in tumor cells from different ATLL patients, however, showed no consistent site of retroviral integration [51]. Thus, a preferred integration site with activation of a specific cellular oncogene does not appear to be the mechanism of transformation in HTLV-I-associated ATLL.

The *tax* gene product, particularly $p40^x$, is currently thought to be the most likely candidate for inducing HTLV-I-associated transformation. A number of mechanisms by which this protein may influence cell transformation have been proposed.

Interleukin-2 (Il-2) is a cellular gene product that plays an important regulatory role in T-cell growth [52]. It has been well documented that HTLV-I-infected nonleukemic cells constitutively express elevated levels of Il-2 and the Il-2 receptor, and that the in vitro proliferation of these cells was dependent on Il-2. This response to exogenous Il-2 led to the proposal of an autocrine or paracrine mechanism for T-cell growth as an early event in HTLV-I-associated leukemogenesis [53,54]. However, some clonal populations of leukemic T-cells derived from ATLL patients were not uniformly dependent on exogenous Il-2 for continued proliferation, even though elevated expression of the Il-2 receptor was still observed in all leukemic clones [53].

More recently, the *tax* gene product, $p40^x$, was shown to *trans*-activate the Il-2 promoter, thereby inducing increased expression of Il-2 receptor and Il-2 [54]. The addition of mitogenic stimuli (specifically phytohemagglutinin *and* phorbol 12-myristate 13-acetate) further increased the level of Il-2 promoter activity [54]. More specifically, the $p40^x$ protein increased binding of a cellular transcription factor found in stimulated T-cells, NF-kB, which in turn increased expression of the IL-2 receptor alpha chain [55]. This finding lends further support to the importance of mitogenic stimuli in the early events of HTLV-I-associated leukemogenesis.

The envelope glycoproteins may also play a role in HTLV-I-associated leukemogenesis. Antibody directed against the N-terminus of human Il-2 (the portion of Il-2 that mediates binding to the Il-2 beta receptor) also cross-reacts with a homologous region of the HTLV-I envelope glycoproteins, gp46 and gp62 [56]. This finding suggests that the HTLV-I envelope glycoproteins may directly interact with the Il-2 receptor to transmit differentiation or mitogenic signals [56].

HTLV-I-infected cells also produce a variety of cytokines that may be implicated in inducing continued cellular proliferation. Primary leukemic T-cells obtained from some ATLL patients were shown to produce high levels of interleukin 1 (Il-1), a cytokine that alters Il-2 expression and may partially explain why leukemic cells have increased expression of the Il-2 receptor [57]. In addition, Il-1 activates osteoclasts, which may explain why hypercalcemia and osteolytic bone lesions are observed in acute ATLL [57]. It should be mentioned that variable expression of Il-1 is observed in long-term cultured ATLL leukemic T-cells, and that the presence of antibodies to Il-1 does not inhibit the spontaneous increase of Il-2 receptors in leukemic T-cells placed in short-term culture. Thus, it is unlikely that Il-1 is directly responsible for the constitutive elevated expression of elevated Il-2 receptor.

Lastly, one group has found that the leukemic B-cells, that were obtained from two Jamaican chronic lymphocytic leukemia patients with high HTLV-I antibody titers produced immunoglobulins (after fusion to a human B-lymphoblastoid cell line) that selectively recognized HTLV-I gp62 and reacted only with HTLV-I infected cells [58]. They concluded that the leukemic B-cells were derived from HTLV-I antigen-committed B-cells that had undergone malignant transformation, and suggested that HTLV-I might play an indirect role in B-cell leukemogenesis.

HIV-1-associated lymphomas

This section will address the AIDS-associated lymphomas, including a description of clinical presentation, and summarize mechanisms proposed to explain the genesis of this class of high-grade B-cell lymphoma. Unlike HTLV-I-associated T-cell malignancies, there has been no direct causal link between HIV-1 and the AIDS-associated B-cell lymphomas. However, there is evidence to suggest that HIV-1 may play several indirect roles in this disease process.

Epidemiology and clinical characteristics of AIDS-associated NHL

Early on in the AIDS epidemic, high-grade non-Hodgkin's lymphoma began to appear in individuals at risk for the development of AIDS. The first article, describing a series of homosexual men with high-grade B-cell lymphoma, was published in 1984 prior to the widespread use of AIDS antibody testing [59]. The type of lymphomas occurring in HIV-1-infected individuals has not changed significantly from that described in this original report; however, the frequency of this disease has increased [60,61].

The lymphomas that have developed in HIV-1-infected individuals have primarily been of intermediate- or high-grade histology and are equally divided into Burkitt's-like small noncleaved, immunoblastic, and large diffuse histiocytic categories. However, all these lymphomas have behaved biologically as high-grade aggressive NHL, and there has been little progress in the develop-

Table 1. Clinical features of AIDS-associated non-Hodgkin's lymphomas

	Reporting Center						
	Multi-Center (59)	USC (62)	Memorial SKI (63)	UCSF (64)	NYU (65)	Pac Med Center (66)	Total (%)
Number of patients	90	63	52	84	20	18	327(100%)
Pathologic classification [67]							
High-grade	56	56	33	65	20	8	238(73%)
Intermediate-grade	26	7	16	19		10	78(24%)
Low-grade	6		3				9(3%)
Chemotherapy response							
Complete	35/66	10/19	17/30	32/59	7/16	4/11	105/201(52%)
Partial/none	31/66	9/19	13/30	27/59	9/16	7/11	96/201(48%)
Survival of CR's							
% NED > 6 mo.	11/35	6/10	9/17	24/31	6/7	4/4	60/104(58%)

Abbreviations:
CR   = Complete response
NED = No evidence of disease

ment of successful therapy. The reports and summaries of clinical experiences with this disease are summarized in table 1.

Several clinical features are characteristic of AIDS-associated lymphomas: 1) there is a 5- to 20-fold increase in the expected frequency of bone marrow and central nervous system involvement, with the frequent occurrence of primary CNS lymphoma; 2) at least one third of patients present with tumors in atypical extranodal sites such as rectum, liver, mouth, heart, and lung; 3) almost three quarters of patients present with stage IV disease, with 'B symptoms' including fever, night sweats, and/or weight loss (however, these symptoms may be associated with the underlying HIV-1-infection); 4) approximately one third of AIDS NHL patients present with lymphoma as their initial manifestation of HIV-1-infection, one third had pre-existing generalized lymphadenopathy, and approximately another one third had a diagnosis of AIDS prior to the development of lymphoma; and 5) the median survival of NHL patients with pre-existing AIDS is approximately two months, compared with a median survival of eight months for all those patients without a pre-existing AIDS diagnosis [64].

Molecular characterization of AIDS-associated NHL

Very little is known about the molecular characteristics of the AIDS-associated lymphomas. Tumor cells are primarily of B-cell origin, and the majority of tumors express cell-surface IgM [68,69]. Immunoglobulin gene rearrangement analyses have only been performed on a few cases of AIDS-associated lymphoma, and suggest that they are primarily monoclonal in origin [70]. More recent studies, however, found that more than 50% of AIDS-associated immunoblastic lymphomas were polyclonal expansions of B-lymphocytes (M.S. McGrath and T. Meeker, unpublished observations). Other studies found that the majority of monoclonal AIDS-associated lymphomas examined for chromosomal translocations contained rearranged c-*myc* genes [70–74] similar to those described in African Burkitt's lymphoma. HIV genes were not present within tumor cells probed by viral molecular hybridization techniques [75], and EBV genomes were present in the DNA of only one third of the lymphomas tested [64,75]. Overall, much more information will be required to allow full molecular characterization of the AIDS-associated lymphomas.

Pathogenesis of the AIDS-related lymphomas

Three broad hypotheses concerning mechanisms by which B-cells might be transformed in association with HIV-1 infection are under investigation. They are 1) HIV-1-induced immunosuppression allows outgrowth of EBV-infected and immortalized B-cells; 2) chromosomal translocation with resultant oncogene activation occurs frequently in lymphomas of HIV-1-infected individuals; and 3) chronic viral antigenic/mitogenic stimulation leads to B-cell overproliferation with the ultimate appearance of lymphoma. These hypotheses will be discussed in the following sections.

HIV-1-induced immunosuppression allows outgrowth of EBV-infected and immortalized B-cells. Immunosuppression secondary to infection with HIV-1 has been well documented [76], and the longer an individual has been infected with HIV-1 the more immunosuppressed he becomes. Immunosuppression in transplant patients has been known for many years to be associated with an increased incidence of NHL [77]. The lymphomas that occur in immunosuppressed transplant patients are primarily associated with Epstein–Barr virus infection [78,79]. Mechanistically, immunosuppression with agents such as steroids and cyclosporin-A are thought to decrease the T-cell control of the polyclonal population of EBV-infected B-lymphocytes. With the removal of T-cell control, the population of polyclonal EBV-infected and immortalized B-cells proliferates with the ultimate monoclonal outgrowth of a highly aggressive lymphoma. EBV infection has also been associated with development of Burkitt's lymphoma in Africa [80,81], although EBV has been found less frequently in the non-AIDS-associated Burkitt's lymphoma in the United States [82,83]. However, it has been difficult to determine whether EBV can initiate B-cell transformation in vivo because Epstein–Barr virus can infect any B-lymphocyte that expresses the complement receptor [84].

Although no large molecular studies have been performed on the AIDS-associated lymphomas, current data indicate that only 30% of these lymphomas contain EBV DNA [64,75]. The role that EBV plays in this 30% of tumors, however, is not clear. A detailed analysis of one case where multiple lymph nodes containing the same clonal B-cell tumor (as assessed by immunoglobulin gene rearrangement analysis) were examined showed EBV to be present in only one of two separate nodes analyzed [85,86]. Thus, although there are increased numbers of circulating B-lymphocytes containing EBV DNA in AIDS patients [87], the role that EBV plays as a direct transforming agent resulting in AIDS lymphomas in vivo is still in question.

Although EBV does not appear to play a major role in the AIDS-associated lymphomas, HIV-1-mediated removal of T-lymphocytes with subsequent immunosuppression may be an important cofactor for lymphoma development. Further studies analyzing control of B-cell proliferation and differentiation in HIV-1-infected individuals will be required to determine the cells and/or factors important in controlling this overstimulated class of cells.

Chromosomal translocation with oncogene activation. Peripheral blood lymphocytes isolated from HIV-1-infected individuals proliferate and differentiate at more than a ten-fold higher rate than B-cells isolated from normal individuals [87,88]. This chronic B-cell stimulation could promote an increased frequency of nonlethal chromosomal mutations that could sometimes occur in DNA regions containing cellular oncogenes. One report demonstrated that c-*myc* translocations can be found in the majority of AIDS-associated NHL [70], and that the 8:14 translocations at the chromosomal break point occurred within the 5' portion of the c-*myc* gene. (This type of chromosomal translocation is discussed in detail elsewhere in this volume and will not be further discussed here). Although c-*myc* translocation with chronic expression of the c-*myc* gene product is an attractive model to explain how B-cells may become transformed in HIV-1-infected individuals, other investigators have found a much lower frequency of c-*myc* translocations than that originally reported [85,89]. Further analysis of other oncogenes in all classes of AIDS-associated lymphoma will be required before the role that oncogene activation might play in this disease process can be defined.

Chronic antigenic/mitogenic stimulation leads to B-lymphocyte overproliferation. Individuals infected with HIV-1 have marked B-lymphocyte function abnormalities [87,88]. The peripheral blood B-lymphocytes from HIV-1-infected individuals display a ten-fold increase in spontaneous proliferation and immunoglobulin secretion. Monoclonal and oligoclonal paraproteins are present in the serum of 3%–15% of AIDS patients [90,91]. B-cell abnormalities are not corrected by the addition of normal helper T-lymphocytes, suggesting that B-lymphocytes from HIV-1-infected individuals have either intrinsic defects or are responding to some proliferative stimulus present in vivo.

Dalla-Favera and colleagues [70] reported the finding of oligoclonal B-cell populations in lymph nodes of individuals prior to the development of monoclonal B-cell malignancies. They hypothesized that multiple clonal expansions of B-lymphocytes coupled with a chromosomal translocation in the c-*myc* gene locus occurred in lymph nodes of some AIDS patients, ultimately allowing the emergence of a truly transformed B-lymphocyte. They speculated that EBV or HIV-1 gene products [92], both of which cause polyclonal B-cell activation, may have been responsible for the polyclonal B-cell proliferation prior to the emergence of a monoclonal transformed B-cell population.

Because HIV-1 was reported to cause polyclonal B-cell activation [92], and continuous HIV-1 replication occurs in infected individuals, we studied a series of HIV-1-infected individuals with paraproteinemias to ask whether those paraproteins represented immunoglobulins produced by premalignant B-cell clones. The question asked was whether HIV-1-infected individuals with paraproteins were predisposed to the development of lymphomas, with the lymphoma arising from the paraprotein-producing B-cell population.

Over the past several years, 11 HIV-1-infected individuals with oligoclonal and monoclonal paraproteins were identified. During a 2- to 3-year period of observation, only one of these individuals developed a high-grade B-cell lymphoma, and during the four months prior to the diagnosis of lymphoma the patient's paraprotein disappeared [93]. Thus none of the HIV-1-infected individuals with paraproteinemias (some as high as 40 gm/L) developed lymphomas during the time period described by Dalla-Favera and coworkers [70] between the presence of oligoclonal B-cells and the development of high-grade B-cell lymphoma.

One characteristic of individuals with paraproteinemias is that their anti-HIV-1 antibody titer is extraordinarily high [90,94]. We characterized one paraprotein to determine whether it was directed against HIV-1 determinants, was specific for an individual HIV-1 protein, or represented a monoclonal antibody. We also evaluated the patient's bone marrow (plasma cells 15%–20% of all cellular elements) to determine whether a monoclonal B-cell population producing this paraprotein was present [94].

Serum from this patient with AIDS-related complex contained 80 gm/L globulin, of which 40 gm/L was contained within an IgG kappa paraprotein. The purified paraprotein had two light chain species, reacted with both *gag* and *pol* HIV-1 gene products, and contained the majority of anti-HIV-1 antibody reactivity present in the serum. Immunoglobulin gene rearrangement analysis failed to reveal a clonal population of plasma cells in this patient's bone marrow. These data clearly demonstrated that this paraprotein was polyclonal in origin. We have since evaluated sera from an additional four HIV-1-infected individuals containing paraproteins, all with high anti-HIV-1 antibody titers (ranging from 1:10,000 to 1:500,000) associated with the purified paraproteins. All of these paraproteins were similarly polyclonal in origin. However, these paraproteins that occur in the sera of HIV-infected individuals have not been associated with an increased incidence of myeloma or lymphoma.

Retroviral proteins may have a role in AIDS-associated lymphomagenesis. In experimental systems, chronic antigenic stimulation has been implicated as a cause of B-cell transformation. For example, the H-2a4bp/wts mouse strain develops high-grade B-cell lymphomas after hyperimmunization with sheep red blood cells (SRBC). Analysis of the lymphoma surface immunoglobulins showed them to be directed against SRBC determinants [95]. Similarly, B-cell lymphomas develop spontaneously in BALB/c mice in association with an endogenous retrovirus and display cell surface IgM directed against retroviral gene products [96]. Although the sequence of events leading to human B-cell transformation in vivo is most likely complex, it is plausible that transformation in some cases can be initiated through chronic antigenic stimulation. However, the presence of anti-HIV-1 determinants on B-cell lymphomas from AIDS patients has not been demonstrated to date.

HIV-1 antigens can cause B-cell proliferation either in a mitogenic or antigen-specific manner [97,98], and anti-HIV-1 antibody titers greater than 1:100,000 are commonly encountered in HIV-1-infected individuals [90]. The finding that the macrophage is a principal target for HIV-1 infection [99] suggests that this population of HIV-1 antigen-presenting cells may serve as a potent stimulus for HIV-1-responsive B-lymphocytes in vivo. No data are currently available concerning the antigenic specificity of the immunoglobulins expressed by AIDS-associated lymphomas.

Alternatively, retroviral-mediated antigenic stimulation could be caused by another retrovirus present in HIV-1-infected individuals. For example, some HIV-1-infected individuals are co-infected with the human T-lymphotropic viruses (HTLV-I, HTLV-II). [100]. HTLV-I has been implicated as the transforming agent, or at least as a predisposing agent, to abnormal T-cell proliferation in HIV-1-infected individuals [101], and in B-cell transformation in a subpopulation of patients infected with HTLV-I alone [58].

Because HTLV-I is a noncytopathic virus, transformation of B-cell mediated through antigenic stimulation can be envisioned to occur through two possible mechanisms. Figure 2a depicts how initiation of the transformation cascade could occur with a cell making its own set of antigens. In this situation, the retrovirus-infected transformed cell would express an immunospecific receptor for a retrovirus determinant, resulting in continuous rounds of proliferation not dissimilar to the Il-2-mediated autocrine model described earlier [53]. Alternatively, an antigen-presenting accessory cell (e.g., macrophage) chronically producing retroviral antigens could cause antigenic

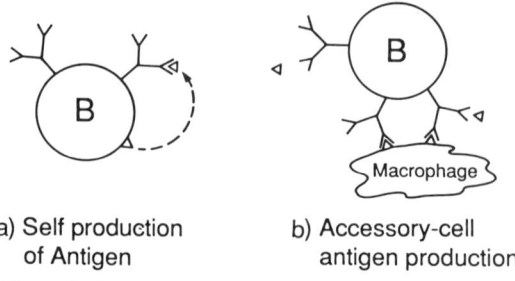

a) Self production of Antigen   b) Accessory-cell antigen production

Figure 2. Retroviral antigen-driven lymphomagenesis.

stimulation indirectly, and responding B-lymphocytes would be unable to escape the chronic stimulus produced by those infected accessory cells (figure 2b). This model does not exclude any of the previously discussed hypotheses of HIV-1-associated B-cell transformation. After antigen-specific activation, any non-lethal genetic mutation, including those described previously, could contribute to in vivo lymphomagenesis. Clearly, more basic investigation of the AIDS-associated lymphomas will be required in order to elucidate all of the factors involved in this disease process.

References

1. Varmus H: Retroviruses. Science 24:1427–1435, 1988.
2. Morgan DA, Ruscetti RW, Gallo RC: Selective in vitro growth of T-lymphocytes from normal human bone marrow. Science 193:17–18, 1976.
3. Sagata N, Yasunaga T, Tsuzuku-Kawamura J, et al.: Complete nucleotide sequence of the genome of bovine leukemia virus: It evolutionary relationship to other retroviruses. Proc Natl Acad Sci USA 82:677–681, 1985.
4. Kalyanaraman VS, Sarngadharan MG, Robert-Guroff M, et al.: A new subtype of human T-cell leukemia virus (HTLV-II) associated with a T-cell variant of hairy cell leukemia. Science 218:571–573, 1982.
5. Rosenblatt JD, Golde DW, Wachsman W, et al.: A second isolate of HTLV-II associated with atypical hairy-cell leukemia. N Engl J Med 315:372–377, 1986.
6. Hahn BH, Popovic M, Kalyanaraman VS, et al.: Detection and characterization of an HTLV-II provirus in a patient with AIDS. In: Gottlieb MS, Groopman JE (eds): Acquired Immune Deficiency Syndrome. New York, Liss, 1984 p 73.
7. Kalyanaraman VS, Narayanan P, Feorino P, et al.: Isolation and characterization of a human T-cell leukemia virus type II from a hemophilia-A patient with pancytopenia. EMBO J 4:1455, 1985.
8. Manzari V, Gismondi A, Barillari G, et al.: HTLV-V: A new human retrovirus isolated in a Tac-negative T-cell lymphoma/leukemia. Science 238:1581–1583, 1987.
9. Barre-Sinoussi F, Chermann JC, Rey F, et al.: Isolation of a T-lymphotropic retrovirus from a patient at risk for Acquired Immune Deficiency Syndrome (AIDS). Science 22:868–871, 1983.
10. Levy JA, Hoffman AD, Kramer SM, et al.: Isolation of lymphocytopathic retroviruses from San Francisco patients with AIDS. Science 25:84–842, 1984.
11. Gallo RC, Salahuddin SZ, Popovic M, et al.: Frequent detection and isolation of cytopathic retroviruses (HTLV-III) from patients with AIDS and at risk for AIDS. Science 224: 50–52, 1984.
12. Haase AT: Pathogenesis of lentivirus infections. Nature 322:130–136, 1986.
13. Uchiyama T, Yodoi J, Sagawa K, et al.: Adult T-cell leukemia: clinical and hematologic features of 16 cases. Blood 5:481–492, 1977.
14. Bunn PA, Schechter GP, Jaffe E, et al.: Clinical course of retrovirus-associated adult T-cell lymphoma in the United States. N Engl J Med 39:257–264, 1983.
15. Catovsky D, Graves MF, Rose M, et al.: Adult T-cell lymphoma-leukemia in Blacks from the West Indies. Lancet i:639–643, 1982.
16. Shimoyama M, Kagami Y, Shimotohno K, et al.: Adult T-cell leukemia/lymphoma not associated with human T-cell leukemia virus type I. Proc Natl Acad Sci USA 83:4524–4528, 1986.
17. Amagasaki T, Momita S, Suzuyama J, et al.: Detection of adult T-cell leukemia-associated antigen in T-cell malignancies in the Nagasaki district of Japan. Cancer 54:274–281, 1984.
18. Kinoshita K, Amagasaki T, Ikeda S, et al.: Preleukemic state of adult T-cell leukemia:

abnormal T-lymphocytosis induced by human adult T-cell leukemia-lymphoma virus. Blood 66:120–127, 1985.
19. Miyoshi I, Kubonishi I, Yoshimoto S, et al.: Type C virus particles in a cord T-cell line derived by co-cultivating normal human cord leukocytes and human leukemic T-cells. Nature 296:770–771, 1981.
20. Poiesz BJ, Ruscetti FW, Gazdar AF, et al.: Detection and isolation to type C retrovirus particles from fresh and cultured lymphocytes of a patient with cutaneous T-cell lymphoma. Proc Natl Acad Sci USA 77:7415–7419, 1980.
21. Popovic M, Sarin PS, Robert-Guroff M, et al.: Isolation and transmission of human retrovirus (human T-cell leukemia virus). Science 219:856–859, 1983.
22. Ishibashi K, Hanada S, Hashimoto S: Expression of HTLV-I in serum of HTLV-I-related subjects and the early detection of overt ATL in HTLV-I carriers. J Immunol 139:159–1513, 1987.
23. Yoshida M: Expression of the HTLV-I genome and its association with a unique T-cell malignancy. Biochim Biophys Acta 97:145–161, 1987.
24. Yoshida M, Miyoshi I, Hinuma Y: Isolation and characterization of retrovirus from cell lines of human adult T-cell leukemia and its implication in the disease. Proc Natl Acad Sci USA 79:231–235, 1982.
25. Wong-Staal F, Hahn B, Manzari V, et al.: A survey of human leukaemias for sequences of a human retrovirus, HTLV. Nature 32:626–628, 1983.
26. Halbert SP, Poiesz B, Friedman-Kien AE, et al.: Quantitative estimation by a standardized enzyme-linked immunosorbent assay of human T-cell lymphotropic virus type I antibodies in adult T-cell leukemia and acquired immune deficiency syndrome. J Clin Microbiol 23:212–216, 1986.
27. Saxinger C, Gallo RC: Methods in laboratory investigation. Application of the indirect enzyme-linked immunosorbent assay microtest to the detection and surveillance of human T-cell leukemia-lymphoma virus. Lab Invest 49:371–377, 1983.
28. White PMB: Comparison of assays for antibody to HTLV-I. J Clin Path 41:70–72, 1988.
29. Robert-Guroff M, Nakao Y, Notake K, et al.: Natural antibodies to human retrovirus HTLV in a cluster of Japanese patients with adult T cell leukemia. Science 215:975–978, 1982.
30. Kalyanaraman VS, Sarngadharan MG, Nakao Y, et al.: Natural antibodies to the structural core protein (p24) of the human T-cell leukemia (lymphoma) retrovirus found in sera of leukemia patients in Japan. Proc Natl Acad Sci USA 79:1653–1657, 1982.
31. Wong-Staal F, Gallo RC: The family of human T-lymphotropic leukemia viruses: HTLV-I as the cause of adult T cell leukemia and HTLV-III as the cause of acquired immunodeficiency syndrome. Blood 65:253–263, 1985.
32. Kondo T, Kono H, Nonaka H, et al.: Risk of adult T-cell leukemia/lymphoma in HTLV-I carriers. Lancet ii:159, 1987.
33. Editorial. HTLV-I comes of age. Lancet i:217–219, 1988.
34. Shimoyama M, Abe T, Miyamoto K, et al.: Chromosome aberrations and clinical features of adult T cell leukemia-lymphoma not associated with human T cell leukemia virus type I. Blood 69:984–989, 1987.
35. Gibbs WN, Lofters WS, Campbell M, et al.: Non-Hodgkin lymphoma in Jamaica and its relation to adult T-cell leukemia-lymphoma. Ann Int Med 16:361–368, 1987.
36. Sato H, Okochi K: Transmission of human T-cell leukemia virus (HTLV-I) by blood transfusion: demonstration of proviral DNA in recipients' blood lymphocytes. Int J Cancer 37:395–4, 1986.
37. Tajima K, Tominaga S, Suchi T, et al.: Epidemiological analysis of the distribution of antibody to adult T-cell leukemia-virus-associated antigen: Possible horizontal transmission of adult T-cell leukemia virus. Gann 73:893–91, 1982.
38. Hino S, Sugiyama H, Doi H, et al.: Breaking the cycle of HTLV-I transmission via carrier mother's milk. Lancet ii:158–159, 1987.
39. Hattori S, Kiyokawa T, Imagawa K-I, et al.: Identification of *gag* and *env* gene products of

human T-cell leukemia virus (HTLV). Virology 136:338–347, 1984.
40. Nam S, Hatanaka M: Identification of a protease gene of human T-cell leukemia virus type I (HTLV-I) and its structural comparison. Biochem Biophys Res Comm 139:129–135, 1986.
41. Hiramatsu K, Nishida J, Naito A, Yoshikura H: Molecular cloning of the closed circular provirus of human T cell leukemia virus type I: a new open reading frame in the *gag-pol* region. J Gen Virol 68:213–218, 1987.
42. Chen ISY, Slamon DJ, Rosenblatt JD, et al.: The *x*-gene is essential for HTLV replication. Science 229:54–58, 1985.
43. Slamon DJ, Shimotohno K, Cline MJ, et al.: Identification of the putative transforming protein of the human T-cell leukemia viruses HTLV-I and HTLV-II. Science 226:61–65, 1984.
44. Slamon DJ, Press MF, Souza LM, et al.: Studies of the putative transforming protein of the type I human T-cell leukemia virus. Science 228:1427–143, 1985.
45. Nagashima K, Yoshida M, Seiki M: A single species of pX mRNA of human T-cell leukemia virus type I encodes transactivation $p4^0x$ and two other phosphoproteins. J Virol 6:394–399, 1985.
46. Inoue J, Seiki M, Yoshida M: Transcriptional ($p40^x$) and post-transcriptional ($p27^{x-III}$) regulators are required for the expression and replication of human T-cell leukemia virus type I genes. Proc Natl Acad Sci USA 84:3653–3657, 1987.
47. Rosenblatt JD, Cann AJ, Slamon DJ, et al.: HTLV-II transactivation is regulated by the overlapping *tax/rex* nonstructural genes. Science 24:916–919, 1988.
48. Kiyokawa T, Seiki M, Iwashita S, et al.: $p27^{x-III}$ and $p21^{x-III}$, proteins encoded by the pX sequence of human T-cell leukemia virus type I. Proc Natl Acad Sci USA 82:8359–8363, 1985.
49. Slamon DJ, Boyle WJ, Keith DE, et al.: Subnuclear localization of the *trans*-activating protein of human T-cell leukemia virus type I. J Virol 62:680–686, 1988.
50. Payne GS, Bishop JM, Varmus HE: Multiple arrangements of viral DNA and an activated host oncogene in bursal lymphomas. Nature 295:209–214, 1982.
51. Hahn B, Manzari V, Colombini S, et al.: Common site of integration of HTLV in cells of three patients with mature T-cell leukemia-lymphoma. Nature 33:253–256, 1983.
52. Smith RA: Interleukin 2. Annu Rev Immunol 2:319–333, 1984.
53. Siekevitz M, Feinberg MB, Holbrook N, et al.: Activation of interleukin 2 and interleukin 2 receptor (Tac) promoter expression by the trans-activator (*tat*) gene product of human T-cell leukemia virus, type I. Proc Natl Acad Sci USA 84:5389–5393, 1987.
54. Maeda M, Arima N, Daioku Y, et al.: Evidence for the interleukin-2 dependent expansion of leukemic cells in adult T-cell leukemia. Blood 7:1407–1411, 1987.
55. Leung K, Nabel GJ: HTLV-I transactivator induces interleukin-2 receptor expression through an NF-kB-like factor. Nature 333:776–778, 1988.
56. Kohtz DS, Altman A, Kohtz JD, Puszkin S: Immunological and structural homology between human T-cell leukemia virus type I envelope glycoprotein and a region of human interleukin-2 implicated in binding the b receptor. J Virol 62:659–662, 1988.
57. Wano Y, Hattori T, Natsuoka M, et al.: Interleukin 1 gene expression in adult T cell leukemia. J Clin Invest 8:911–916, 1987.
58. Mann DL, DeSantis P, Mark G, et al.: HTLV-I-associated B-cell CLL: Indirect role for retrovirus in leukemogenesis. Science 236:113–116, 1987.
59. Ziegler JL, Beckstead J, Volberding P, Abrams DI, et al.: Non-Hodgkin's lymphoma in 90 homosexual men. Relation to generalized lymphadenopathy and the acquired immunodeficiency syndrome. N Engl J Med 311:565, 1984.
60. Biggar RJ, Horm J, Melbye M, Goedert J: Cancer trends among young single men in the SEER Registries of the United States. Abstract presented at the International Conference on AIDS, June 23–25, 1986, Paris, France, p 31.
61. Harnly ME, Swan SH, Holly EA, Keltner A, Pardian N: Temporal trends in the incidence of non-Hodgkin's lymphoma and selected malignancies in a population with a high

incidence of acquired immunodeficiency syndrome (AIDS). Am J Epidemiol 128:261–267, 1988.
62. Levine AM, Gill PS: Oncology 1:41, 1987.
63. Lowenthal DA, Straus DJ, Campbell SW, Gold JWM, Clarkson BD, Koziner B: AIDS-related lymphoid meoplasia. The Memorial Hospital experience. Cancer 61:2325–2337, 1988.
64. Kaplan LD, Abrams DI, Feigal E, McGrath MS, Kahn J, Neville P, Ziegler J, Volberding PA: AIDS associated non-Hodgkin's lymphoma in San Francisco. JAMA, in press.
65. Odajnyk C, Subar M, Dugan M, et al.: Clinical features and correlation with immunopathology and molecular biology in a large group of patients with AIDS-associated small non-cleaved cell lymphoma (SNCL), Burkitt's and non-Burkitt's type. Blood 68 (Suppl 1):131a, 1986.
66. Bernandez MA, Grant KM, Rodvien R: Lymphoma (L) in a population with or at risk for AIDS—a single institution experience. Blood 68 (Suppl 1):121a, 1986.
67. Rosenberg SA, et al.: Cancer 49:2112, 1982.
68. Levine AM, Gill PS, Meyer PR, Burkes RL, Ross R, Dwarsky RD, et al.: Retrovirus and malignant lymphoma in homosexual men. JAMA 254:1921–1925, 1985.
69. Levine AM, Meyer PR, Begandy MK, et al.: Development of B cell lymphoma in homosexual men. Clinical and immunologic findings. Ann Int Med 100:7, 1984.
70. Pelicci P-G, Knowles DM, Arlin ZA, Wieczorek R, Luciw P, Dina D, Basilico C, Dalla-Favera R: Multiple monoclonal B-cell expansions and c-*myc* oncogene rearrangements in acquired immune deficiency syndrome-related lymphoproliferative disorders. J Exp Med 164:2049–2060, 1986.
71. Petersen JM, Tubbs RR, Savage RA, et al.: Small non-cleaved B cell Burkitt-like lymphoma with chromosome (8;14) translocation and Epstein-Barr virus nuclear-associated antigen in a homosexual man with acquired immunodeficiency syndrome. Am J Med 78: 141, 1985.
72. Magrath IT, Erikson J, Wang-Peng, J, et al.: Synthesis of kappa light chains by cell lines containing an 8:22 chromosomal translocation derived from a male homosexual with Burkitt's lymphoma. Science 22:1094, 1983.
73. Wang-Peng J, Lee EC, Sieverts R, Magrath IT: Burkitt's lymphoma in AIDS: cytogenetic study. Blood 63:818, 1984.
74. Chaganti RSK, Jhanwar SC, Koziner B, Arlin Z, Mertelsmann R, Clarkson BD: Specific translocations characterize Burkitt's-like lymphoma of homosexual men with the acquired immunodeficiency syndrome. Blood 61:1265, 1983.
75. Feigal EG, Lekas P, Beckstead JH, Reyes G, Kaplan L, McGrath MS: Evidence for coinfection with HTLV-I and HIV in AIDS risk group patients with high-grade non-Hodgkin's lymphoma. In: Biolognesi D (ed): Human Retroviruses, Cancer, and AIDS. Approaches to Prevention and Therapy. New York, Liss, 1988, p 213–228.
76. Lane HC, Fauci AS: Immunologic abnormalities in the acquired immunodeficiency syndrome. Annu Rev Immunol 3:477–500, 1985.
77. Purtilo DT, Tatsumi E, Manolov G, Manolova Y, Harada S, Lipscomb H, Krueger G: Epstein-Barr Virus as an etiological agent in the pathogenesis of lymphoproliferative and aproliferative diseases in immune deficient patients. Int Rev Exp Path 27:114–183, 1985.
78. Hanto DW, Gajl-Peczalska KJ, Frizzera G, Arthru DC, Balfour HH, McGlain K, Simmons RL, Najarian JS: Epstein-Barr Virus (EBV) induced polyclonal and monoclonal B-cell lymphoproliferative diseases occurring after renal transplantation. Ann Surg 198: 356–369, 1983.
79. Purtilo DT, Sakamoto K, Saemundsen AK, Sullivan JL, Synnerholm A-C, Anvret M, et al.: Documentation of Epstein-Barr virus infection in immunodeficient patients with life-threatening lymphoproliferative diseases by clinical, virological, and immunopathological studies. Cancer Res 41:1226–1236, 1981.
80. de-The G, Geser A, Day NE, et al.: Epidemiological evidence for causal relationship

between Epstein-Barr virus and Burkitt's lymphoma from Ugandan prospective study. Nature 274:756, 1987.
81. Whittle HC, Brown J, Marsh K, et al.: T-cell control of Epstein-Barr virus-infected B cells is lost during P. Falciparum malaria. Nature 312:449, 1984.
82. Zeigler J, McGrath MS: Lymphoma in HIV positive individuals. In: Magrath I (ed): Non-Hodgkin's Lymphoma. London, Edward Arnold, Ltd., in press.
83. Pelicci P-G, Knowles DM, Magrath I, Dalla-Favera R: Chromosomal breakpoints and structural alterations of the c-*myc* locus differ in endemic and sporadic forms of Burkitt's lymphoma. Proc Natl Acad Sci USA 83:2984–2988, 1986.
84. Rickinson AB: Cellular immunological responses to the virus infection. In: Epstein MA, Achong BG (eds): The Epstein-Barr Virus: Recent Advances. New York, John Wiley & Sons, 1986, pp 77–125.
85. Brown NA, Liu C-R, Feigal EG, McGrath MS: Evidence that Epstein-Barr virus can infect a metastatic B-lymphoma lineage as a passenger virus. Submitted.
86. McGrath MS, Lifson JD, Weissman IL: The role of immunospecific receptors in human lymphoid neoplasia. Abstract presented at the International Conference on AIDS, June 12–16, 1988, Stockholm, Sweden, #7601.
87. Birx DL, Redfield RR, Tosato G: Defective regulation of Epstein-Barr virus infection in patients with acquired immunodeficiency syndrome (AIDS) or AIDS-related disorders. N Engl J Med 314:874, 1986.
88. Yarchoan R, Redfield RR, Broder S: Mechanisms of B cell activation in patients with acquired immunodeficiency syndrome and related disorders. J Clin Invest 78:439–447, 1986.
89. Meeker T, McGrath MS: Submitted.
90. Nath N, Wunderlich C, Darr FW, et al.: Immunoglobulin level in donor blood reactive for antibodies to human immunodeficiency virus. J Clin Microbiol 25:364–369, 1987.
91. Heriot K, Hallquist AE, Tomar RH: Paraproteinemia in patients with acquired immunodeficiency syndrome (AIDS) or lymphadenopathy syndrome (LAS). Clin Chem 31:1224, 1985.
92. Pahwa S, Pahwa R, Saxinger C, et al.: Influence of the human T-lymphotropic virus/lymphadenopathy-associated virus and functions of human lymphocytes: Evidence of immunosuppressive effects and polyclonal B-cell activation by banded viral and lymphocyte preparations. Proc Natl Acad Sci USA 82:8198–8202, 1985.
93. Ng V, Jacobson MD, Khayam-Bashi H, McGrath MS: Coincident disappearance of a paraprotein with the development of lymphoma in an HIV infected male. N Engl J Med 318:1761, 1988.
94. Ng V, Hwang KM, Reyes GR, Kaplan LD, Khayam-Bashi H, Hadley WK, McGrath MS: High titer anti-HIV antibody reactivity associated with a paraprotein spike in a homosexual male with AIDS related complex (ARC). Blood 71:3197–3201, 1988.
95. Bishop GA, Arnold IW, Haughton G: Antigen-specific B cell tumors of mice. CRC Crit Rev Immunol 6:105–21, 1986.
96. McGrath MS, Tamura GS, Weissman IL: Receptor mediated leukemogenesis: Murine leukemia virus interacts with BCL_1 lymphoma cell surface IgM. JMCI 3:243–253, 1987.
97. Schnittman SM, Lane HC, Higgins SE, Folks T, Fauci AS: Direct polycloncal activation of human B-lymphocytes by the acquired immunodeficiency virus. Science 233:1084–1086, 1986.
98. Yarchoan R, Redfield R, Broder S: Mechanisms of B cell activation in patients with acquired immunodeficiency syndrome and related disorders. Contribution of antibody-producing B-cells, of Epstein-Barr virus-infected B-cells, and of immunoglobulin production induced by human T-cell lymphotropic virus, type III/lymphadenopathy-associated virus. J Clin Invest 78:439–447, 1986.
99. Crowe S, Mills J, McGrath MS: Quantitative immunocytofluorographic analysis of CD4 surface antigen expression and HIV infection of human peripheral blood monocyte/

macrophages. AIDS Res Human Retroviruses 3(2):135–145, 1987.
100. Robert-Guroff M, Weiss SH, Giron JA, Jennings AM, Ginsburg H, Margolis I: Prevalence of antibodies to HTLV-I, -II, and -III, in intravenous drug abusers from an AIDS endemic region. JAMA 255:3133, 1986.
101. Harper ME, Kaplan MIT, Marselle LM, et al.: Concomitant infection with HTLV-I and HTLV-II in a patient with TB lymphoproliferative disease. N Engl J Med 315:1703, 1986.

12. The human DNA tumor viruses: Human papilloma virus and Epstein–Barr virus

Nancy Raab-Traub

Introduction

Viruses and cancer

Many DNA viruses are able to transform cells in culture or induce tumors in experimental animals. However, proving a causal association between infection with a specific human virus and the development of cancer has been difficult because most of the viruses are ubiquitous infectious agents, whereas a malignancy is apparently a rare outcome of infection that develops many years after initial infection. Moreover, neoplasia develops during latent or persistent infections with the viruses, making it difficult to determine whether viral functions are critical to the development of cancer or essential to the latent state.

The DNA tumor viruses are classified into four families: the papovaviruses, adenoviruses, herpesviruses, and hepadnaviruses. In humans, particular members of the papilloma viruses, herpesviruses, and hepadnaviruses have been linked to specific malignancies.

The simian papovavirus was the first virus of primate origin shown to have oncogenic potential in that it could transform fibroblasts in vitro and induced fibrosarcomas when inoculated into newborn hamsters. However, neither SV40 nor the related human papovaviruses, JC and BK, have been associated with malignancies in the natural hosts of the viruses. However, research on SV40 has been instrumental in characterizing potential mechanisms of growth transformation. The transforming gene encoded by SV40, large T-antigen, is the best characterized virally-encoded potential oncogene. The recent demonstration of binding between T-antigen and the human retinoblastoma gene indicates that virally encoded products may interfere with cell growth regulation, leading to the development of human cancer [1].

Human papilloma viruses (HPVs) are structurally classified as belonging to the papovavirus family. Human papilloma virus was initially discovered in warts by electron microscopy but has been difficult to study because of the inability to cultivate the virus in vitro. However, the molecular cloning and characterization of papilloma viral genomes has revealed the existence of multiple distinct viral genotypes. Compelling molecular data link specific HPV strains with several types of human cancer [2,3]. HPV genomes of types 16 and 18 have been detected in greater than 80% of cervical cancers by molecular hybridization techniques and have also been detected in hyperplasias and preneoplastic lesions [4]. Specific changes in viral DNA structure and expression distinguish the malignant cells. In addition, viral genes that are consistently expressed at elevated levels in malignant tissues have been shown to have transforming capacity in experimental systems. This suggests that HPVs like SV40 may alter cellular growth through expression of a particular viral function.

Epidemiologic evidence that indicated shared risk factors for cervical carcinomas with sexually transmitted disease were initially interpreted to implicate herpes simplex infection (HSV) [5]. However, prospective epidemiologic studies of women at risk for the development of cervical cancer did not disclose a connection between HSV-2 infection and the cancer. The shared risk factor with sexually transmitted disease is now thought to represent infection with HPV. Moreover, in contrast with the detection of HPV genome, HSV genomes or gene products could not be consistently detected in the malignant tissue. However, the ability of herpesviruses to establish latent infections and the potential interaction of viral functions with cellular control mechanisms may still allow HSV to contribute in some way to the development of cancer [6].

Human cytomegalovirus (HCMV) is implicated in the aggressive form of Kaposi's sarcoma, which occurs with high frequency in patients with acquired immunodeficiency syndrome (AIDS) [7]. The association is suggested by the fact that male homosexuals with AIDS frequently have active HCMV infections and tend to develop Kaposi's sarcoma, whereas hemophiliacs with AIDS do not have active HCMV infections and do not develop Kaposi's sarcoma. However, the detection of HCMV DNA in Kaposi's sarcoma is inconsistent, suggesting that although HCMV infection may be involved in the initiation of transformation, the presence of the virus is not essential to maintain the neoplastic state [8]. Alternatively, the detection of HCMV may indicate that some Kaposi's sarcomas are sites of latent infection or sites of HCMV replication.

The human B-lymphotrophic herpesvirus, Epstein–Barr virus (EBV), is the etiologic agent of the benign lymphoproliferative disease, infectious mononucleosis, and B-cell lymphomas that develop in the immunocompromised [9,10]. It is also implicated in the African endemic form of Burkitt's lymphoma (BL) and in nasopharyngeal carcinoma (NPC) in that the viral genome is consistently detected within the malignant cells [11,12]. Unlike the other human herpesviruses, infection with EBV is predominantly nonlytic and efficiently induces growth transformation of B-lymphocytes both in vitro and in vivo [13]. Within the infected, growth-transformed lymphocytes, specific viral functions are continuously expressed in each infected cell [14].

Some of these gene products most likely function in regulating viral expression and replication [15]. Others may also alter cellular growth regulation. Expression of particular viral genes can alter human B-cell growth properties in vitro and can transform rodent cells, conferring tumorigenicity in nude mice [16,17]. Thus the acute transforming capacity of EBV is likely due to the effects of expression of specific viral genes.

Human hepatitis B virus (HBV) is associated with hepatocellular carcinoma (HCC), which develops with greatly elevated risk in patients with chronic HBV infection [18]. Similarly, HCC develops in woodchucks chronically infected with the related hepadnavirus of woodchucks. Viral genomes can be detected not only within the tumor tissue but also within adjacent noncancerous tissue. Structural analyses of viral integrative events have not revealed a preferred integration site nor identified potential cellular oncogenes whose expression is altered by HBV integration [19]. Since a virally encoded transforming gene has not yet been identified, it has been suggested that perhaps viral integration at critical sites may alter expression of transformation-associated genes.

Of the human DNA viruses that are implicated in the etiology of malignancies, compelling epidemiologic and molecular data suggest that HPV and EBV are contributing and probable causative agents in the development of specific cancers. Moreover, infection of human cells in vitro with these agents induces transformation. Although the process that promotes the development of malignancy in a rare cell from the many that are infected is unknown, considerable biochemical and molecular biologic data have been gathered and have begun to illuminate the transforming capacities of these agents. Therefore, because of the ability of HPV and EBV to transform cells in culture and because of their compelling association with human cancer, this chapter will review the molecular epidemiologic data, the biochemical analyses of viral DNA structure and viral expression, and the biologic properties of HPV and EBV genes in transformation.

Human papilloma virus

Pathogenesis

Papilloma viruses are ubiquitous infectious agents that induce hyperplastic growths and tumors in animals and humans. In humans, papilloma virus (HPV) infection induces genital warts or condylomas and oral and laryngeal papillomas [20]. Viral genomes are also detected in precancerous, neoplastic growths, termed cervical intraepithelial neoplasias (CINs), and in squamous-cell carcinomas of the vulva, penis, cervix, larynx, and oral cavity [21].

The greatest risk factor for developing condylomas, CIN, and cervical cancer correlates with the number of sexual partners and suggests that cervical carcinoma, like condyloma, is a sexually transmitted disease [22]. Other epidemiologic data reveal that spouses of individuals with cervical or penile cancer have a three-fold increased risk of also developing cancer [23].

Cervical carcinoma develops at a site in the cervix where immature metaplastic cells differentiate into mature squamous epithelium or columnar epithelium [24]. Both condyloma and CIN contain atypical cells, called koilocytes, that have irregular nuclear borders, multiple nuclei, and vacuolization of the cytoplasm [25]. The CIN lesions are marked by a more disordered pattern of growth, significantly increased numbers of mitotic figures, and aneuploidy. The degree of severity of the CIN lesion corresponds with decreased differentiation. In contrast, replication of HPV is linked to the differentiated state of the cell with classic crystalline arrays of HPV in the terminally differentiated keratin-producing cells in condyloma [26]. In vivo, the growth of condylomas is controlled such that they develop to some point and remain constant or regress. In contrast, CINs progress and eventually evolve into invasive carcinomas [27].

Viral DNA structure

The papilloma virus is a small icosahedral virion with a double-stranded covalently closed circular DNA genome of approximately 8 kilobase-pairs (kb). There is extensive sequence divergence among the papilloma viruses with at least 50 distinct genotypes [28]. Although the general organization of open reading frames within the HPV genomes is conserved, the HPV types display considerable variation in restriction endonuclease recognition sites and extensive sequence divergence. The distinct genotypes of HPV correlate with disease phenotypes such that HPV types 6 and 11 are detected in benign genital condylomas, whereas HPV 16 and 18 are associated with most CINs and all squamous-cell carcinomas. HPV 6 and 11 DNAs are rarely detected in cervical cancer [27].

In most condylomas, the viral DNA is a replicating extrachromasomal episome with production of infectious virus in differentiated cells. The relative abundance of viral DNA as indicated by in situ hybridization is more intense in superficial cells, which suggests that these terminally differentiated cells are a site of viral replication. However, viral DNA can also be detected at low levels near the basement membrane [27]. In contrast, in carcinomas, it is difficult to detect HPV 16 or 18 DNA by in situ hybridization, which is a relatively insensitive technique. Detection of viral DNA by Southern blot hybridization suggests that a small number of copies of HPV DNA integrate into the host DNA [29]. Integration appears to be random within the host genome. In several of the cervical carcinoma cell lines that contain HPV 16 or 18 DNAs, partial or multiple copies have integrated at random fragile chromosomal sites. However, within the viral genome, integration interrupts the E2 open reading frame, suggesting a specificity for the viral site of integration [30]. The lack of E2 expression could alter expression of those viral functions that are regulated by the E2 transcriptional transactivator. In the cervical carcinoma cell lines and primary biopsies that contain partial HPV genomes, the regulatory regions and the E6 and E7 regions are consistently retained.

HPV transcription in infected tissues

The transcriptional pattern of HPV is similar to that of bovine papilloma virus (BPV), which has been characterized in more detail [30]. The E2 ORF of HPV 16 encodes a transcriptional regulatory factor that activates an enhancer element in the upstream regulatory region (URR) [31]. In addition to this enhancer element, a glucocorticoid-responsive element and a keratinocyte-specific enhancer have also been identified in the URR [32,33].

Transcription in condylomas, CINs, and cervical carcinomas has been analyzed using probes for in situ hybridization that represented specific HPV open reading frames (ORFs) or through cDNA sequence analysis. Transcription of HPV-6 and HPV-11 in condyloma tissue is considerably more abundant than that of HPV-16 in CIN [4]. In the basal layers of CIN, the early E4 and E5 ORFs are the most abundantly expressed viral genes, with lower levels of transcription from the E6/E7 ORF. Late gene expression was only detectable in the terminally differentiated cells in both condyloma and CIN.

In contrast, in most cervical carcinomas and derived cell lines, the most abundant transcripts are derived from E6/E7 without expression of late viral functions [34]. Primer extension analyses and cDNA sequencing have identified the E6 mRNA, a spliced E6, and the E7 mRNA in most samples [35,36]. Studies of transcription in benign and malignant lesions have suggested that E7 overproduction and the spliced E6 message may be characteristic of HPV-16- and HPV-18-associated carcinomas. Transcription of both E6 and E7 is regulated by the E2 products. Therefore the integration and disruption of E2 in cervical carcinoma probably results in the deregulation of E6 and E7 expression.

The spliced E6 message is thought to only be transcribed from the oncogenic HPV variants, HPV-16 and HPV-18, which contain splice donor and acceptor sites in the E6 ORF that are not present in HPV-6 or HPV-11. It is thought that the spliced E6 allows for more efficient translation of the E7 ORF [37].

Identification of transforming genes

In transformation assays with BPV, the E5 and E6 ORFs have been identified as two independent transforming genes [38]. The E5 gene product is a 44-amino-acid membrane protein that can stimulate DNA synthesis in cultured cells. The BPV E6 protein is found in both membrane and nuclear fractions.

Both HPV-16 and HPV-18 can transform established rodent cells such as NIH-3T3 and Rat-1 cells [39]. Transfection of HPV-16 or HPV-18 can also induce transformation of human fibroblasts or keratinocytes. This property has been mapped to the E6/E7 region [40]. The data suggests that E7 is important for transformation and immortalization, whereas E6 contributes to anchorage independence. In addition, HPV-16 can transform primary rodent cells in conjunction with the *ras* oncogene [41]. These data, in conjunction with the observation that the most abundant viral protein in cervical cancers is the E7 protein, suggest that E7 is a critical viral transforming gene.

It has recently been demonstrated that the E7 gene has conserved domains with the adenovirus E1a gene and that, similarly to E1a, E7 can *trans*-activate the adenovirus E2 promoter [42]. The transcriptional *trans*-activation capacity of E7 may be central to its ability to alter cellular growth regulation and is likely to be involved in the malignant progression characteristic of infection with oncogenic HPVs. The fact that expression of E7 is consistently detected in CIN and cervical carcinomas suggests that E7 expression may be continuously required for the malignant phenotype.

Remarkably, the adenovirus E1a gene and the HPV E7 gene have both been shown to bind to the retinoblastoma gene, as does the SV40 large T-antigen [43]. This suggests that despite the diversity of viral genotypes and infectious processes, there may be a common transformation pathway through the retinoblastoma gene.

Epstein–Barr virus

Pathogenesis

Burkitt's lymphoma. The Epstein–Barr virus (EBV) was first identified in cultures of B-lymphocytes that were cultured from an unusual lymphoma, originally described by Dennis Burkitt [44]. Burkitt's lymphoma (BL) is a childhood disease, usually appearing as a mass in the jaw. The tumor is rare and appears sporadically in most countries, but is endemic in the equatorial belt of Africa. EBV DNA is consistently detected in the endemic African variety of the lymphoma but is only present in 10% to 20% of the sporadic form [45]. Patients with EBV-associated BL have elevated antibody titers to the viral capsid antigen (VCA) and early replicative functions or early antigen (EA) [46].

Subsequent seroepidemiology with the new virus revealed that infection with the virus was universal. In equatorial Africa, more than 90% of infants are infected postpartum in the first year of life. Primary infection with EBV is usually silent, with the classic syndrome of infectious mononucleosis (IM) characteristic of primary infection of adolescents.

Both the endemic and rare sporadic forms of BL have characteristic chromosomal translocations (8;14, 8;22, 2;8). These translocations involve the immunoglobulin (Ig) heavy and light chain loci on chromosomes 14, 2, and 22, and the c-*myc* oncogene on chromosome 8 [47]. The translocation of c-*myc* seems to alter its expression, possibly by placing the gene in proximity to Ig regulatory sequences such as the Ig heavy chain enhancer or through changes within c-*myc* non-coding sequences that alter transcriptional control mechanisms [48,49].

Lymphoproliferative syndrome. The importance of the immune system in controlling the proliferation of EBV-infected B-lymphocytes is compellingly revealed in patients with genetic or acquired immunodeficiency and allograft recipients. The X-linked lymphoproliferative syndrome (XLP) is a rare fatal disease that arises from the inability to handle EBV infection. Without prior immunologic difficulties, after primary EBV infection, the patients may develop relentless mononucleosis, invasive lymphoid infiltration, and lymphomas of Burkitt's type and immunoblastic sarcomas [50].

Malignant EBV-containing lymphomas are also detected in ataxia-telangiectasia and Wiskott–Aldrich syndromes (WA). In allograft recipients, polyclonal invasive B-cell lymphoproliferations occasionally develop [10]. The proliferations may subside with decreased immunosuppressive therapy, although in some patients fatal monoclonal lymphomas develop from the initially polyclonal proliferation. The immune deficiences of XLP and WA and the likelihood of development of lymphoproliferative syndrome during immunosuppression with cyclosporin reveal the importance of T-cell surveillance in controlling EBV-infected B-cell proliferation and also underscore the potent capacity of EBV to induce cell proliferation. Similarly, in acquired immunodeficiency syndrome (AIDS), EBV-associated lymphoproliferations are frequently detected. Surprisingly, these include Burkitt's lymphomas with the characteristic translocations, which are rarely seen in allograft recipients [51].

Nasopharyngeal carcinoma. Carcinoma of the posterior nasopharynx (NPC) is a malignancy of epithelial cells that is endemic in southern China. The disease also occurs with elevated incidence in Alaskan Eskimos and in parts of northern Africa. It occurs sporadically at low incidence in Caucasians in the Western world. Patients with NPC have characteristic elevated EBV IgA antibody titers to viral replicative antigens, suggesting that viral reactivation and replication accompanies the appearance of the tumor. Unlike BL, the disease is consistently associated with EBV, and EBV DNA is detected in all NPC specimens from both endemic and sporadic cases [52]. The structure of the EBV DNA, as discussed in the following section, predicts that NPC, like BL, is a monoclonal cellular proliferation in which viral infection preceded outgrowth.

Other tumors of epithelial origin are also linked to EBV infection. EBV genomes have been detected in laryngeal, supraglottal, and parotid gland carcinomas. These tissues represent a subset of epithelial cells, the members of which have their origin in the primitive oropharynx [53,54].

Molecular biology

EBV DNA structure. EBV is unique among the herpesviruses in that there are no cell lines that can be infected in vitro resulting in virus replication. Rather, infection of primary B-lymphocytes induces the ability to grow

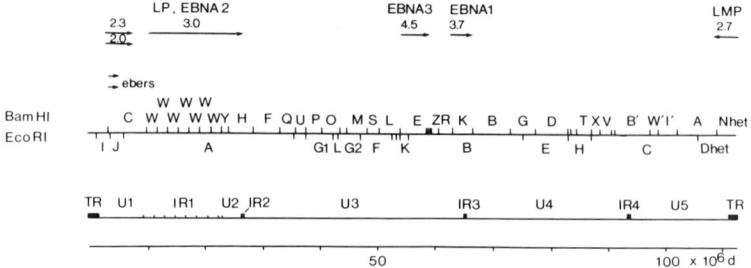

Figure 1. Epstein–Barr virus DNA structure and viral transcription in latently infected lymphocytes. Structural features of the EBV genome, including the direct tandem repeats at the termini (TR) and the direct, internal repeats (IR1, 2, 3, 4), are indicated. The BamHI and EcoRI restriction endonuclease fragments are designated. The size and direction of transcription of the mRNAs specific for each EBV polypeptide expressed in latently infected lymphocytes are indicated above the encoding DNA sequences.

indefinitely in vitro without lytic infection [13]. EBV-infected B-cell lines can be established from infected tissues including nodal tissue from Burkitt's lymphoma, infectious mononucleosis, and from the peripheral blood of previously infected people. Most of the biochemistry and molecular biology has been determined through the study of such B-cell lines [14]. In some of the cell lines, a small percentage of the cells will produce virus. The virus produced by most cell lines can then be used to infect B-cells obtained from uninfected individuals or from umbilical cord blood to establish permanent cell lines.

Within the virion, the EBV genome is a linear double-stranded DNA molecule of 172×10^3 nucleotide base-pairs (bp) [55]. Homologous direct, tandemly repeated sequences of approximately 500 bp are located at the termini of EBV (TR), and several other sets of direct tandem repeats are located internally (IR1, IR2, IR3, IR4) [56] (figure 1). The number of terminal repeats (TR) at the two ends of the genome varies between individual viral DNA molecules such that after digestion with restriction enzymes, the terminal fragments are heterogeneous in size, varying by increments of 500 bp, and form a ladder array on gels or Southern blots (figure 2) [57].

After infection and entry into the cell, the two ends of the linear genome join through the TR sequences, which produces the intracellular episomal form of the virus. Most infected cells contain multiple copies of the EBV episome, which is replicated by the host cell polymerase in an episomal form. The circularization of the genome produces fused terminal restriction enzyme fragments that can be distinguished from the linear forms by their larger size and can be identified by probes representing unique DNA adjacent to the TR from either the left or right ends of the linear genome (figure 2). In EBV DNA from monoclonal lymphomas and from NPC and carcinoma of the parotid gland, a single fused terminal fragment was detected [57]. The detection of a single fused terminal fragment, despite the variability that is

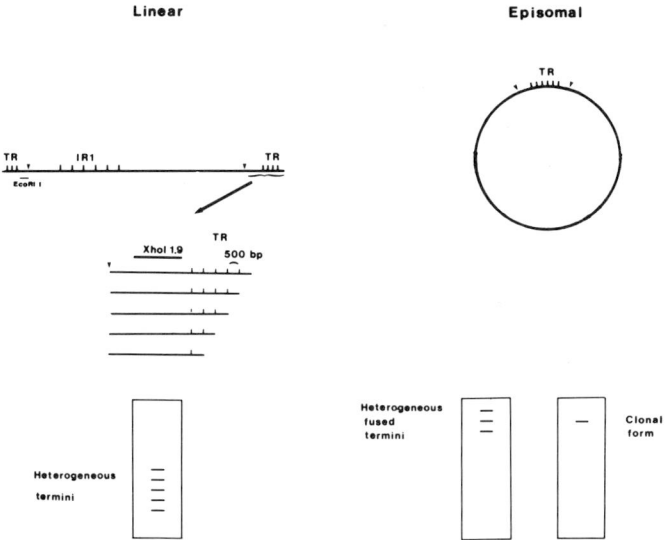

Figure 2. The structure of the termini of EBV. The positions of the Xho I 1.9 kb and EcoRI I fragments, which represent unique DNA adjacent to the 500-bp repeated sequences located at each terminus (TR), are designated. The Xho I 1.9-kb fragment and the EcoRI I fragment each identify a distinct array of terminal fragments in restriction enzyme digestions of linear virion DNA. These fragments differ in size by increments of approximately 500 base-pairs and result from varying numbers of copies of TR in each terminal fragment. Circularization of the linear DNA through the TR produces the intracellular episomal form of Viral DNA. Restriction endonuclease digestion produces fused terminal restriction enzyme fragments that hybridize to probes from both ends of the genome. A single fused terminal fragment is detected in clonal cell lines established at low multiplicities of infection and in malignancies associated with EBV.

possible in this fragment, revealed that the viral episomes in all of the cells were identical and suggested that the epithelial malignancies, NPC and carcinoma of the parotid gland, were also monoclonal proliferations. This observation suggested that the structure of the EBV termini could be used as an indicator of the cellular clonality of the proliferation. In addition, as lytic viral replication and the synthesis of linear viral DNA produces heterogeneous terminal restriction enzyme fragments, the detection of ladder arrays of terminal fragments identifies tissues that contain some lytically infected cells.

The detection of a single clonal episomal fused terminal fragment in both NPC and BL suggests that EBV did not infect the neoplasias secondarily, in that the infection of multiple cells would produce multiple, distinct episomal populations, but rather that EBV infection preceded the cellular proliferation. In the endemic area of southern China with a high incidence of NPC, intensive screening programs identified a type of nasopharyngeal mucosal lesion, atypical hyperplasia of the epithelium, that has a significant propensity to develop into NPC. EBV DNA was detected in all of the atypical hyperplasias. Analysis of the EBV terminal fragment revealed that most of the hyperplasias were apparently focal reactivations of EBV with clonal EBV episomes (N. Raab-Traub, unpublished). These data reveal that the premalignant lesions that precede the development of NPC are induced by EBV infection.

Patients with AIDs develop hairy leukoplakia, a lesion on the side of the tongue that contains EBV virions [58]. Analysis of the EBV terminal fragments reveals abundant ladder arrays representing the linear termini in these tissues (figure 3). These lesions respond to acyclovir therapy and apparently represent an example of a lytic infection with EBV. Interestingly, these tissues contain abnormal koilocytic cells that were originally interpreted as a co-infection with EBV and HPV. Subsequent studies have revealed that hairy leukoplakia does not contain HPV. In situ hybridization has detected EBV DNA and abundant transcription of the EBV latent membrane protein in the koilocytes. The detection of EBV DNA and viral transcription in the koilocytes suggests that lytic infections with HPV or EBV may have similar cytopathology (N. Raab-Traub, unpublished).

Integrated copies of EBV have been detected in some cell lines [59]. The sequence of the viral/cellular junction fragments has been analyzed in the BL cell line, Namalwa, and has revealed that the entire EBV genome had integrated into chromosome 1, via the TR, with both duplication and deletion of cellular sequences at the site of integration. In a cell line established in vitro, a similar integrative event occurred on chromosome 4. The lack of detectable homology between the two sites suggests the lack of a unique integration site.

Viral expression in latent infection. Most lymphocytes infected with EBV do not produce virus. Rather, as a consequence of infection, they are induced to proliferate continuously in culture. In these latently infected lymphocytes in vitro, at least eight polyadenylated mRNAs and two nonpolyadenylated RNAs are transcribed (figure 1) [14].

Five of the mRNAs encode components of the EBV nuclear antigen, EBNA. Most human antisera with antibodies to EBNA have reactivity to the protein encoded by an open reading frame (ORF) within the BamHI K fragment of EBV, EBNA1. The 3.7-kb mRNA that encodes EBNA1 is intricately spliced and originates 70 kb upstream from a promoter within the large internal repeat sequence, IR1. In some BL cell lines a different promoter, which is located approximately 5 kb 5' to the IR1 promoter within the short, unique DNA (U_S), may function as the EBNA promoter [60]. Transcripts from the IR1 or U_S promoters are differentially spliced to the five mRNAs that encode the EBV nuclear antigens.

The origin of replication for the plasmid form of the viral genome (oriP) has been identified within the BamHI C fragment at the left end of the genome [15]. In the presence of the EBNA1 protein that binds to sequences within oriP, DNA linked to oriP will be replicated as an extrachromosomal plasmid. Therefore, EBNA1, which acts in *trans* to maintain the replication of the EBV episome, is fundamental to latent infection.

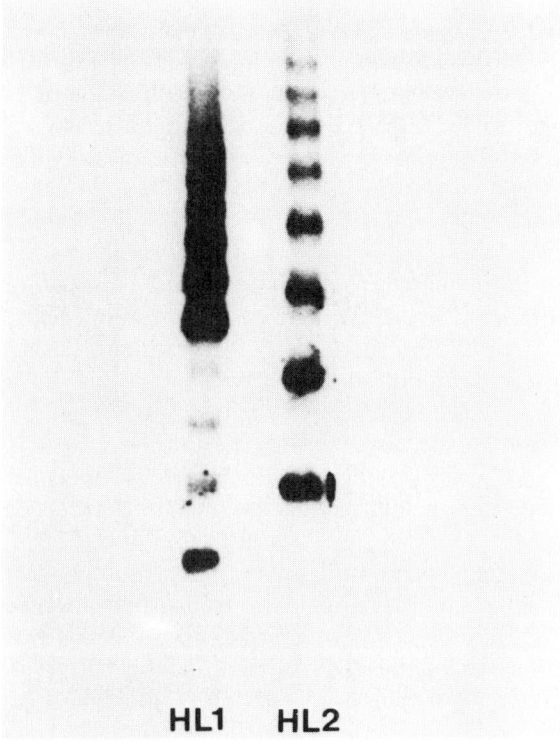

HL1   HL2

Figure 3. The structure of the EBV terminal fragments in hairy leukoplakia of the tongue. The right terminal EBV BamHI fragments were identified in DNA extracted from two specimens of hairy leukoplakia tissue by hybridization with a probe representing unique DNA from the right end of the genome adjacent to the terminal repeats. Abundant ladder arrays of fragments that differed in molecular weight by constant increments were identified in each specimen. Detection of ladder arrays of fragments that can be distinguished by hybridization with probes from either end of the genome are indicative of linear virion DNA. The structure of the EBV termini in hairy leukoplakia suggests that this lesion represents a lytic infection with EBV.

A second nuclear protein, EBNA2, is encoded by a 3.0-kb mRNA transcribed from the BamHI W, Y, and H fragments of EBV. Nontransforming strains of EBV, which are produced by the HR1 and Daudi cell lines, are deleted for the sequences that encode EBNA2. HR1 is a subclone of the Jijoye cell line, which produces virus that is transformation-competent and retains the EBNA2 encoding sequences [61]. Superinfection of the latently infected Raji cell line with HR1 virus produces Raji:HR1 recombinant virus, which has regained EBNA2 encoding sequences and can transform B-cells [62].

The mRNA that encodes EBNA2 is bicistronic and encodes another nuclear antigen that is encoded by multiple copies of two exons within IR1 and additional sequences within BamHI Y [60]. The protein is heterogeneous in molecular weight, varying in size by increments reflecting differing numbers of copies of the IR1 exons. This protein has been referred to as leader protein (LP) or EBNA 4 [63]. LP may also be important in transformation in that the nontransforming isolate, HR1, is also deleted for part of LP.

Two allelic forms of EBNA2 have been identified. The DNA sequences and the predicted amino acid sequences are highly divergent [64]. The 2A form appears to be more prevalent, although 2B isolates have been detected in BL and NPC. EBNA2B variants of EBV are less efficient in transformation of B-lymphocytes, and cell lines established after infection with EBNA2B strains grow poorly in culture. Human antisera may contain reactivity to either form of EBNA2. It is surprising that a protein apparently essential for transformation would be so divergent. Interestingly, EBNA2B variants predominate in the lytic infection, hairy leukloplakia of the tongue (N. Raab-Traub, unpublished). This suggests that strain variation may contribute to the pathology of this specific disease.

Three mRNAs of approximately 4.5 kb, transcribed from the BamHI E fragment, encode the nuclear proteins, which are termed EBNA3A, 3B, and 3C, or EBNA 3, 5, and 6. The three differentially spliced mRNAs contain similarly sized, somewhat homologous ORFs within the BamHI E fragment. Their role in latent infection or in growth transformation is presently unknown [14].

Sequence analyses of the cDNAs that encode EBNA 1, 2, 3A, 3B, 3C, and LP indicate that in lymphoid cell lines established from BL all of the transcripts originate from a common promoter in the large internal repeated sequence, IR1, and are transcribed rightward. The transcripts are then differentially spliced into the specific mRNAs. In some cell lines established in vitro, transcription initiates two kilobases 5' to the IR1 promoter within the short unique DNA [60].

Two additional mRNAs of 2.3 and 2.0 kb have been identified in latently infected lymphocytes. The protein products encoded by these mRNAs have not yet been identified. However, sequence analysis of cDNAs representing these mRNAs revealed that the transcripts are initiated at the right end of the linear EBV genome and are transcribed rightward, splicing across the TR of the episomal form of the genome, with coding sequences predominantly formed from exons at the left end of the linear EBV genome [65].

The only mRNA in latent infection that is transcribed from right to left off the opposite DNA strand of the virus encodes the latent membrane protein. This hydrophobic protein contains six alpha-helical domains envisaged as winding through the cell membrane [66]. The 60-kDa protein has been identified in the membrane fraction and on the surface of latently infected lymphocytes. The protein is phosphorylated on serine and threonine residues shortly after synthesis and complexes with the intermediate filament cytoskeletal protein, vimentin, forming patches in the membrane. Protease cleavage studies have revealed a cytoplasmic orientation for the hydrophilic amino and carboxy termini and that the only extracellular component is the first outer reverse turn.

Identification of transforming functions. Although direct transfection of DNA from BL into established rodent cell lines failed to identify a transforming gene, transfer of the LMP gene under the control of heterologous promoters transformed Rat-1 cells as assayed by loss of contact inhibition, development of anchorage independence, and tumorigenicity in nude mice [16]. The effects of LMP on Rat-1 cells suggest that LMP is an important component of EBV-induced transformation.

Transformation of primary lymphocytes after gene transfer of specific EBV functions has not yet been attained. However, many of the effects of EBV infection of lymphocytes occur after infection of EBV-negative American BL cells. The infected cells continuously express the viral genes expressed in latent infection, grow in tight clumps, and express high levels of B-cell activation antigens. Expression of LMP under the control of the Moloney Murine Leukemia virus promoter did not alter the growth patterns or cellular phenotype. However, the level of LMP expression was considerably lower than actual LMP expression under the control of its own regulatory sequences as detected in transformed lymphocytes or in NPC tissue. When LMP was expressed from the metallothionein promoter at levels similar to EBV-infected lymphocytes, the growth phenotype of transfected lymphocytes was dramatically altered. LMP expression increased cell size and induced plasma membrane ruffling, expression of lymphocyte activation markers, CD23 and transferrin receptor, and TGF-beta responsiveness [67]. A partially deleted form of LMP, expressed in permissively infected cells and lacking the amino terminus and the first four transmembrane domains, did not aggregate in patches, complex with the cytoskeleton, or alter lymphocyte growth. This suggests that the cytoskeletal interaction may be essential to LMP transforming activity [67].

Interestingly, expression of the EBNA2 gene also induced transcription of the B-cell activation antigen, CD23, and induced cell clumping [17]. However, EBNA2 had little effect on growth of Rat-1 cells, where its expression only decreased serum dependence. Several studies have suggested that EBNA2 expression is not detected in NPC tissue and may be lymphoid-specific [68]. Since EBV strains that are deleted for EBNA2 cannot transform lymphocytes in vitro, the specific induction of CD23 expression by EBNA2 may be fundamental to EBV-induced transformation of lymphocytes.

As multiple EBV genes are continuously expressed in all EBV-transformed lymphocytes, it is likely that LMP and some of the EBV nuclear antigens complement and cooperate in induction of transformation and may also complement cellular oncogenes such as c-*myc*.

Summary

HPV and EBV are common infectious agents that persist after primary infection in a latent state with occasional shedding of virus. Therefore, one of the fundamental questions in the etiology of those cancers that are linked to infection with such ubiquitous viruses is why cancer develops in a few people when many are infected. Because only a small subset of infected people will develop specific cancers, it has been suggested that the presence of the viral genomes in the malignancies merely indicates a persistent or latent infection. However, if the viral infection was not an etiologic factor in the development of the specific cancers, then one would predict that the proportion of cancers that contained the viral genome would reflect the proportion of infected people and that the same cancers could develop in uninfected people. The sporadic detection from nonendemic areas of Burkitt's lymphoma without EBV initially suggested that EBV infection was not etiologic. However, the rate of incidence of BL in infected populations of children is disproportionately greater than the very low incidence in uninfected children, which suggests that EBV infection is an important contributing factor. Moreover, the development of EBV-induced lymphomas in the immunocompromised and the consistent detection of EBV in specific epithelial malignancies such as NPC suggest that EBV infection is essential in the induction of specific cancers. Similarly, the consistent detection of particular HPV types in certain types of cancer suggests that HPV is also an etiologic factor.

There are several strikingly similar aspects of infection with HPV and EBV. In latent infection, both of the viral genomes persist as an extrachromosomal episome with an origin of replication that is activated by binding to a virally encoded polypeptide. The state of viral infection appears to be linked with the state of cellular differentiation such that latent infections are activated into a replicative state as the cells differentiate. Moreover, elevated levels of expression of the putative transforming genes are linked to transformation. However, perhaps most importantly, the malignancies are clonal with regard to the viral infection; HPV-associated malignancies have unique integrative events and EBV-associated malignancies have clonal episomal forms. This reveals that the specific cancers are clonal cellular proliferations that developed after viral infection.

In vitro, the initially polyclonal cell lines produced by EBV infection rapidly evolve to oligoclonality or monoclonality. This could be due to a slightly faster rate of growth such that the progeny of one clone rapidly predominate. Similarly, in vivo, in a population of proliferating cells there would be continual clonal evolution such that those cells predominate that develop genetic changes conferring a growth advantage.

The potential role of HPV and EBV in oncogenesis concurs with the belief that oncogenesis is a multistep process in which changes in the expression or function of multiple genes result in uncontrolled cellular proliferation. Experimental support for this process includes the observation that the complementary action of two distinct cellular oncogenes, viral or cellular, is required for transformation of primary cells. However, even in transgenic mice in which activated *ras* and c-*myc* are expressed from heterologous promoters, the clonal tumors develop in a stochastic manner, suggesting that additional genetic changes are involved. Both EBV and HPV infection can induce the initial proliferation, but an important remaining question is whether they also contribute to the genesis of subsequent genetic changes. The ability of these agents to maintain the viral genome without inducing cell death, to integrate into cellular DNA, and to *trans*-activate expression of cellular genes are properties that could change genetic structure and alter the expression of cellular genes.

References

1. DeCaprio JA, Ludlow JW, Figge J, Shew JY, Huang CM, Lee WH, Marsilio E, Paucha E, Livingston DM: SV40 large tumor antigen forms a specific complex with the product of the retinoblastoma gene. Cell 54:275–283, 1988.
2. Gissman L, Wolnik L, Ikenberg H, Koldovsky U, Schnurch HG, zur Hausen H: Human papillomavirus types 6 and 11 sequences in genital and laryngeal papillomas and in some cervical cancers. Proc Natl Acad Sci USA 80:560–563, 1983.
3. Boshart M, Gissman L, Ikenberg H, zur Hausen H: A new type of papillomavirus DNA from a cervical carcinoma and its prevalence in cancer biopsy samples from different geographic regions. EMBO J 3:1151–1157, 1984.
4. Crum CP, Mitao M, Levine RU, Silverstein SJ: Cervical papillomavirus segregate within morphologically distinct precancerous lesions. J Virol 54:675–681, 1985.
5. Graham S, Rawls W, Swanson M, McCurtis J: Sex partners and herpes simplex virus type 2 in the epidemiology of cancer of the cervix. Am J Epidemiology 115:729–735, 1982.
6. zur Hausen H: Human genital cancer: synergism between two viruses or synergism between a virus infection and initiating events? Lancet: 1370–1372, 1982.
7. Huang ES, Davis MG, Baskar JF, Huong SM: Molecular epidemiology and oncogenicity of human cytomegalovirus. In: Harris CC (ed): Biochemical and Molecular Epidemiology of Cancer. New York, Alan R. Liss, 1986, pp 323–343.
8. Giraldo G, Beth E, Huang ES: Kaposi's sarcoma and its relationship to cytomegalovirus (CMV) III. CMV DNA and CMV early antigens in Kaposi's sarcoma. Int J Cancer 26: 23–29, 1980.
9. Henle G, Henle W, Diehl V: Relation of Burkitt tumor associated herpes-type virus to infectious mononucleosis. Proc Natl Acad Sci USA 59:94–101, 1968.
10. Hanto DW, Gajl-Peczalska KJ, Frizzera G, Arthur DC, Balfour HH, McClain K, Simmons RL, Najerian JS: Epstein-Barr virus (EBV) induced polyclonal and monoclonal B-cell lymphoproliferative disease occurring after renal transplantation: clinical, pathologic, and virologic findings and implications for therapy. Ann Surg 198:356–369, 1983.
11. Nonoyama M, Pagano JS: Homology between Epstein-Barr virus DNA and viral DNA from Burkitt's lymphoma and nasopharyngeal carcinoma determined by DNA–DNA reassociation kinetics. Nature 242:44–47, 1973.
12. Raab-Traub N, Flynn K, Pearson G, Huang A, Levine P, Lanier A, Pagano JS: The differentiated form of nasopharyngeal carcinoma contains Epstein-Barr virus DNA. Int J Cancer 39:25–29, 1987.
13. Pope J, Horne M, Scott W: Transformation of fetal human leukocytes in vitro by filtrates of a human leukemic cell line containing herpes-like virus. Int J Cancer 3:857–866, 1968.
14. Dambaugh T, Hennessy K, Fennewald S, Kieff E: The virus genome and its expression in latent infection. In: Epstein MA, Achong, BG (eds): The Epstein-Barr Virus: Recent Advances. London, William Heinemann Medical Books LTD, 1986, pp 13–45.
15. Yates JL, Warren N, Sugden B: Stable replication of plasmids derived from Epstein-Barr virus in various mammalian cells. Nature 313:812–815, 1985.
16. Wang D, Liebowitz D, Kieff E: An EBV membrane protein expressed in immortalized

lymphocytes transforms established rodent cells. Cell 43:831–840, 1985.
17. Wang F, Gregory C, Rowe M, Wang D, Rickinson A, Kieff E: Epstein-Barr virus nuclear protein 2 specifically induces high surface expression of the B cell activation antigen, CD23. Proc Natl Acad Sci USA 84:3452–3456, 1987.
18. Beasley R, Lin C, Huang L: Hepatocellular carcinoma and hepatitis B virus: a prospective study of 22, 707 men in Taiwan. Lancet 2:1129, 1981.
19. Tiollais P, Pourcel C, Dejean A: The hepatitis B virus. Nature 317:489–495, 1985.
20. Williams MG, Howardson AF, Almeida JD: Morphologic characterization of the virus of the human common wart (verruca vulgaris). Nature 189:895–897, 1961.
21. Zoler ML: Human papilloma virus linked to cervical (and other) cancers. JAMA 249:2997–2999, 1983.
22. Kessler H: Venereal factors in human cervical cancer: evidence from marital clusters. Cancer 39:1912–1919, 1977.
23. Kessler H: Human cervical cancer as a venereal disease. Cancer Res 36:783–791, 1976.
24. Richart RM: Cervical intraepithelial neoplasia. In: Sommers, SC (ed): Pathology Annual New York, Appleton Century Crofts, 1973, pp 301–328.
25. Winkler B, Crum CP, Fujii T: Koilocytic lesions of the cervix: the relationship of mitotic abnormalities to nuclear DNA content. Cancer 53:1081–1087, 1987.
26. Strauss MJ, Shaw EW, Bunting H, Melnick JL: Crystalline virus-like particles from skin papilloma characterised by intramuscular inclusion bodies. Proc Soc Exp Biol Med 72:46–51, 1949.
27. Nuovo G, Crum CP, Silverstein S: Papillomavirus infection of the uterine cervix. Micro Path 3:71–78, 1987.
28. Faras AJ, Kryzysek RA, Ostrow RS, Watts SL, Smith DM, Anderson DI, Quick CA, Pass F: Genetic variation among papilloma viruses. Ann NY Acad Sci 354:60–79, 1980.
29. Durst M, Gissman L, Ikenberg H, zur Hausen H: A papillomavirus DNA from a cervical carcinoma and its prevalence in cancer biopsy samples from different geographic regions. Proc Natl Acad Sci USA 80:3812–3815, 1983.
30. Matsukura T, Kanda T, Furuno A, Yoshikawa H, Kawana T, Yoshike K: Cloning of monomeric human papillomavirus type 16 integrated within cell DNA from a cervical carcinoma. J Virol 58:979–982, 1986.
31. Phelps WC, Howley PM. Transcriptional transactivation by the human papillomavirus type 16 E2 gene product. J Virol 61:1630–1638, 1987.
32. Cripe TP, Haugen TH, Turk, OP, Tabatabai F, Schmid, PG, Durst M, Gissman L, Roman A, Turek LP: Transcriptional regulation of the human papillomavirus-16 E6-E7 promoter by a keratinocyte-dependent enhancer and by viral E2 transactivator and repressor gene products: implications for cervical carcinogenesis. EMBO J 6:3745–3753, 1987.
33. Gloss B, Bernard HU, Seedorf K, Kiock G: The upstream regulatory region of the human papilloma virus-16 contains an E2 protein-independent enhancer which is specific for cervical carcinoma cells and regulated by glucocorticoid hormones. EMBO J 6:3735–3743, 1987.
34. Baker CC, Phelps WC, Lindgren V, Braun MJ, Gonda MA, Howley PM: Structural and transcriptional analysis of human papillomavirus type 16 sequences in cervical carcinoma cell lines. J Virol 61:962–971, 1987.
35. Smotkin D, Wettstein FO: Transcription of human papillomavirus 16 early genes in a cervical cancer and a cancer-derived cell line and identification of the E7 protein. Proc Natl Acad Sci USA 83:4680–4684, 1987.
36. Schneider-Gadicke A, Schwarz E: Different human cervical carcinoma cell lines show similar transcription patterns of human papillomavirus type 18 early genes. EMBO J 6:2285–2292, 1986.
37. Schwartz E, Freese UK, Gissman L, Mayer W, Roggenbuck B, Stemlau A, zur Hausen H: Structure and transcription of human papillomavirus sequences in cervical carcinoma cells. Nature 314:111–113, 1985.
38. Howley P, Schlegel R: Papillomavirus transformation. In: Salzman NP, Howley PM (eds): The Papillomaviruses. New York, Plenum Press, 1987.

39. Yasumoto S, Burkhardt AL, Doniger J, DiPaolo JA: Human papillomvirus type 16 DNA-induced malignant transformation of NIH 3T3 cells. J Virol 57:572–577, 1986.
40. Bedell MA, Jones KH, Laimins LA: The E6–E7 region of human papillomavirus type 18 is sufficient for transformation of NIH 3T3 and Rat-1 cells. J Virol 61:3635–3640, 1987.
41. Matlaschewski G, Schneider J, Banks L, Jones N, Murray A, Crawford L: Human papillomavirus type 16 DNA cooperates with activated ras in transforming primary cells. EMBO J 6:1741–1746, 1987.
42. Phelps WC, Lee CL, Munger K, Howley PM: The human papillomavirus type 16 E7 gene encodes transactivation and transformation functions similar those of adenovirus E1A. Cell 53:539–547, 1988.
43. Buchkovich KJ, Whyte P, Dyson N, Horowitz JM, Friend SH, Raybuck M, Weinberg RA, Harlow E: The transforming proteins of three DNA tumor viruses interact with the retinoblastoma gene product. Abstract #1. Cold Spring Harbor Meeting: SV40, Polyoma, and Adenoviruses. August 10–14, 1988.
44. Epstein MA, Achong BG, Barr YM: Virus particles in cultured lymphoblasts from Burkitt's lymphoma. Lancet 1:702–703, 1964.
45. Pagano JS, Huang ES, Peine P: Absence of Epstein-Barr viral DNA in Burkitt's lymphoma. N Engl J Med 289:1395–1399, 1973.
46. Henle W, Henle G: Seroepidemiology of the Epstein-Barr virus. In: Epstein MA, Achong BG (eds): The Epstein-Barr Virus, Berlin, Springer-Verlag, 1979, pp 62–78.
47. Erikson J, Finan J, Croce CM: Translocation of immunoglobulin VH genes in Burkitt's lymphoma. Proc Natl Acad Sci USA 79:5611–5615, 1982.
48. Pelicci PG, Knowles DM, Magrath I, Dalla-Favaera R: Chromosomal breakpoints and structural alterations of the c-*myc* locus differ in endemic and sporadic forms of Burkitt lymphoma. Proc Natl Acad Sci USA 83:2984–2988, 1986.
49. Zajac-Kaye M, Gelman, E, Levens, D: A point mutation in the c-*myc* locus of a Burkitt's lymphoma abolishes binding of a nuclear protein. Science 240:1776–1780, 1988.
50. Purtilo DT: Hypothesis: pathogenesis and phenotoype of an X-linked lymphoproliferative syndrome. Lancet 2:882–885, 1976.
51. Pelicci PG, Knowles DM, Arlin ZA, Wieczorek R, Lciw P, Dina D, Basilico C, Dalla-Favera R: Multiple monoclonal B-cell expansions and c-*myc* oncogene rearrangements in acquired immune deficiency syndrome-related lymphoproliferative disorders. Implications for lymphomagenesis. J Exp Med 164:2049–2058, 1986.
52. Desgranges C, Wolf H, de The' G, Shanmugaratnam K, Ellouz R, Cammoun N, Klein G, zur Hausen H: Nasopharyngeal carcinoma X. Presence of Epstein-Barr virus genomes in epithelial cells of tumors from high and medium risk areas. Int J Cancer 16:7–15, 1975.
53. Saemundsen AK, Albeck H, Hansen JPH: Epstein-Barr virus nasopharyngeal and salivary gland carcinomas in Greenland Eskimos. Br J Cancer 46:721–728, 1982.
54. Brichacek B, Hirsch J, Sibl O, Vilikusova E, Vonka V: Association of some supraglottic laryngeal caracinomas with EBV virus. Int J Cancer 32:193–197, 1983.
55. Baer R, Bankier A, Biggin M, Dienenger P, Farrell P, Gibson T, Hatfull G, Hudson G, Satchwell S, Sequin C, Tuffnell P, Barrell B: DNA sequence and expression of the B95–8 Epstein-Barr virus. Nature 310:207–211, 1984.
56. Dambaugh T, Beisel C, Hummel M, King W, Fennewald S, Cheung A, Heller M, Raab-Traub N, Kieff E: Epstein-Barr virus (B95–8) DNA. VII. Molecular cloning and detailed mapping of EBV (B95–8) DNA. Proc Natl Acad Sci USA 77:2999–3003, 1980.
57. Raab-Traub N, Flynn K: The structure of the termini of the Epstein-Barr virus as a marker of clonal cellular proliferation. Cell 47:883–889, 1986.
58. Greenspan JS, Greenspan D, Lennette E, Abrams DI, Conant MA, Petersen V, Freese VK: Replication of Epstein-Barr virus within the epithelial cells of oral 'hairy' leukoplakia an AIDs associated lesion. N Engl J Med 313:1564–1571, 1985.
59. Matsuo T, Heller, M, Petti L, O'Shiro E, Kieff E: Persistence of the entire Epstein-Barr virus genome integrated into human lymphocyte DNA. Science 226:1322–1325, 1984.
60. Sample J, Hummel M, Braun D, Birkenbach M, Kieff E: Nucleotide sequence of messenger

RNAs encoding Epstein-Barr virus nuclear proteins reveals a probable transcriptional initiation site. Proc Natl Acad Sci USA 83:6096–6100, 1986.
61. Rabson M, Gradoville L, Heston L, Miller G: Non-immortalizing P3JHR-1 Epstein-Barr virus: a deletion mutant of its transforming parent, Jijoye. J Virol 44:834–844, 1982.
62. Skare J, Farley J, Strominger JL, Fresen K, Cho MS, zur Hausen H: Transformation by Epstein-Barr virus requires DNA sequences in the region of BamHI fragments Y and H. J Virol 55:286–297, 1985.
63. Rowe D, Farrell P, Miller G: Novel nuclear antigens recognized by human sera in lymphocytes latently infected with Epstein-Barr virus. Virology 156:153–162, 1987.
64. Dambaugh T, Hennessey K, Chamnankit L, Kieff E: U2 region of Epstein-Barr virus DNA may encode Epstein-Barr nuclear antigen 2. Proc Natl Acad Sci USA 81:7632–7636, 1984.
65. Laux G, Perricaudet M, Farrell PJ: A spliced Epstein-Barr virus gene expressed in immortalized lymphocytes is created by circularization of the linear viral genome. EMBO J 7:769–774, 1988.
66. Fennewald S, van Santen V, Kieff E: Nucleotide sequence of an mRNA transcribed in latent growth-transforming virus infection indicates that it may encode a membrane protein. J Virol 51:411–419, 1984.
67. Wang D, Liebowitz D, Wang F, Gregory C, Rickinson A, Larson R, Springer T, Kieff E: Epstein-Barr virus latent infection membrane protein (LMP) alters lymphocyte morphology, adhesion, and growth: deletion of the amino terminus abolishes activity. J Virol 62:4173–4184, 1988.
68. Young L, Dawson C, Clark D, Rupani H, Busson P, Tursz T, Johnson A, Rickinson A: Epstein-Barr virus gene expression in nasopharyngeal carcinoma. J Gen Virol 69:1051–1065, 1988.

13. Molecular biology of the human retinoblastoma gene

Yuen Kai T. Fung, Anne T'ang, and Theresa L. Thompson

The recessive nature of cancer

The notion that genetic damage is the underlying cause of cancer comes from two apparently contradictory lines of evidence on the nature of carcinogenesis. On the one hand, many genomic changes found in malignant cells, such as point mutations, amplification, translocation, and various other rearrangements induced chemically or by retroviruses, have been shown to result in the activation of a set of genes termed oncogenes [1]. These genes, when introduced into target cells either as part of a virus of by DNA transfection can confer neoplastic transformation on the target cells. The existence of these oncogenes suggests that tumorigenicity may be dominant in nature. On the other hand, there is equally compelling evidence to suggest that recessive genomic changes may underlie the neoplastic phenotype of tumor cells.

One line of evidence for the recessive nature of tumorigenesis comes from somatic cell hybrid studies. Harris, Klein, and their colleagues were the first to demonstrate conclusively that stable suppression of malignancy can be achieved by fusion between malignant and nonmalignant cells [2,3]. Stable suppression of tumorigenicity and of the tumorigenic phenotype was also demonstrated in human cancer by the fusion of human malignant cells with normal human cells [4]. When rare tumorigenic segregants were isolated, a detailed chromosome analysis of these cells invariably revealed that specific chromosome(s) were lost in the tumorigenic segregants. It is therefore the presence of certain specific chromosomes (contributed by the normal parental cells) that are involved in the suppression of tumorigenicity in the hybrid. The observations that different tumorigenic cells can complement each other in suppression of the tumorigenic phenotype suggests that different chromosomes are involved in controlling the tumorigenic expression in different cancer cells. Taken together, these studies imply that a loss of genetic material that has a tumor-suppression function is involved in the development of cancer. Further support of this notion came from the recent finding that introduction of a normal chromosome 11 can suppress tumorigenicity in certain tumor cells [6,7].

A second line of evidence for a role of recessive genetic damage in tumor development comes from studies of a number of familial pediatric tumors such as retinoblastoma (RB) and Wilms' tumor. Retinoblastoma is a malignant intraocular childhood tumor of the retina that can occur in utero but rarely beyond the age of seven. Like many human cancers, retinoblastoma occurs in sporadic and hereditary forms. Most unilateral cases are nonhereditary. Bilateral cases, however, are always hereditary, with the mutation that predisposes to the development of retinoblastoma being transmitted in a dominant Mendelian fashion. It should be pointed out that at the cellular level, the predisposing mutation is recessive in nature because inheritance of the germ-line mutation is not sufficient for the tumor to develop. Based on the statistical analysis of clinical observations, Knudson has proposed that the development of retinoblastoma requires two mutational events (two hits) [8]. In hereditary cases, although the germ-line mutation is present in all cells, a second somatic mutation in a target retinoblast is required for tumor development.

What is the nature of these two mutational events? The first clue came from cytogenetic studies. Karyotypic analysis of lymphocytes or fibroblasts from retinoblastoma patients revealed the presence of a constitutional deletion in the long arm of chromosome 13 in some of the patients. Although there are variations in the size of the deletions, they all encompass the chromosomal region 13 q14 [5,9]. Further evidence that the first hit involves 13 q14 comes from studies done on the enzyme esterase D. A tight linkage between the retinoblastoma gene locus and esterase D gene locus has been demonstrated in families with the hereditary form of retinoblastoma [10,11]. In all the deletion cases examined, the esterase D enzyme was found to be reduced to 50% of normal in constitutional cells [18]. It was therefore hypothesized that the mutation of the gene or a group of genes encoded in this region represents the first mutational event in the hereditary form of retinoblastoma.

Initial cytogenetic data also implicated chromosome 13q 14 as the target for the second mutation. Partial or total deletions were frequently observed in retinoblastomas from patients with two apparently karyotypically normal chromosome 13s. Analysis using DNA probes, which can detect restriction fragments length polymorphism (RFLP) in specific regions of chromosome 13, provided more precise evidence for the involvement of this DNA region in the second hit. By a comparison of the constitutional and tumor genotype (defined by RFLPs on chromosome 13), it was shown that in the tumor, the wild-type chromosome 13 was lost, leaving the chromosome 13 with the deletion in the tumor cells. Examination of the RFLP patterns in a number of other retinoblastomas shows that the reduction to hemizygosity or homozygosity of part or all of chromosome 13 appeared to be a common event in the development of retinoblastoma [13].

The two mutational events (two hits) therefore act by inactivating or eliminating the two alleles of the tumor-suppressor gene on chromosome 13. Mitotic nondisjunction and recombination appear to be common mechanisms whereby the remaining wild-type allele is eliminated, resulting in hemizygosity of all the loci on the chromosome that carries the first hit. Subsequent duplication of this chromosome results in homozygosity.

The availability of DNA probes that can detect RFLP in specific chromosomal regions has allowed a detailed analysis of the involvement of particular chromosomes or chromosomal regions in different types of cancer. Already RFLP studies have allowed the mapping of chromosomal losses in various solid tumors that have so far escaped detection by cytogenetic studies. For example, losses of a gene or genes in the short arm of chromosome 11 have been detected in Wilms' tumor, rhabdomyosarcoma, and hepatoblastoma [14]. In many different types of tumors, multiple chromosomal loci losses are involved. For example, in colorectal carcinoma, reduction to homozygosity of part or all of chromosomes 5q, 17p, 18q, 22, and others has been reported [15]. Taken together, these data tend to support the concept that tumorigenicity behaves as a recessive genetic trait and that the loss of genetic information (tumor-suppressor genes) is a necessary step in the development of cancer. The isolation and characterization of the various putative tumor-suppressor genes will no doubt provide information on the nature of tumor suppression. At present, only two recessive cancer genes have been isolated: the lethal [2] giant larvae of Drosophila melanogaster [16] and the human retinoblastoma gene [17,18,21].

Isolation of the human retinoblastoma gene

The localization of the putative retinoblastoma gene to chromosome region 13q 14 set the stage for its eventual isolation. Given the lack of information about the putative RB gene other than its location and visible deletions in some tumors, the most logical choice of strategy for isolation was that of chromosomal walking. The 13q 14.1 region, however, is at least 6000 kb. The enormous size as well as the probability of many unclonable regions makes chromosomal walking of such magnitude seem impractical. To get around this problem, random probes free of highly repetitive sequences were isolated from the chromosome-13-specific library LL13NS01 obtained from Lawrence Livermore laboratory. The idea was to saturate the chromosomal 13q 14.1 region with as many probes as possible as starting points for the walking, such that each probe would be used to walk only a short distance. To do this, we made use of two hamster–human hybrid cell lines. Each of these cell lines was made by fusion of a hamster cell line to fibroblasts of patients with visible deletions in the chromosome 13q 14.1 region. DNA clones from the chromosome 13 library containing DNA inserts within the chromosomal region 13q 14.1 were identified by the absence of hybridization to the DNA of these hybrid cell lines. Since the deletion endpoints map to different positions in each of the cell lines, we reasoned that only the probes closest to the RB gene would be absent from both these cell lines.

Several probes were isolated in this fashion. Two other probes, H2–42 and

H3-8 [19], isolated using a similar strategy and kindly provided to us by Dr. Samuel Latt, were also used. Since the esterase D and the putative RB loci are both located in 13q 14.1, we also isolated a full-length esterase D cDNA clone to use as a probe. Regardless of which probe was used as a starting point for walking, we almost invariably encountered unclonable regions after several hundred kb. The H3-8 probe was found to be absent from all the libraries we made in our laboratory as well as from those obtained from several other laboratories. We reasoned that the absence of the H3-8 probe, as well as other unclonable regions we encountered, was due to the fact that it is located in a region that is easily deleted. We therefore chose to walk across these regions by cloning shorter, overlapping restriction fragments detected with the walking probes. The insert size of each clone obtained was verified by hybridization of the clone to genomic blots. We were surprised to isolate a probe pG4-4, which was located very near H3-8 and which also hybridizes to a hamster sequence. This sequence similarity between human and hamster immediately suggested to us that the genomic fragment containing the pG4-4 probe sequence also contained the coding sequence of the gene. Hybridization of pG4-4 to Northern blots of several immortalized human fetal retinal cell lines revealed a 4.7-kb message RNA. Using pG4-4 as a probe, we subsequently isolated several cDNA clones, the longest of which was 4.73kb. At the same time [20], the conservation of DNA sequence between human and other animal species was also noticed by S. Friend and his colleagues in R. Weinberg's laboratory at MIT and by T. Dryja at Harvard. Using the H3-8 probe, they isolated a 4.7-kb cDNA. A comparison of the two cDNA restriction maps indicated that the same cDNA clone had been isolated. Later, using an RB probe from T. Dryja's group, Lee and his colleagues reproduced these results by isolated several shorted versions of the cDNA clone [21].

Structural evidence for the authenticity of the retinoblastoma gene

Evidence to support the contention that the isolated cDNA corresponds to the putative RB gene has been derived mostly from structural analysis of the corresponding genomic locus. The RB-1 locus is very complicated. It is divided into 27 exons distributed over at least 200 kb [22] (figure 1). The last exon is the largest (1889 bp) and contains the C-terminal coding sequences as well as a large 3' untranslated region. The cDNA sequence, together with the genomic sequence of the promotor region, is shown in figure 2. In the 5' upstream region, three promotor binding sites for the transcription factor Sp1 are found. That this region has promotor activity is confirmed by ligation of a bacterial chloramphenical acetyltransferase (CAT) gene to its 3' end. CAT activity could be detected in cells transfected with this plasmid.

The lack of TATA and CCAAT boxes and the presence of Sp1 sites amidst an extremely G+C-rich (70%) background is characteristic of the promotors

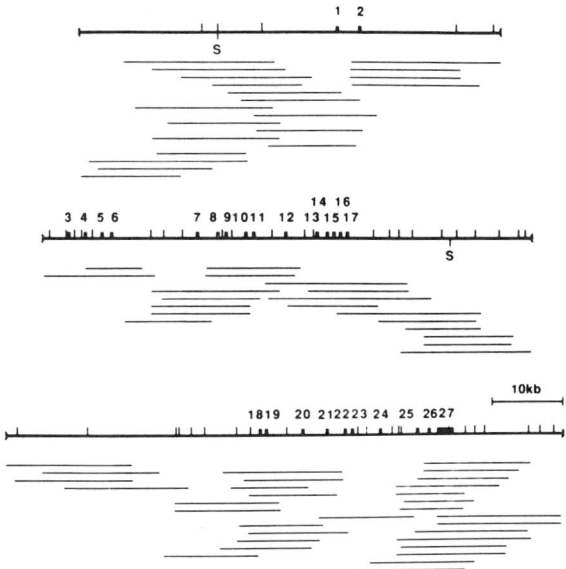

Figure 1. Genomic organization of the RB-1locus. *Hind* III sites are represented by vertical lines. Individual exons are shown as numbered black boxes. Overlapping lambda phage clones are shown as horizontal lines beneath the restriction map. Gaps ( ) represent uncertainty in the size of intron restriction fragments. S, Sal1 site.

found in a number of housekeeping genes, such as hypoxanthine guanine phosphoribosyltransferase gene [28], and a number of genes related to growth regulation, such as c-K-*ras*, c-H-*ras*, and the EGF receptor [29,35,36].

Using the cDNA as a probe, structural abnormalities were detected in the DNA of certain retinoblastoma samples, including those with visible deletions in the 13q 14.1 region. It should be noted that since a cDNA probe was used, only structural aberrations of exon-containing restriction fragments would be detectible; structural aberrations involving very small exons may not be detected. This would also apply to point mutations or extremely small deletions in the exon or at the splice junctions. However, even with these limitations, many examples of structural aberrations involving all or part of the RB-1 locus have been documented [17,18,21]. These structural changes include homozygous total deletions as well as 3' deletions [17,18,21]. However, it is the detection of homozygous internal deletions in some of the retinoblastoma samples that provided the definitive proof of the authenticity of the retinoblastoma gene [18]. Approximately 40% of the 40 cases of retinoblastoma examined show some form of structural aberration at the RB locus by Southern blot analysis (figure 3). However, virtually 100% of the retinoblastoma samples analyzed have no normal RB transcript. Instead, the RB transcript is either totally absent, or presented in a truncated form in the retinoblastoma (regardless of whether an abnormality can be detected at the DNA level).

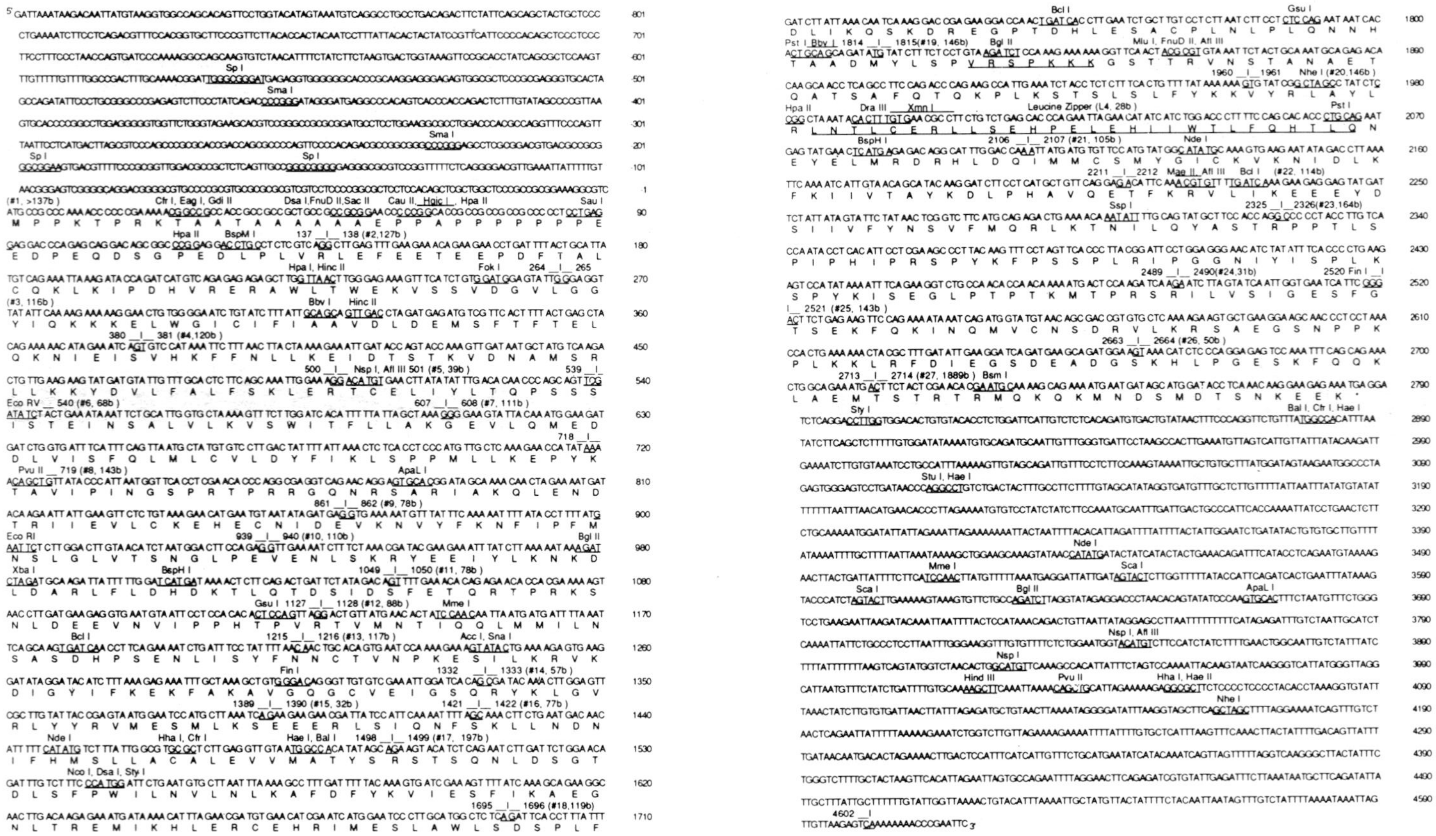

Figure 2. The RB-1 cDNA sequences including part of the genomic sequence immediately 5' of cDNA. The A residues in the ATG translation iniations codon is described as nucleotide position #1. The three Sp1 binding sites are shown underlined. The amino acids of the longest reading frame are shown immediately below each of the coding sequence. The nuclear translocation signal and the leucine zipper are underlined.

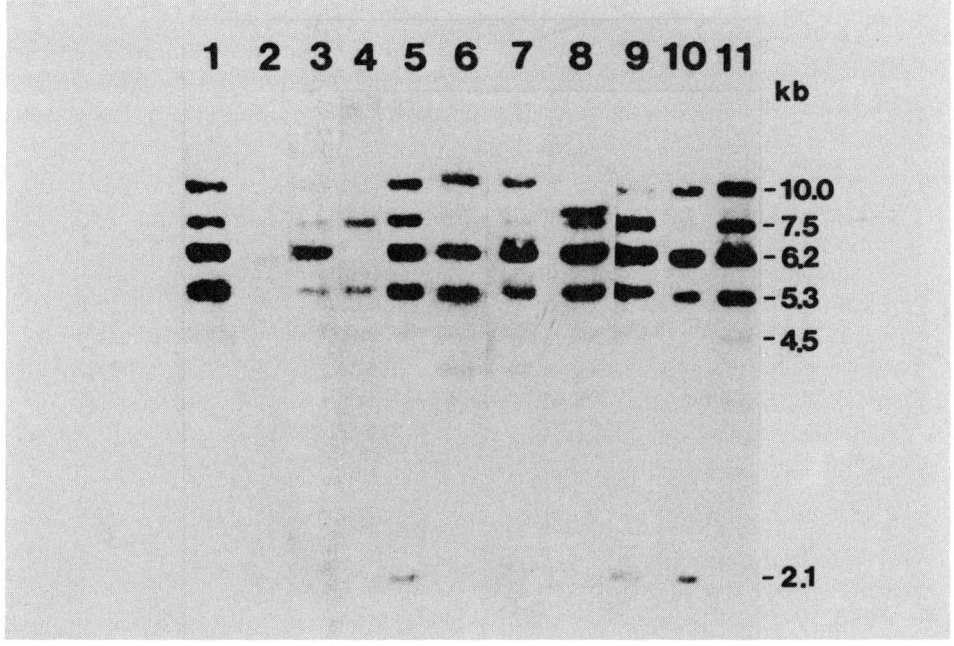

Figure 3. Southern blot analysis of *Hind* III genomic DNA from normal cell (lane 1) retinoblastomas and their constitutional cells (lanes 2–9, 11), and an osteosarcoma (lane 10). The probe used was PG 3.8M, a subclone of the EcoRI 3.8-kb fragment of the cDNA clone. Lane 1, normal control human fibroblast; Lane 2, LA-RB128B (hereditary retinoblastoma); Lane 3, LA-RB128B-F (fibroblast); Lane 4, LA-RB165 (sporadic retinoblastoma); Lane 5, LA-RB165-F (fibroblast); Lane 6, LA-RB74 (hereditary retinoblastoma) Lane 7, LA-RB74-F (fibroblast); Lane 8, LA-RB151 (hereditary retinoblastoma); Lane 9, LA-RB151-F (fibroblast); Lane 10, OHS50 (osteosarcoma); Lane 11, LA-RB73 (sporadic retinoblastoma).

Analysis of the RB locus has resulted in the verification of the two-hit hypothesis at the molecular level. As shown in figure 3, in several bilateral cases where mutations were detected as homozygous deletions of part or all of the RB gene, identical structural changes were readily detected in one of the RB-1 alleles in the fibroblasts of the patients. Normal RB transcripts were readily detected even when only a single copy of the wild-type gene remained in the fibroblasts. In contrast, in the unilateral case with no familial history of retinoblastoma, the two mutational events were detected only in the tumor and not in fibroblasts. These data taken together are consistent with the course of mutational events proposed in the two-hit hypothesis. Aside from providing evidence for the identity of the RB gene, the detection of internal homozygous deletions in RB alleles helps to confirm the recessive nature of retinoblastoma tumorigenesis. Moreover, the ability to detect germ-line structural deletions in the fibroblasts of some patients with bilateral retinoblastoma indicates that the isolated gene may be useful for diagnostic purposes.

Involvement of the retinoblastoma gene in various human cancers

One of the most interesting aspects of hereditary childhood solid tumors is the frequent clinical association of different tumors. In the case of retinoblastoma, it is well documented [23] that surviving patients with the familial form of retinoblastoma are at increased risk for other specific types of nonocular primary malignancies, such as soft-tissue sarcoma, osteosarcoma, and melanoma [23,24,25]. RFLP analysis of the genotypes of normal and tumor cells from osteosarcoma patients [26,27] revealed that reduction to homozygosity of part of chromosome 13 including the 13q 14 region is a common event in osteosarcoma, not only in patients with the hereditary forms of retinoblastoma, but also in patients with no known familial history of retinoblastoma. This suggests that a single pleiotropic recessive locus is the link between retinoblastoma and osteosarcoma. Using the RB gene cDNA as a probe, a homozygous internal deletion and truncated RB transcript were detected in an osteosarcoma from a patient with a prior history of retinoblastoma. Internal deletions, as well as 3' deletions, have been detected in about 25% of osteosarcomas from patients that have no prior history of retinoblastoma predisposition [17,18,30].

While breast tumors have seldom been associated with retinoblastoma, mothers of children with osteosarcoma are at higher risk for breast tumors [19]. A loss of heterozygosity on chromosome 13q has previously been reported in human ductal breast tumors. Using the RB cDNA as a probe, structural aberrations of the retinoblastoma locus were observed in 25% of breast tumor cell lines, and in 7% of primary tumors. These changes include homozygous internal deletions and total deletion of the RB-1 locus. Interestingly, a duplication of an exon was observed in one of the cell lines [31]. In all cases, structural changes either resulted in the absence or truncation of the RB-1 transcript.

Structural rearrangements of the human retinoblastoma gene locus have recently been demonstrated in two other adult cancers: small-cell lung cancer [32,33] and transitional-cell bladder tumor [34]. Harbour et al. [32] observed structural abnormalities within the RB gene in one of eight primary small-cell lung carcinomas (SCLC), 4 out of 22 SCLC cell lines, and 1 out of 4 pulmonary carcinoid lines. Similarly, Yakota et al. have examined 9 small-cell lung carcinoma cell lines; none express RB protein [33].

In 2 of 12 primary transitional-cell bladder carcinoma and in 3 of 8 bladder tumor cell lines, inactivation of the retinoblastoma gene can be detected either at the DNA, RNA, or protein level [34]. A summary of the involvement of the retinoblastoma gene in various malignancies is presented in figure 4. A close inspection of the structural aberrations in these various malignancies indicates that there are certain hot spots for rearrangement in the retinoblastoma cDNA sequence. Structural analysis of the cDNA reveals the presence of 15 dyad symmetrical elements, distributed in 6 exons, #1, #4, #10, #16, #17 and #27. Eight of these sequences are in the 3' untranslated

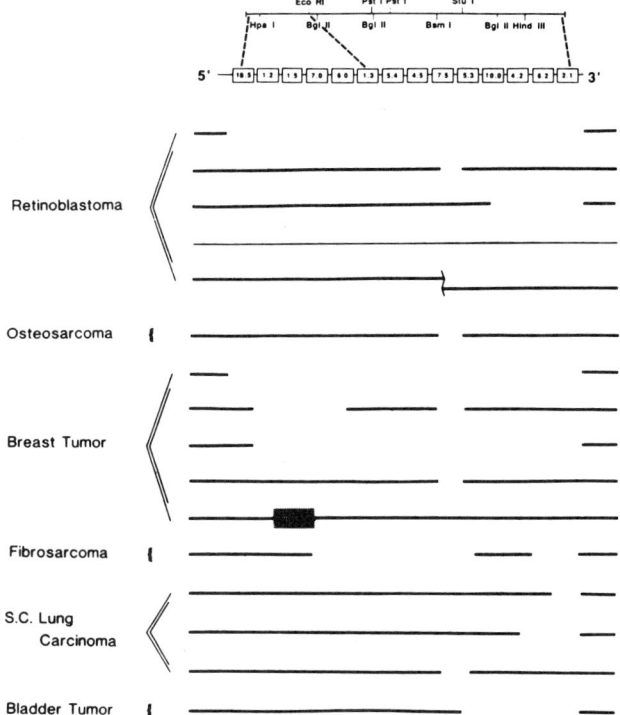

Figure 4. Schematic representation of a summary of structured aberrations of the RB gene in various malignancies, including homozygous internal deletions, homozygous total deletions, homozygous 3' deletions, translation, and amplification. A restriction map of the 4.7-kb cDNA clone of the RB gene is shown at the top. The linear order of the *Hind* III restriction fragments detectable with cDNA probes is shown below. Each of the boxes represents a discrete *Hind* III fragment the size (kilobases) of which is indicated by the number in the box.

region of exon #27, and 6 of the 7 remaining elements are in the translated region. The positions of such sequences, relative to the deletions discussed above, tend to suggest that they could be potential recombination hot spots. There appears to be a clustering of dyad-symmetrical elements in exons #16 and #17; moreover, exon #17 also contains an inverted repeat sequence. Both of these exons, contained in a 7.5-kb *Hind* III restriction fragment (figure 5), have been designated as hot spots for deletion because they are frequently involved in gross structural rearrangements.

Structure and function of the retinoblastoma gene product

Sequence analysis of the cDNA indicated that the longest reading frame encodes a protein of 928 amino acids. Preliminary results using rabbit antisera prepared against a tryp E-RB fusion protein, a protein of an apparent mole-

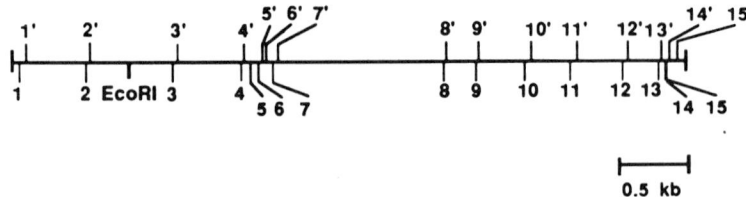

Figure 5. Distribution of dyad-symmetrical elements in the RB-1 cDNA. The RB-1 cDNA is represented as a horizontal line. Each pair of numbers above and below the horizontal line represents the two halves of a hyad symmetry.

cular mass of 110,000 to 114,000 can be immunoprecipitated (39). Furthermore, the RB protein can be metabolically labeled with ^{32}P-phosphate, indicating that it is a phosphoprotein. Similar results were obtained by us, and others, using rabbit antisera prepared against oligopeptides synthesized according to the sequence of various portions of the RB gene. Antisera prepared against either synthetic oligopeptides or bacterially expressed peptides can immunoprecipitate a protein of approximately 105 kDa. As shown in figure 6, the 105-kDa protein can be modified to about 116 kDa. The metabolic labeling with ^{35}S-methionine and ^{32}P-phosphate indicated that the 105 kDa protein is the native form of RB protein. The smear above it, however, is the phosphorylated form of the RB protein.

Nuclear localization

A close inspection of the cDNA sequence reveals the presence of a stretch of amino acids at position 609 to 615 (VRSPKKK) that is reminiscent of the nuclear translocation signal found in SV40 large T-antigen and in Polyoma large T-antigen. This implies that the RB protein is a nuclear protein. Lee and his colleagues have reported the detection, by immunostaining, of the RB protein in the nuclei of some cells [39]. Subcellular localization by fractionation of cellular components also located the RB gene product in the nuclear fraction. Using column chromatography of the RB protein on single-strand as well as double-strand DNA cellulose columns, it was shown that the RB protein can be retained under low salt conditions on the column [39], indicating that under certain conditions, the RB protein may be able to bind to DNA or that it is associated with DNA-binding proteins under those conditions. It was reported earlier [21] that the RB protein has a putative zinc finger structure that is characteristic of some DNA-binding proteins. However, a close inspection of the cDNA sequence failed to reveal any convincing evidence that such a zinc finger motif exists.

Leucine zipper

Recently, a hypothetical structure common to a new class of DNA-binding proteins has been described. The hypothetical structure was derived from

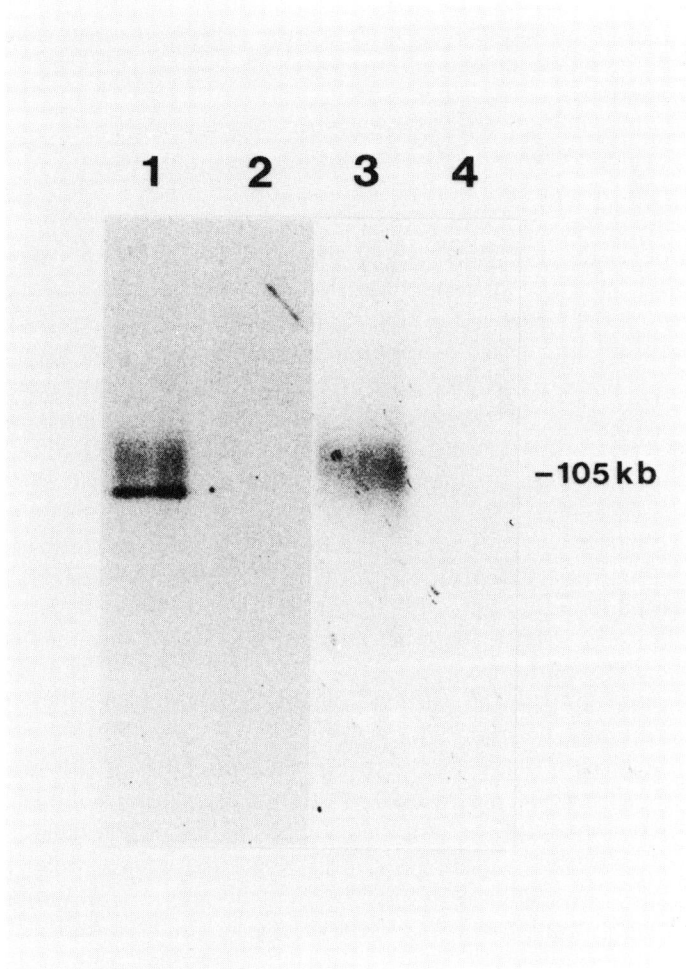

Figure 6. Immunoprecipitation of the RB protein by antisera prepared against RB oligopetides (KKLRFDIEGSDEADGS). The human cell line SW613 labeling with ^{35}S-methionine (lane 1) shows the 105-kDa native protein as a sharp band and the phosphorylated form as a smear above. Labeling with ^{32}phosphoric acid (lane 3) shows only the smear pattern of the phosphorylated protein. Lanes 2 and 4 are the same as 1 and 3, respectively, except that the antiserum used was preabsorbed with the immunizing oligopeptide.

stretches of amino acid sequence motif common to several DNA-binding proteins, among them the oncogenes c-*myc*, N-*myc*, L-*myc*, and the transcription factors GCN4 and C/EBP [40]. The common motif is the periodic repetition of leucine residues. In the DNA-binding domain of C/EBP, for example, leucine appears at every seventh position over a region of 35 amino acids. When the amino acid sequence of this region is displayed on a schematic α helix, it was noticed that one side of the hypothetical helix was predominantly composed of leucine, while the other was composed of amino acids with charged side chains and uncharged polar side chains.

It was hypothesized that such a structural motif could allow the leucine residues from one α-helix to interdigitate with those of a second α-helix, forming a molecular zipper between two polypeptides. It was predicted that dimerization in this manner may allow a protein complex to recognize specific DNA sequences. It is interesting to note that, besides being homoduplex, the leucine zipper can potentially allow dimerization between two dissimilar DNA-binding proteins. It is possible that association between the two oncogene products of *fos* and *jun* may represent a heterodimer formed by the interdigitation of their leucine zippers.

A close inspection of the amino acid sequences of the human retinoblastoma gene cDNA revealed the presence of just such a leucine zipper motif from amino acid 661 to 689 (LNTLCELLSEHPELEHIIWTLFQHTLQ). An α-helix wheel display [40] of this stretch of amino acids is shown in figure 7. A comparison of this RB domain with that of C/EBP and GCN4 revealed that the sequence conservation is not limited to the leucine zipper side of the helix. It is remarkable to note that the amino acids residues R667, E674, T681, and Q688, which all face the same side of the RB α-helix domain, are conserved relative to those in C/EBP (with the minor exception of glutamic acid, E674, being replaced by glutamine, Q, in C/EBP). In addition, the positions of R667, L669, and E671 are conserved in L-*myc*, E671 in N-*myc*, I 679 in v-*fos*, and E674 and Q688 in v-*jun*. The positions of the amino acid residues E676, E666, and S670 in RB are found to be the conserved in the transcription factor GCN4. In general, amino acid position conservation is more prominent between RB and C/EBP as well as GCN4. This observation raised the interesting questions of whether the RB protein exists as a dimer in the cell and whether it can complex with the other leucine-zipper-containing proteins, such as the *myc* protein families or the transcription factors, and thereby exert its effect. The close resemblance of this leucine zipper domain in RB and C/EBP suggests that the RB protein may regulate the transcription of certain genes. It may do that either on its own or by complexing with other leucine-zipper-containing proteins.

Association with oncoproteins

While it is still not known whether RB protein and the *myc* families or protein can form heterodimers, association between the RB protein and two viral proteins has been demonstrated [37,38]. Yu and Branton [41], as well as Ed Harlow and his colleagues [42], have previously observed an association of the adenovirus EIA protein with a whole spectrum of host-cell proteins of molecular mass ranging from 28 kDa to 300 kDa. Of these, the most predominant are 105 kDa, 107 kDa, and 300 kDa. It was observed that mutations in the EIA protein that abolish its ability to bind these three

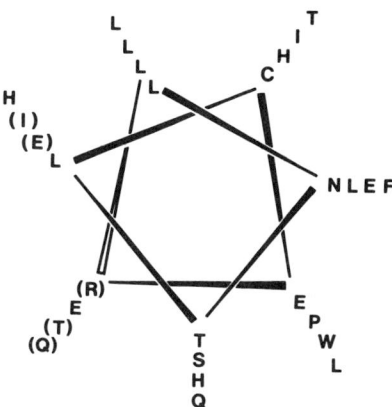

Figure 7. α-helical wheel analysis of the leucine zipper found in the RB protein as described [40]. L, leucine; C, cystein; H, histidine; I, isoleucine; T, threonine; N, asparagine; E, glutamic acid; F, phenylatamine; P, proline; W, tryptophan; S, serine; Q, glutamine; R, arginine.

host proteins also destroy its ability to cooperate with the oncogene *ras* in transcription of primary baby-rat kidney cells. Using antisera prepared against oligopeptides of the RB protein, P. Whyte in Ed Harlow's laboratory succeeded in demonstrating an association of the RB protein with the EIA protein [37]. Comparative peptide mapping revealed that the 105 kDa host protein brought down with the antibodies was in fact the RB protein.

Structural similarities between EIA and SV40 large T-antigen, as well as the *myc* protein, have been described previously [43,44]. In fact, in transformation assays, a region of 18 amino acids in the SV40 large T protein can substitute for the 19-amino-acid transforming domain of the EIA protein [43]. The N-terminal portion of this 19-amino-acid sequence is required for EIA protein binding to the RB protein. As predicted, using anti-RB serum, an association between RB protein and the SV40 large T-antigen was demonstrated [38]. The region of similarity between SV40 large T and EIA domain 2 was shown to be necessary for the association with the RB protein. Moreover, mutants of SV40 larg T unable to transform cells also failed to bind to the RB protein.

The fact that the domain required for transformation is also required for these viral proteins to bind to RB protein implies that at least part of the transforming functions of these viruses is due to their inhibition of the normal function of the RB protein. Conversely, one can speculate that the normal function of the RB protein at the cellular level is one of antiproliferation or prevention of cooperation with *ras* oncogene (or its equivalent genes) in bringing about tumorigenesis. In other words, the RB gene is either a senescence gene that may confer mortality upon specific cell types, or it is a gene that interferes with the cell's ability to respond to the signal of an activated *ras* (or equivalent) gene. In either case, the effect of the RB gene would be one of suppression of tumorigenicity.

Physiological role of the retinoblastoma gene in cells

In order to define the role of the RB gene in the suppression of tumor development, we have recently attempted to introduce an intact copy of the RB gene into various human tumor cell lines that have suffered homozygous inactivation of the RB gene. A plasmid, PRbE, was constructed such that the RB cDNA was ligated to upstream 5' RB-1 promotor sequences. In this plasmid, the cDNA is under the control of the RB-1 gene transcription promotor. As a control, we constructed a similar plasmid, PRbC, but deleted the translation initiation site. Both plasmids carry the neomycin gene. Transfection of the control plasmid PRbC into the above-mentioned cell lines resulted in G418-resistant cell lines that were otherwise identical to the parental cell lines. Transfection with the full-length RB cDNA under its own promoter (PRbE plasmid) elicited several different observed responses:

1. Many of the cell lines became senescent soon after transfection with PRbE. The numerous G418-resistant colonies grew to about 50–200 cells after three weeks and then stopped proliferating. In contrast, cells transfected with the control plasmid PRbC became G418-resistant and proliferated to the same extent as the parental cell lines.
2. Some cell lines grew equally well whether they were transfected with PRbC or PRbE. These cell lines seem to be unaffected by the presence or absence of the transfected RB gene.
3. Several cell lines changed their growth properties when transfected with PRbE but not PRbC. The cells grow very slowly with a doubling time of 80 hours instead of the normal 20 hours observed with the parental cells. The cell morphology also changed. In general, the cells tend to lie side by side along the long axis of the cell.

It is perhaps not surprising that different cells can respond to the RB gene differently. For example, immunostaining of a tissue section of the normal mammary gland shows that only a specific subset of the different cell types that make up the organ express RB protein (Fung, unpublished). This tissue specificity of the RB gene is consistent with the fact that the RB gene is not the only tumor-suppressor gene in the cell.

The study of the RB gene at this juncture is reminiscent of the study of the retroviral oncogenes in the late 1970s. Since that time, more than three dozen oncogenes have been discovered. In the coming decade, we should witness the isolation and characterization of more tumor-suppressor genes.

References

1. Bishop JM: The molecular genetics of cancer. *Science* 235:305–311, 1987.
2. Harris H, Miller OJ, Klein G, Worst P, Tachibana T: (Suppression of malignancy by cell fusion. *Nature* 223:363–368, 1969.

3. Wiener, F, Klein G, Harris H: The Analysis of Malignancy by cell fusion. III. Hybrids between diploid fibroblasts and other tumor cells. *J Cell Sci* 8:681, 1971.
4. Stanbridge EJ: Suppression of malignancy in human cells. Nature 260: 17–20, 1976.
5. Yunis JJ, Ramsay N: Retinoblastoma and subband deletion of chromosome 13. Am J Dis Child 132:161, 1978.
6. Saxon PJ, Srivatsan ES, Stanbridge EJ: Introduction of human chromosome 11 via microcell transfer controls tumorigenic expression of HeLa cells. EMBO J 5:3461–3466, 1986.
7. Weissman BE, Saxon PJ, Pasquale SR, Jones GR, Geiser AG, Stanbridge EJ: Introduction of a normal human chromosome 11 into a Wilms' tumor cell line controls its tumorigenic expression. Science 236:175–180, 1987.
8. Knudson, AG: Mutation and cancer: Statistical study of retinoblastoma. Proc Natl Acad Sci USA 68:820–823, 1971.
9. Ward P, Packman S, Loughman W, Sparkes, M, Sparkes R, McMahon A, Gregory T, Ablin A: Location of the retinoblastoma susceptibility gene(s) and the human esterase D locus. J Med Genet 21:92, 1984.
10. Sparkes RS, Murphree, AL, Lingua RW, Sparkes, MC, Field LL, Funderburk, SJ, Benedict WF: Gene for hereditary retinoblastoma assigned to human chromosome 13 by linkage to esterase D. Science 219;971, 1983.
11. Connolly MJ, Payne RG, Johnson G, Gallie BL, Allerdice PW, Marshall, WH, Lawton RD: Familial, *EsD*-linked, retinoblastoma with reduced penetrance and variable expressivity. Hum Genet 65:122, 1983.
12. Sparkes RS, Sparkes MC, Wilson MG, Towner JW, Benedict W, Murphree AL, Yunis JJ: Regional assignment of genes for human esterase D and retinoblastoma to chromosome band 13q14. Science 208:1042, 1980.
13. Cavenee WK, Dryja TP, Philips RA, Benedict WF, Godbout R, Gallie BL, Murphree AL, Strong LC, White RL: Expression of recessive alleles by chromosomal mechanisms in retinoblastoma. Nature (London) 305:779–784, 1983.
14. Koufos A, Hansen MF, Copeland NG, Jenkins NA, Lampkin BC, and Cavenee WK: Loss of heterozygosity in three embryonal tumours suggests a common pathogenetic mechanism. Nature 316:330–334, 1985.
15. Vogelstein B, Fearon ER, Hamilton SR, Kern SE, Preisinger AC, Leppert M, Nakamura Y, White, R, Smits AMM, Bos JL: Genetic alterations during colorectal-tumor development. N Engl J Med 319:525, 1988.
16. Mechler BM, McGinnis W, Gehring WJ: Molecular cloning of lethal (2) giant larvae, a recessive oncogene of Drosophila melanogaster. EMBO J 4:1551–1557, 1985.
17. Friend SH, Bernards R, Rogelj S, Weinberg RA, Rapaport JM, Albert DM, Dryja TP: A human DNA segment with properties of the gene that predisposes to retinoblastoma and osteosarcoma. Nature (London) 323:643–646, 1986.
18. Fung YK, Murphree AL, T'Ang A, Qian J, Hinrichs SH, Benedict WF: Structural evidence for the authenticity of the human retinoblastoma gene. Science 236:1657–1661, 1987.
19. Hartley AL, Birch JM, Marsden HB, Harris M: Breast cancer risk in mothers of children with osteosarcoma and chondrosarcoma. Br J Cancer 54:819, 1986.
20. Fung YK, T'ang A, Thompson TL: Findings reported at the American Academy of Ophthalmology, New Orleans, November 12, 1986.
21. Lee WH, Bookstein R, Hong F, Young LJ, Shew JY, Lee E: Human retinoblastoma susceptibility gene: Cloning, identification and sequence. Science 235:1394–1399, 1987.
22. Tang A, Wu KJ, Liu WY, Hashimoto T, Shi XH, Mihara K, Takahashi R, Zhang FH, Chen YY, Du C, Qian J, Lin YG, Murphree AL, Qiu WR, Benedict WF, Thompson T, Fung YK: Genomic organization of the human retinoblastoma gene. Oncogene, in press.
23. Abramson DH, Ellsworth RM, Kitchin FD, Tung G: Second nonocular tumors in retinoblastoma survivors. Are they radiation induced? Ophthalmol 91:1351, 1984.
24. Schimke RN, Lowman JT, Cowan GAB: Retinoblastoma and osteogenic sarcoma in siblings. Cancer 34:2077, 1974.
25. Gordon H: Family studies in retinoblastoma. Birth Defects Orig Art Ser 10(10):185, 1974.

26. Hansen MF, Koufos A, Gallie BL, Phillips RA, Fadstad O, Brogger A, Gedde-Dahl T, Cavenee WK: Tumor suppressors: Recessive mutations that lead to cancer. Proc Natl Acad Sci USA 82:6216–6220, 1985.
27. Dryja TP, Rapaport JM, Epstein J, Goorin AM, Weichselbaum R, Koufos A, Cavenee WK: Chromosome 13 homozygosity in osteosarcoma without retinoblastoma. Am J Hum Genet 38:59–66, 1986.
28. Melton DW, Konecki DS, Brennard J, Caskey CT: Structure, expression, and mutation of the hypoxanthine phosphoribosyltransferase gene. Proc Natl Acad Sci USA 81:2147–2151, 1984.
29. Ishii S, Xu YH, Stratton RH, Roe BA, Merlino GT, Pastan I: Characterization and sequence of the promoter region of the human epidermal growth factor receptor gene Proc Natl Acad Sci USA 82:4920–4924.
30. Friend SH, Horowitz JM, Gerber MR, Wang XF, Bogenmann E, Li FP, Weinberg RA: Deletions of a DNA sequence in retinoblastomas and mesenchymal tumors: Organization of the sequence and its encoded protein. Proc Natl Acad Sci USA 84:9059–9063.
31. T'Ang A, Varley JM, Chakraborty S, Murphree AL, Fung YK: Structural rearrangement of the retinoblastoma gene in human breast carcinoma. Science 242:263–266, 1988.
32. Harbour JW, Lai SL, Whang-Peng J, Gazdar AF, Minna JD, Kaye FJ: Abnormalities in structure and expression of the human retinoblastoma gene in SCLC. Science 241:353–357, 1988.
33. Yokota, Akiyama T, Fung YK, Benedict WF, Namba Y, Hanaoka M, Wada M, Terasaki T, Shimosato Y, Sugimura T, Terada M: Altered expression of the retinoblastoma (RB) gene in small-cell carcinoma of the lung. Oncogene 3:471–475, 1988.
34. T'Ang A, et al.: Unpublished, 1989.
35. Ishii S, Merlino GT, Pastan I: Promotor region of the human Harvey ras proto-oncogene: Similarity to the EGF receptor proto-oncogene promotor. Science 230:1378–1381, 1985.
36. Holfman, EK, Trusko SP, Freeman N, George D: Structural and functional characterization of the promotor region of the mouse c-Ki-*ras* gene. Mol Cell Biol 7:2592–2596, 1987.
37. Whyte P, Buchkovich KJ, Horowitz JM, Friend SH, Raybuck M, Weinberg RA, Harlow E: Association between an oncogene and an anti-oncogene: the adenovirus EIA proteins bind to the retinoblastoma gene product. Nature 334:124–129, 1988.
38. Decaprio JA, Ludlow JW, Figge J, Shew JY, Huang CM, Lee WH, Marsilio E, Paucha E, Livingston DM: SV40 large tumor antigen forms a specific complex with the product of the retinoblastoma susceptibility gene. Cell 54:275–283, 1988.
39. Lee WH, Shew JY, Hong FD, Sery TW, Donoso LA, Young LJ, Bookstein R, Lee EYH: The retinoblastoma susceptibility gene encodes a nuclear phosphoprotein associated with DNA binding activity. Nature 329:642–645, 1987.
40. Landschulz WH, Johnson PF, McKnight SL: The leucine zipper: A hypothetical structure common to a new class of DNA binding Proteins. Science 240:1759–1764, 1988.
41. Yee S, Branton PE: Detection of cellular proteins associated with human adenovirus type 5 early region 1A polypeptides. Virology 147:142–153, 1985.
42. Harlow E, Whyte P, Franza BR, Schley C: Association of adenovirus early region 1A Proteins with cellular polypeptides. Mol Cell Biol 6:1579–1589, 1986.
43. Moran E: A region of SV40 large T-antigen can substitute for a transforming domain of the adenovirus EIA products. Nature 334:168–170, 1988.
44. Figge J, Webster T, Smith TF, Paucha E: Prediction of similar transforming regions in simian virus 40 large T, adenovirus EIA, and *myc* oncoproteins. J Virol 62:1814–1818, 1988.

14. Therapeutic applications of oncogenes

James W. Larrick and Edison Liu

Oncogene research and cancer treatment

It is hoped that understanding the fundamental mechanisms of oncogenesis will lead to novel and more rational treatments of cancer. Explorations into the differences between the growth kinetics of cancerous and normal tissues have already given us cell-cycle-dependent chemotherapeutic agents. The development of the oncogene concept, depicting tumorigenesis as perturbations in individuals genes, has further raised expectations for therapeutic advances. Conceivably, methods might be devised to directly inhibit the activity of individual transforming genes. In this chapter, we will describe current work using our knowledge of oncogenes in cancer therapy, and discuss possibilities for therapeutic applications. Whereas the diagnostic and monitoring functions of oncogenes are already being used in contemporary medicine, the therapeutic applications that will be discussed remain hypothetical. The possibilities, however, are intriguing in that anti-oncogene therapeutics represent a conceptually novel approach to cancer treatment.

Oncogenes as prognostic markers in cancer therapy

Cancer patients are frequently stratified according to clinical parameters in order to tailor their cancer therapy. For example, the separation of patients with acute leukemia into those with lymphocytic leukemia and those with myelocytic leukemia is important, since the optimal treatment for each form is different. Even in a particular disease, the identification of patients with good and poor prognostic potential is helpful, since more aggressive therapy may be needed to achieve cures in the poor prognostic group.

Oncogenes are prognostic markers in certain human cancers. N-*myc* amplification is an independent determinant in predicting a poor outcome in childhood neuroblastoma. Those children with amplification of N-*myc*, regardless of stage, will have a shorter survival [1,2]. Thus current therapeutic efforts are concentrated on intensifying treatment in this poor prognostic group. The *bcr/abl* rearrangement in chronic myelogenous leukemia (CML) occurs within

Benz, C. and Liu, E., (eds.), Oncogenes. © 1989 Kluwer Academic Publishers.
ISBN 0-7923-0237-0. All rights reserved.

a 6-kb DNA segment on chromosome 22 called the breakpoint cluster region (*bcr*) [3,4]. Those with breakpoints in the 5' portion of the *bcr* appear to have a longer chronic phase than those with breakpoints in the 3' portion [5,6]. Presently the only cure for CML is bone marrow transplantation during the chronic phase, which is a therapy with considerable morbidity and mortality. Because certain individuals may survive for many years and even decades with the disease [7] on minimal therapy, the timing of the bone marrow transplantation becomes critical. Transplanation too early in the course of the disease may result in premature death from therapy-related complications. Transplantations too late in the disease, when the patient is entering blast crisis, result in greatly reduced cure rates. Thus Southern blot determination of the location of the *bcr/abl* breakpoint may help clinicians decide the optimal timing for the bone marrow transplantation. Similarly, patients with myelodysplasia (a preleukemic condition) progress to acute leukemia at very different rates. Recently, mutations in the *ras* proto-oncogenes have been detected in approximately 30% of such patients, with some studies showing early development of acute leukemia in those harboring aberrant *ras* alleles [8,9]. Bone marrow transplantation may be curative in limited circumstances [10] and would be applied only to those with a poor prognosis. Thus the presence of a *ras* mutation, besides providing prognostic information for the physician and the patient, may possibly be used one day to help identify patients with the myelodysplastic syndrome who will benefit from an early bone marrow transplantation. Approximately 10%–20% of acute lymphocytic leukemias (ALL) have *bcr/abl* rearrangments either of the ALL type or of the CML type (see chapter 10). Childhood ALL can be cured by chemotherapy, but 30%–50% will relapse. Since CML has never been cured by conventional chemotherapy, it is speculated that ALL patients with *bcr/abl* rearrangments will be in the relapsing group. In fact, children with Philadelphia-chromosome-positive ALL have a significantly greater relapse rate than other ALL cases [11].

Other oncogenes have been associated with malignancies, but the relevance of these associations to prognosis has not been ascertained. Nevertheless, work is proceeding to determine their utility in cancer therapy. In diffuse large-cell lymphoma (DLCL), chemotherapy is curative in 50%–60% of patients. Of these patients, 15%–28% harbor a *bcl*-2 rearrangement that is commonly seen in follicular lymphomas [12,13]. In contrast, follicular lymphomas are not curable even with intensive therapy. If DLCL patients with *bcl*-2 rearrangments originate as follicular lymphomas, then it is anticipated that these patients will not be cured with aggressive chemotherapy, a potentially important prognostic point that demands more study. Amplification of HER-1/*neu*, *int*-2, or *myc* have been seen in breast cancer [14,15,16], but the significance of each event in the primary disease is unclear [17,18]. The possibility exists that the presence of any gene amplification may indicate increased genetic plasticity of the tumor cells, and thus a greater potential of these cells to develop drug resistance or increased tumorigenicity [19]. Therefore, in metastatic breast cancer, the presence of gene amplification may be an indicator of a shorter remission duration. Again, the veracity of this speculation awaits experimental proof.

Oncogenes as markers of response to therapy

The efficacy of any therapy can immediately be determined by reduction in tumor burden. Cures cannot occur without drastic decreases in tumor cell number. In most situations, light microscopic and biochemical methods are insensitive in detecting minimal residual disease. An activated oncogene, however, may be used as a marker of cancer cells, and response to therapy can be monitored using this marker. Acute myelogenous leukemia patients with *ras* mutations who fail to eliminate the aberrant allele after induction chemotherapy will not achieve a complete response and therefore will not be cured by the chemotherapeutic regimen [20]. Detection of residual tumor using oncogene markers has been employed in monitoring the effects of treatment in myelodysplasia [21], CML [22], and lymphomas [23]. In another approach, the expression of growth-related oncogenes has been used as a predictor of chemotherapeutic efficacy. It has been found that *myc* expression quickly decreases as leukemic cells die after in vitro exposure [24]. Patients whose cells did not exhibit such a reduction of proto-oncogene expression did not achieve remissions. Thus oncogenes can be used not only as markers of residual disease, but also as markers of chemosensitivity.

Antibody-directed therapy

Antibodies against oncoproteins

The best example of a cell surface oncogene product that might serve as a target for monoclonal antibody directed therapies is the *neu* proto-oncogene. The human *neu* gene, also called HER-2 or c-*erb*B-2, encodes a polypeptide of 185 kDa with a transmembrane topology similar to the epidermal growth factor receptor (EGF-R; see chapter 6). A single point mutation in the gene that encodes the transmembrane portion of the molecule accounts for activation of the *neu* proto-oncogene in mice [25,26,27]. In humans, amplification of *neu* is seen in a proportion of breast adenocarcinomas and head and neck squamous carcinoma [16,17,28]. Antibodies binding the *neu* oncogene product inhibit the in vitro and in vivo growth of cells expressing this protein [25,29]. Efforts to optimize the tumor cell kill of the anti-*neu* antibodies show that monoclonals of certain IgG subclasses were more effective than others in suppressing tumor growth [30]. Furthermore, combinations of monoclonals are synergistic in their anti-tumor effects. Despite the ability of these monoclonal antibodies to suppress tumor growth, they are incapable of eradicating established *neu*-expressing tumors in athymic nude mice: once the monoclonals were discontinued, the tumors grew to kill the animals. Though cure could not be demonstrated, the dramatic reductions in tumor growth are sufficiently exciting to warrant further investigation. Conceivably, attachment of toxins such as ricin A may further increase the therapeutic efficacy of the anti-oncoprotein monoclonal antibodies [31,32,33]. This is particularly attractive with anti-*neu* antibodies since rapid internalization of these monoclonals, which occurs after binding, would augment the transport of the conjugated toxins into *neu*-expressing cells [34,35].

Antibodies may also be exploited for their ability to bind autocrine growth factors [36]. For example, antibodies have been shown to block the growth in vitro and in vivo of small-cell lung carcinoma cells by binding bombesin, an autocrine growth factor released by these cells [37]. Because bombesin possesses various normal metabolic functions, the effects of depriving normal cells of this growth factor remain unknown but are of concern.

In some cases, anti-growth-factor antibodies have been found to be ineffective. Neutralizing antibodies to the oncogene *sis* (the oncogene homologue of the platelet-derived growth factor) will not block growth in culture of *sis*-transformed cell lines [38]. It has been suggested that this lack of effect may be the result of intracellular stimulation of growth by this factor, thus preventing the antibody access to its target.

Antibodies, directed against transformation-associated protein products

Malignant T- and B-cells frequently express lineage- and clonal-specific markers on their cell surfaces. For T-cells these markers are the T-cell receptors, and for B-cells, they are surface immunoglobulins. Levy and coworkers [39] have shown that anti-idiotype antibodies can identify a malignant clone of T- or B-cells. In a limited number of cases, treatment of B-cell lymphoma patients with anti-idiotype antibodies has resulted in clinical remissions [39, 40]. However, in most cases, tumor cells escape recognition by the anti-idiotype antibodies by accumulating mutations within the immunoglobulin variable regions [41]. Escape of aberrant clones has remained a consistent problem for antibody therapy in malignant lymphomas, and serves as a warning against undue optimism when applying this form of treatment against other targets such as oncogenes.

Antibodies may be directed against other transformation-associated proteins. Transferrin-receptor expression is generally increased in rapidly growing cells, including malignant cells. Antitransferrin-receptor monoclonal antibodies with attached toxins are capable of killing cells in vitro overexpressing the transferrin receptor [32].

Increased levels of proteolytic enzymes such as collagenases as well as serine proteases have been associated with some malignant tumors and tumor cell lines. An important proteolytic activity associated with neoplastic cells results from the cascade initiated by the generation of plasmin from serum plasminogen by the protease plasminogen activator (PA). PA production and the generation of plasmin correlate with growth in agar, tumorigenicity of viral transformants, and the tumorigenicity of malignant melanoma cells, though increased PA production is not required for transformation. Low concentrations of a monoclonal antibody against PA inhibited the morphological changes associated with Rous sarcoma virus transformation of chick embryo fibroblasts [42]. The monoclonal antibody inhibited the degradation of extracellular matrix, and the effect mediated by PA released from the tumor cells.

Therapeutic interventions against oncogene-related processes

Anti-ras therapeutics

Because of the high prevalence of *ras* mutations in human cancers, and the importance of this proto-oncogene in normal cellular function, interventions designed to interrupt *ras* action are conceptually attractive therapeutic possibilities.

The importance of *ras* in the induction and maintenance of the transformed state is underscored by experiments where the phenotype of *ras*-transformed cells was reverted to the normal state by microinjection of anti-*ras* antibodies [43]. Furthermore, other microinjection experiments have shown that inhibition of normal *ras* function prevents proliferation of cells transformed by oncogenes attached to the plasma membrane, such as *fms*, *fes*, and *src* [44]. Thus successful anti-*ras* therapeutics may have a wide range of action.

Since the intracellular introduction of anti-*ras* antibodies is not a practical therapeutic approach, other means of interrupting *ras* function are necessary. It is known that the Na^+/K^+ – ATPase inhibitor, ouabain, is 100–1000 times more toxic to *ras*-transformed cells than to their nontransformed counterparts [45,46]. This sensitivity is augmented in alkaline pH, or by co-incubation with Na^+, K^+ ionophores, and occurs to the same degree in v-*fes*- and *met*-transformed cells but to a lesser extent in cells transformed by v-*src*, v-*mos*, and c-*myc* [47,48]. Clearly, ouabain cannot be used as a chemotherapeutic agent due to the systemic (mainly cardiac) effects of the drug. However, it is conceivable that a less toxic ouabain analogue might be synthesized that could safely be employed in intact animals. More importantly, these studies demonstrate that *ras*-transformed cells are more sensitive to ionic stress and that membrane ion pumps may serve as new targets for cancer therapeutics.

The recent discovery of the GTPase activating protein (GAP) provides another link in the transformation pathway in which novel therapies can intervene [49]; see chapter 4). GAP may either be the effector protein for *ras* function or a necessary cofactor. In either case, agents that interrupt GAP action or the GAP/*ras* interaction have the potential of becoming important anti-*ras* agents. Such agents, however, are presently unknown, and their development awaits further understanding of GAP function.

There is evidence that *ras* may play a regulatory role in the phosphatidylinositol (PI) pathway [57]. Fibroblasts transformed by *ras* oncogenes exhibit elevated steady states of phophatidylinositol-4, 5-biphosphate (PIP_2), 1,2-diacylglycerol (DAG), and inositol-1, 4,5-triphosphate (IP_3) [50]. Furthermore, overexpression of the N-*ras* proto-oncogene augments PI turnover in cells treated with growth factors such as bombesin and bradykinin [51]. In every case, the increase in intracellular DAG also stimulates protein kinase C (PKC) activity. Agents that perturb this signal transduction pathway, especially those that block PKC function, may have anticancer activity and conceivably will have more effect on cells harboring a mutant *ras* gene. Agents such as adriamycin [52], tamoxifen [53], and m-AMSA [54] are known inhibitors of protein kinase C and are currently used in cancer chemotherapy. Staurosporine, a microbial alkaloid and an inhibitor of PKC, inhibits the growth of leukemic cells in culture, but its most striking effect is the augmentation of differentiation of HL-60 cells by compounds such as retinoic acid, dibutyryl cyclic AMP, and dihydroxyvitamin D_3 [55]. Agents that induce differentiation have been used in antileukemic therapy with limited success [68]. This suggests that the coupling of PKC inhibitors with other antineoplastic agents might prove efficacious.

Protein mimetics

Protein mimetics are molecules synthesized and designed to mimic or block the function of proteins. In the case of the growth receptors, molecules can be identified that inhibit the binding of a given ligand to its receptor. Recently, inhibitors of substance P, a peptide related to bombesin, have been synthesized and shown to inhibit the growth of small-cell carcinoma cells in vitro [56]. Theoretically, a similar approach can be applied to other growth-factor/growth-factor-receptor complexes, though the practical implementation of these approaches will prove difficult: the receptors may be mutated so as to be constitutively activated (e.g., EGFR, perhaps *neu*), or the growth factor receptor may be so vital to the function of normal cells that systemic administration of a growth factor inhibitor will be too toxic.

Anti-tyrosine kinase inhibitors

Compounds such as quercetin and genistein that inhibit protein tyrosine kinase activity have been described, but their lack of specificity as kinase inhibitors and their toxicity have precluded their use in vivo [58,59]. Umezawa and colleagues characterized a compound, erbstatin, isolated from an actinomycete that specifically inhibits the autophosphorylation of the EGF receptor on the surface of A431 epidermoid carcinoma cells [60]. Chemical modifications of this benzylidene malonitrile-based compound results in a number of derivatives with highly specific anti-EGFR activity: EGF-dependent cell proliferation is specifically inhibited, whereas EGF-independent proliferation is not affected [61]. The synthesis of such oncogene-specific inhibitors may allow for the fine-tailoring of cancer therapies in the future.

Antisense oligonucleotide therapeutics

Single-stranded mRNA is capable of hybridizing with a single-stranded oligonucleotide with a complementary sequence. In some c ses, this antisense oligonucleotide can inhibit the ultimate expression of the target gene's protein by mechanisms that may involve activation of RNAse H, a cellular enzyme that destroys RNA hybridized to DNA. Antisense oligonucleotides have been shown to inhibit cellular processes in vitro [62,63,64,69]; however, a major obstacle had been the relative inability of charged oligonucleotides to pass through the cell membrane. This problem has been partly solved by the use of noncharged and nonhyrolyzable methylphosphonate oligonucleotides [62]. Using antisense oligonucleotides, viral expression has been curtailed [62,63,64] and *myc* action attenuated [64]. More recently, antisense oligonucleotides against c-*myb* inhibited in vitro colony growth of normal hematopoietic precursors [66], and oligonucleotides against proliferating cell nuclear antigen (PCNA) were able to reduce the proliferative rate of cells in vitro [70]. Thus there is mounting evidence supporting the applicability of this approach to altering cell growth [71]. Conceptually, a panel of antisense oligonuleotides each directed to different portions of a critical oncogene or to a group to oncogenes can be applied to a tumor with the hope that the simultaneous attenuation of expression of these oncogenes will kill the malignant cells. Practical future applications of such antisense therapeutics will be in tumors localized to the skin or confined to a body cavity. In this respect, Miller and Ts'o [72] report that when applied as a cream, antisense oligonucleotides against HSV-1 immediate early mRNA 4 and 5 were able to prevent the emergence of herpetic lesions in ears of infected mice.

Anti-cancer vaccines

Can the protein products of oncogenes be used for immunogens? When the behavior of oncogenes in cancer is better understood, it may be possible to predict which oncogene perturbations occur most commonly in certain subgroups. High-risk individuals could be vaccinated, particularly if the oncoproteins are expressed on the cancer cell surface. In at least one model case, surface expression of the oncoprotein was not necessary for successful vaccination. In utero administration of the carcinogen ethylnitrourea (ENU) followed by the tumor promoter butylated hydroxyl toluene (BHT) in mice leads to development of lung adenocarcinomas and T-cell lymphomas. These tumors are associated with increased expression of *raf*-1, an oncogene coding for an intracellular protein kinase. When animals were immunized with the v-*raf* protein, the time to tumor development after birth was significantly delayed, though the ultimate mortality rate was unchanged [65].

The most practical anticancer vaccines may prove to be antiviral vaccines, since the most prevalent cancers worldwide are caused by viruses. Perinatal hepatitis B infection followed by chronic active hepatitis and cirrhosis is strongly associated with hepatocellular carcinoma. It is hoped that the development of effective and relatively inexpensive hepatitis B vaccines will break the maternal-perinatal infection cycle and significantly reduce the incidence of liver cancer. Because of the long latency period between HBV infection and development of liver cancer, observation over many years will be necessary before the efficacy of these vaccines can be established. Other examples of human viruses closely associated with cancers include Epstein–Barr virus with lymphomas and nasopharyngeal carcinomas, cytomegalovirus with Kaposi's sarcoma, papilloma virus with cervical, laryngeal, and esophageal cancers, and the human T-cell lymphotropic viruses with adult T-cell leukemia.

Though there is little experience with human anticancer vaccines, work on veterinary vaccines to prevent cancers is encouraging. Vaccines against the retrovirus feline leukemia virus reduce the incidence of leukemia/lymphoma in cats, and bovine papilloma virus vaccines prevent genital warts in cattle [66,67].

Perspectives

The utility of oncogenes in the classification of human cancers and in monitoring cancer therapy is clear. The future of anti-oncogene-based therapies, however, is uncertain. This uncertainty comes from the increasing awareness that the structural differences between the proto-oncogenes and their transforming counterparts, the oncogenes, are frequently miniscule, and that proto-oncogenes play important functions in normal cell growth and differentiation. Thus therapies that can distinguish the normal from the transforming oncoproteins will be difficult to develop, and such therapies may damage normal cells by interfering with proto-oncogene function. Anti-oncogene therapeutics, therefore, possess all the inherent problems of current chemotherapeutic agents. Nevertheless, they represent a conceptual advance in rational therapeutic design: treatments are formulated to attack specific biochemical changes in malignant cells induced by the presence of activated oncogenes.

Though cures may not be accomplished with individual anti-oncogene therapeutics, neither are cures found using single-agent chemotherapy. Thus the effectiveness of antioncogene agents will be maximized when used in combination with other modalities. In this manner, anti-oncogene therapeutics will expand the armamentarium available to the cancer therapist.

References

1. Seeger RC, Brodeur GM, Sather H, et al.: Association of multiple copies of the N-*myc* oncogene with rapid progression of neuroblastoma. N Engl J Med 313:1111–1117, 1985.
2. Brodeur GG, Seeger RC, Schwab M, et al.: Amplification of N-*myc* in untreated human neuroblastoma correlates with advanced disease stage. Science 224:1121–1124, 1984.
3. Heisterkamp N, Stephenson JR, Groffen J: Localization of the c-*abl* oncogene adjacent to a translocation breakpoint in chronic myelocytic leukemia. Nature 306:239–242, 1983.
4. Bienerhassett GT, Further ME, Anderson A, Burns JP, et al.: Clinical evaluation of a DNA probe for the Philadelphia translocation in chronic myelogenous leukemia. Leukemia 2:648–657, 1988.
5. Schaefer-Rego K, Dudek H, Popenoe D, et al.: CML patients in blast crisis have breakpoints localized to a specific region of the bcr. Blood 70:448–455, 1987.
6. Mills KI, MacKenzie ED, Birnie GD: The site of the breakpoint within *bcr* is a prognostic factor in Philadelphia-positive CML patients. Blood 72:1237–1241, 1988.
7. Kantarjian HM, Smith TL, McCredie KB, et al.: Chronic myelogenous leukemia: a multivariate analysis of the associations of patient characteristics and therapy with survival. Blood 66:1326–1335, 1985.
8. Liu E, Hjelle B, Morgan R, Hecht F, Bishop JM: Mutations of the Kirsten *ras* protooncogene in myelodysplastic syndrome. Nature 330:186–188, 1987.
9. Hirai H, Kobayashi Y, Mano H, et al.: A point mutation at codon 13 of the N-*ras* oncogene in myelodysplastic syndrome. Nature 327:430–432, 1987.
10. Appelbaum FR, Storb R, Ramberg RE, et al.: Treatment of preleukemic syndromes with marrow transplantation. Blood 60:92–96, 1987.
11. Ribeiro RC, Abromowitch M, Raimondi SC, Murphy SB, Behm F, Williams DL: Clinical and biological hallmarks of the Philadelphia chromosome in childhood acute lymphoblastic leukemia. Blood 70:948–953, 1987.
12. Weiss LM, Warnke RA, Sklar J, Cleary M: Molecular analysis of the t(14;18) chromosomal translocation in malignant lymphomas. N Engl J Med 317:1185–1189, 1987.
13. Aisenberg AC, Wilkes BM, Jacobson JO: The bcl-2 gene is rearranged in many diffuse B-cell lymphomas. Blood 71:969–972, 1988.
14. Varley JM, Walker RA, Casey G, Brammar WJ: A common alteration to the int-2 protooncogene in DNA from primary breast carcinomas. Oncogene 3:87–91, 1988.
15. Escot, C, Theillet C, Lidereau R, Spyratos F, Champeme M, Gest J, Callahan R: Genetic alteration of the c-*myc* protooncogene in primary human breast carcinomas. Proc Natl Acad Sci USA 83:4834–4838, 1986.
16. Slamon DJ, Clark GM, Wong S, Levin WJ, Ullrich A, McGuire WL: Human breast cancer: correlation of relapse and survival with amplification of the HER-1/*neu* oncogene. Science 235:177–182, 1987.
17. van der Vijver M, van de Bersselaar R, Devilee P, Cornelisse C, Peterse J, Nusse R: Amplification of the *neu* (c-*erb*B-2) oncogene in human mammary tumors is relatively frequent and is often accompanied by amplification of the linked c-*erb*A oncogene. Mol Cell Biol 7:2019–2023, 1987.
18. Varley JM, Swallow JE, Brammar WJ, Whittaker JL, Walker RA: Alterations of either c-*erb*B-2 (neu) or c-*myc* protooncogenes in breast carcinomas correlate with poor short-term prognosis. Oncogene 1:423–430, 1987.
19. Lippman ME: Oncogenes and breast cancer. N Engl J Med 319:1281–1282, 1988.
20. Senn HP, Tran-Thang C, Wodnar-Filipowicz A, Jiricny J, Fopp M, Gratwohl A, Signer E, Weber W, Moroni C: Mutation analysis of the N-*ras* protooncogene in active and remission phase of human acute leukemias. Int J Cancer 41:59–64, 1988.
21. Layton DM, Mufti GJ, Lyons J, Janssen JWG, Bartram CR: Loss of *ras* oncogene mutation in a myelodysplastic syndrome after low dose cytarabine therapy. N Engl J Med 318:1468–1469, 1988.

22. Kawasaki ES, Clark SS, Coyne MY, Smith SD, Champlin R, Witte ON, McCormick FP: Diagnosis of chronic myeloid and acute lymphocytic leukmias by detection of leukemia specific mRNA sequences amplification in vitro. Proc Natl Acad Sci USA 85:5698–5702, 1988.
23. Lee MS, Chang KS, Cabanillas E, et al.: Detection of minimal residual cells carrying the t(14;18) by DNA sequence amplification. Science 237:175–178, 1987.
24. Venturelli D, Lange B, Narni F, Selleri L, Mariano MT, Torelli U, Gewirtz AM, Calabretta B: Prognostic significance of short term effects of chemotherapy on MYC and histone H3 mRNA levels in acute leukemia patients Proc Natl Acad Sci USA 85(10):3590–3594, 1988.
25. Drebin JA, Link VC, Stern DF, Weinberg RA, Greene MI: Down-modulation of an oncogene protein product and reversion of the transformed phenotype by monoclonal antibodies. Cell 41:695–706, 1988.
26. Akiyama T, Sudo, Ogawara T, et al.: The product of the human c-*erb*B-2 gene: 185 kilodalton glycoprotein with tyrosine kinase activity. Science 232:1644–1646, 1986.
27. Bargman C, Hung MC, Weinberg R: Multiple independent activations of the *neu* oncogene by a point mutation altering the transmembrane domain of p185. Cell 45:649–657, 1986.
28. Semba K, Kamata N, Toyoshima K, Yamamoto T: A v-*erb*B related protooncogene, c-*erb*B-2 is distinct from the c-*erb*B-1 epidermal growth factor gene and is amplified in a human salivary gland adenocarcinoma. Proc Natl Acad Sci USA 82:6497–6501, 1985.
29. Drebin JA, Link VC, Weinberg RA, Greene MI: Inhibition of tumor growth by a monoclonal antibody reactive with an oncogene encoded tumor antigen. Proc Natl Acad Sci USA 83:9129–9133, 1986.
30. Drebin JA, Link VC, Greene MI: Monoclonal antibodies reactive with distinctive domains of the *neu* oncogene-encoded p185 molecule exert synergistic anti-tumor effects in vivo. Oncogene 2:273–277, 1988.
31. Vitetta ES, Korlick KA, Miyama-Inaba M, et al.: Immunotoxins: A new approach to cancer therapy. Science 219:644–650, 1983.
32. Taetle R, Castagnola J, Mendelsohn J: Mechanisms of growth inhibition by anti-transferrin receptor monoclonal antibodies. Cancer Res 46:1759, 1986.
33. Fitzgerald DJ, Willingham MC, Pastan I: Antitumor effects of an immunotoxin made with Pseudomonas extoxin in a nude mouse model of human ovarian cancer. Proc Natl Acad Sci USA 83:6627–6633, 1986.
34. Ceriani RL, Blank EW, Peterson JA: Experimental immunotherapy of human breast carcinomas implanted in nude mice with a mixture of monoclonal antibodies against human milk fat globule components. Cancer Res 47:532–540, 1987.
35. Reisfeld RA: Immunochemical characterization of human tumor antigens. Semin Oncol 13:153–164, 1984.
36. Sporn MB, Roberts AB: Autocrine growth factors and cancer. Nature 313:745–747, 1985.
37. Cuttita F, Carney DN, Mulshine J, et al.: Bombesin-like peptides can function as autocrine growth factors in human small cell lung cancer. Nature 316:823–826, 1985.
38. Williams LT: The sis gene and PDGF. Cancer Surv 5:223–241, 1986.
39. Levy R, Stratte P, Link M, et al.: Monoclonal antibodies to human lymphocytes: clinical application in therapy of leukemia. In: Kennett RH, Bechtold KB, McKearn TJ (eds): Monoclonal Antibodies and Functional Cell Lines. New York, Plenum Press, 1984, p 193.
40. Meeker TC, Lowder J, Maloney DG, Miller RA, Thielemans K, Warnke R, Levy R: A clinical trial of anti-idiotype therapy for B cell malignancy. Blood 65:1349–1363, 1985.
41. Cleary ML, Meeker TC, Levy S, Lee E, Trela M, Sklar J, Levy R: Clustering of extensive somatic mutations in the variable region of an immunoglobulin heavy chain gene from a human B cell lymphoma. Cell 44:97–106, 1986.
42. Sullivan LM, Quigley JP: An anticatalytic monoclonal antibody to avian plasminogen activator: its effect on behavior of RSV-transformed chick fibroblasts. Cell 45:905–915, 1986.
43. Feramisco JR, Clark R, Wong G, Arnhein N, Milley R, McCormick F: Transient reversion of *ras* oncogene-induced cell transformation by antibodies specific for amino acid 12 of *ras* protein. Nature 314:639–642, 1985.

44. Smith MR, DeGudicibus SJ, Stacey DW: Requirement for c-*ras* proteins during viral oncogene transformation. Nature 320:540–543, 1986.
45. Noda M, Selinger Z, Scolnick E, Bassin R: Flat revertants isolated from Kirsten sarcoma virus-transformed cells are resistant to the action of specific oncogenes. Proc Natl Acad Sci USA 80:5602–5606, 1983.
46. Benade L, Talbot N, Hardy K, Tagliaferri P, Card J, Noda M, Najam N, Bassin R: Ouabain sensitivity is linked to *ras*-transformation in human HOS cells. Biochem Biophys Res Comm 136:807–814, 1986.
47. Wany SY, Bassin RH, Racker E: Effect of high K+ hypertonicity and ouabain on MeAIB uptake and on growth of c-*myc* and v-*ras* transfected rat fibroblasts. Oncogene 3:53–57, 1988.
48. Talbot N, Tagliaferri P, Yanagihara K, Rhim JS, Bassin RH, Benade LE: A pH-dependent differential cytotoxicity of ouabain for human cells transformed by certain oncogenes. 3:23–26, 1988.
49. Trahey M, McCormick F: A cytoplasmic protein stimulates normal N-*ras* p21 GTPase but does not affect oncogenic mutants. Science 238:543–545, 1987.
50. Fleischman LF, Chahwala SB, Cantley L: *Ras*-transformed cells: altered levels of phosphatidylinositol-4, 5-biphosphate and catabolites. Science 231:407–410, 1986.
51. Wakelam MJO, Davies SA, Houslay MD, McKay I, Marchall CJ, Hall A: Normal p21 N-*ras* couples bombesin and other growth factor receptors to inositol phosphate production. Nature 323:173–176, 1986.
52. Wise BC, Glass DB, Jen Chou CH, Raynor RL, Katoh N, Schatzman RC, Turner RS, Kibler RF, Kuo JF: Phospholipid-sensitive Ca2+-dependent cis protein kinase from heart. II. Substrate specifity and inhibition by various agents. J Biol Chem 257:8489–8495, 1982.
53. Horgan K, Cooke E, Hallett MB, Mansel RE: Inhibition of protein kinase C mediated signal transduction by tamoxifen. Biochem Pharmacol 35:4463–4465, 1986.
54. Hannun YA, Bell RM: Aminoacridines, potent inhibitors of protein kinase C. J Biol Chem 263:5124–5131, 1988.
55. Okazaki T, Kato Y, Mochizuki T, Tashima M, Sawada H, Uchino H: Staurosporine, a novel protein kinase inhibitor, enhances HL-60 cell differentiation induced by various compounds. Exp Hematology 16:42–48, 1988.
56. Woll OJ, Rozengurt E: (D-Arg^1,D-Phe^5,D-Trp^{7,9},Leu^{11}) substance P, a potent bombesin antagonist in murine Swiss 3T3 cells, inhibits the growth of human small cell lung cancer cells in vitro. Proc Natl Acad Sci USA 85:1859–1863, 1988.
57. Barbacid, M: *Ras* genes. Annu Rev Biochem 56:779–827, 1987.
58. Graziani J, Erikson E, Erikson RL: The effect of quercetin on the phosphoryl activity of the Rous sarcoma virus transforming gene product in vitro and in vivo. Eur J Biochem 135:583–589, 1983.
59. Akiyama T, Ishida J, Nakagawa S, Ogawara J, Watanabe SI, et al.: Genistein, a specific inhibitor of tyrosine-specific protein kinases. J Biol Chem 262:5592–5595, 1987.
60. Umezawa H, Imoto M, Sawa T, Isshiki K, Matsuda N, et al.: Studies on a new epidermal growth factor-receptor kinase inhibitor, erbstatin, produced by MH 435-hF3. J Antibiotics 39:170–173, 1986.
61. Yaish P, Gazit A, Gilon C, Levitzki A: Blocking of EGF-dependent cell proliferation by EGF receptor kinase inhibitors. Science 242:933–935, 1988.
62. Smith CC, Autrelion L, Reedy MP, et al.: Antiviral effect of an oligonucleotide methylphosphonate complementary to the splice junction of herpes simples virus type 1 immediate early pre-mRNAs 4 and 5. Proc Natl Acad Sci USA 83:2787–2791, 1986.
63. Zamecnik PS, Goodchild J, Taguchi Y, Sarin PS: Inhibition of replication and expression of human T-cell lymphotropic virus type III in cultured cells by exogenous synthetic oligonucleotides complementary to viral RNA. Proc Natl Acad Sci USA 83:4143–4146, 1986.
64. Holt JT, Redner RL, Nienhuis AW: An oligomer complementary to c-*myc* mRNA inhibits proliferation of HL60 promyelocytic cells and induces differentiation. Mol Cell Biol 8:963–973, 1988.

65. Rapp UR, Cleveland JL, Storm SM, Beck TW, Huleihel M: Transformation by *raf* and *myc* oncogenes. In: Aaronson SA, Bishop JM, Surgimura T, Terada M, Toyashimi K, Vogt PK (eds): Oncogenes and Cancer. Japan Scientific Press/VNU Scientific Press, 1987, pp 6–26.
66. Haffer KN, Sharpee RL, Beckenhauer WH: Feline leukemia vaccine protection against viral latency. Vaccine 5:237–240, 1987.
67. Pfister H: Human papilloma virus and genital cancer. Adv Cancer Res 48:113–147, 1987.
68. Koeffler HP: Induction of differentiation of human acute myelogenous leukemia cells: Therapeutic implications. Blood 62:709–721, 1983.
69. Gewirtz AM, Calabretta B: A c-*myb* antisense oligodeoxynucleotide inhibits normal human hematopoiesis in vitro. Science 242:1303–1306, 1988.
70. Jaskalski O, DeRiel JK, Mercer WE, Calabretta B, Baserga R: Inhibition of cellular proliferation by antisense oligodeoxynucleotides to PCNA cyclin. Science 240:1544–1546, 1988.
71. van der Krol AR, Mol JNM, Stuitje AR: Modulation of eukaryotic gene expression by complementary RNA and DNA sequences. Biotechniques 6:958–976, 1988.
72. Miller PS, Ts'o POP: A new approach to chemotherapy based on molecular biology and nucleic acid chemistry: Matagen (masking tape for gene expression). Anti-Cancer Drug Design 2:117–128, 1987.

Index

abl oncogene, 21, 127, 152
Acquired immunodeficiency syndrome (AIDS)
 Epstein-Barr virus (EBV)-associated lymphoproliferations in, 291
 human immunodeficiency viruses (HIV-1, HIV-2) in, 267
 Kaposi's sarcoma in, 286
 non-Hodgkin's lymphoma (NHL) associated with, 273–279
Acute lymphocytic leukemia (ALL), 14, 105, 244–245, 251, 254
Acute myelogenous leukemia (AML), 14, 105, 251, 255
Acute nonlymphocytic leukemia (ANLL), 253
Adenocarcinomas
 breast cancer and, 205
 epidermal growth factor receptor (EGFR) and, 154
 lung (ADCL), 210–212
 oncogene activation in, 200
Adenovirus E1A
 c-myc oncogene and, 51
 protein-transforming activity in, 11
 ras oncogenes and, 99
 retinoblastoma gene and, 315
 src oncogenes and, 131, 133
Adenoviruses, 11, 285
Adenyl cyclase
 ras oncogenes and, 102
 transduction and, 6–8
Adult T-cell leukemia lymphoma (ATLL), 267, 268–273
AIDS, *see* Acquired immunodeficiency syndrome (AIDS)
Aplysia rho gene, and *ras* oncogene, 79, 97, 98
AP1 transcription factor, 9–10
APUD cells, 223
Astrocytoma, 223
Ataxia-telangiectasia, 291
Avian erythroblastosis virus (AEV), and epidermal growth factor receptor (EGFR), 146–147
Avian leukemia virus (AVL), 11, 43
Avian myeloblastosis virus, 251

Basal cell carcinomas, 224
B-cell lymphoma, 268, 272
bcl-1 oncogene, 14
bcl-2 oncogene, 14, 250–251
Bladder cancer, 14, 220–221
 DNA analysis of, 221
 epidermal growth factor receptor (EGFR) and, 154, 155
 experimental models of, 220
 ras oncogenes and, 105
 retinoblastoma gene in, 310
B-lymphocytes
 bcl-2 protein in lymphoma and, 250
 c-myc oncogene and, 46
 human immunodeficiency virus type 1 (HIV-1) and, 275
 N-*myc* oncogene and, 53
B-*myc* oncogene, 37, 58
Brain cancers, 222–223
Breast cancer, 14, 199, 205–209
 DNA analysis of, 206–208
 epidermal growth factor receptor (EGFR) and, 155
 experimental models of, 205–206
 oncogene activation in, 203–204
 RNA analysis of, 208–209
 scr oncogenes and, 134
 transforming growth factor α (TGF α), 184
Burkitt's lymphoma
 c-myc oncogene and, 44, 45, 47, 208, 248–249
 Epstein-Barr virus (EBV) and, 249–250, 275, 286, 290–291

c-abl oncogene
 chronic myelogenous leukemia (CML) and, 242–246
 gastric cancer and, 213
 sarcomas and, 225
 tyrosine kinase and, 18

c-*bas* oncogene, 225
Calcium
  epidermal growth factor receptor (EGFR) and, 153
  transduction and, 6, 8–9
Calmodium, and transduction, 6, 9
cAMP, and transduction, 6–8
Carcinogenesis, *see* Oncogenesis
Cell culture, 35
Cell proliferation, 3–10
  cancerous phenotype in, 10
  cell cycle in, 33–34
  growth factors in, 4–5
  transmembrane signal transduction in, 5–10
c-*erb*-A oncogene, 19, 20
c-*erb*B-1 oncogene, 204
  bladder cancer and, 221
  breast cancer and, 205, 208
  colorectal cancer and, 214
  gastric cancer and, 213
  head and neck cancers and, 222
  hematopoietic malignancies and, 251
  lung cancer and, 211
  pancreatic cancer and, 217
  renal cancer and, 220
  vulvar cancer and, 218
c-*erb*B-2 oncogene
  breast cancer and, 199, 205, 206, 208–209
  gastric cancer and, 213
  lung cancer and, 211
Cervical cancer, 219, 287–288, 289
c-*fes* oncogene, 208
c-*fgr* oncogene, 121, 122
  oncogenesis and, 131
  tyrosine kinase genes and, 123, 124
c-*fms* oncogene, 170, 218
  breast tumors and, 208
  hematopoietic malignancies and, 251, 252, 254
c-*fos* oncogene
  breast cancer and, 208
  colorectal cancer and, 215, 216
  sarcomas and, 225
  thyroid cancers and, 222
  transcription and, 9, 19, 20
Chain termination method, 28–30
Childhood cancers, 225–227
Choriocarcinoma, 218
Chronic myelogenous leukemia (CML), 14, 18
  c-*abl* oncogene in, 242–246
  progression from chronic to blast-phase in, 245–246
c-*jun* oncogene, 19, 20
Cloning techniques for DNA, 30–32
c-*mos* oncogene, 213, 214
c-*myb* oncogene, 19
  breast cancer and, 207
  hematopoietic malignancies and, 251

leukemogenesis and, 251
c-*myc* oncogene, 37–52
  breast cancer and, 204, 205, 206, 207–208
  Burkitt's lymphoma and, 44, 45, 47, 208, 248–249
  cervical cancer and, 219
  colorectal cancer and, 214, 215, 216
  discovery of, 37–38
  esophageal cancer and, 212
  gastric cancer and, 213
  human immunodeficiency virus type 1 (HIV-1) in B cells and, 276
  liver cancer and, 218
  lung cancer and, 210, 211
  mRNA of, 41
  normal function of, 47–52
  oncogenesis and, 43–47, 131, 199, 204
  open reading frame (ORF) of, 38–39
  prostatic cancer and, 220
  protein of, 42–43
  ras oncogenes and, 99
  renal cancer and, 220
  sarcomas and, 225
  testicular cancer and, 219
  thyroid cancers and, 222
  transcription and, 9, 19, 20, 39–40
  transforming growth factor β (TGF β), 189
  Wilms' tumor and, 226
c-*neu* oncogene protein, 16, 226
Coding sequences, 26
Colony stimulating factor-1 (CSF-1), 16
  epidermal growth factor receptor (EGFR) and, 145
  hematopoietic malignancies and, 252, 254
  platelet-derived growth factor (PDGF) and, 169, 170–171
Colorectal cancer, 14, 214–217
  DNA analysis of, 215–216
  experimental models of, 214–215
  oncogene activation in, 200
  protein analysis of, 216–217
  ras oncogenes and, 105
  RNA analysis of, 216
  src oncogenes and, 134
  uterine cancer and, 218
Consensus DNA, 26
c-*raf* oncogene, 219, 220, 222
c-*ras* oncogene, and colorectal cancer, 214
c-*rel* oncogene, 19
c-*sis* oncogene, 171, 223, 225
c-*src* oncogene, 121, 122
  cervical cancer and, 219
  epidermal growth factor receptor (EGFR) and, 152
  oncogenesis and, 131, 132
  phosphorylation and, 128–130
  primary translation product and, 124–125, 127
  transcription and, 123
  tyrosine kinase genes and, 123, 124

c-*yes* oncogene, 121, 122
 oncogenesis and, 131
 transcription and, 123
 tyrosine kinase genes and, 123, 124
Cystadenocarcinoma, ovarian, 218
Cytomegalovirus, 286

dbl oncogene, 14
Diacylglycerol (DAG)
 epidermal growth factor receptor (EGFR) and, 152
 ras oncogenes and, 102
 transduction in normal cells and, 6, 9
Dideoxynucleotides, and DNA sequencing studies, 30
Diffuse B-cell lymphoma, 14
Diffuse large-cell lymphoma, 250–251
Dimethylbenzathrene (DMBA)
 breast cancer and, 205
 skin carcinoma and, 201
Dimethylhydrazine, and colorectal cancer, 214
DMSO, and c-*myc* oncogene, 48–49
DNA
 cell culture studies of, 35
 cloning of, 30–32
 growth factors in cell replication and, 4
 molecular biology studies of, 27–34
 polymerase chain reaction (PCR) with, 32–34
 protein studies of, 34–35
 replication of, 3, 4
 restriction endonucleases and, 27
 restriction fragment length polymorphism (RFLP) analysis of, 27–28
 RNA splicing and, 26
 sequencing of, 28–30
 Southern hybridization studies of, 27
 transcription and, 25–26
 transfection of, 36
DNA tumor viruses, 11, 285
Double minutes, with c-*myc* oncogene, 46

EGF, *see* Epidermal growth factor (EGF)
Embryonal cell carcinoma, 219
Endometrial carcinoma, 218
Enhancer sequences, 9
Enhancers, 26
Epidermal growth factor (EGF)
 breast cancer and, 209
 mechanism of action of, 150–156
 normal cell replication and, 4, 5
 oncogenes with growth factors similar to, 16
 pancreatic cancer and, 217
 ras oncogenes and, 99
 structure of, 148–149
 transforming growth factors (TGFs) and, 177, 178, 185
Epidermal growth factor receptor (EGFR), 143, 144–146
 bladder cancer and, 221
 carcinogenesis and, 154–155
 cervical cancer and, 219
 colorectal cancer and, 217
 hematopoietic malignancies and, 251, 253
 lung cancer and, 210, 212
 mechanism of action of, 150–156
 neu gene and, 147–147
 ovarian cancer and, 219
 poxvirus growth factors and, 150
 transforming growth factor (TGF) and, 149
 v-*erb*B oncogene and, 146–147
 vulvar cancer and, 218
Epidermoid cancer, 14
Epstein-Barr virus (EBV), 286–287, 290–297
 Burkitt's lymphoma and, 249–250, 275, 286, 290–291
 chronic myelogenous leukemia (CML) and, 245–246
 c-*myc* oncogene and, 46
 molecular biology of, 291–297
 nasopharyngeal carcinoma (NPC) and, 291
 non-Hodgkin's lymphoma (NHL) associated and, 275–276
 pathogenesis of, 290–291
*erb*B oncogene, 146–147, 154, 199
ERBB2 gene, 147
Erythroleukemia
 c-*myc* oncogene and, 48
 retroviruses and, 248
Esophageal cancer
 epidermal growth factor receptor (EGFR) and, 154, 155
 oncogenes in, 212
Estrogen, and breast cancer, 184, 206
ets oncogene, and hematopoietic malignancies, 251, 253
Ewing's sarcoma, 200, 224–225
Exons, 26
Expression libraries, 34

Familial polyposis coli, 200
Feline sarcoma virus (FeSV), 16
fes oncogene, 251, 252
Fibroadenoma, 209
Fibroblast growth factor (FGF), 16
Fibroblasts
 c-*scr* oncogene and, 130
 ras oncogenes and, 80–81, 99
 transforming growth factor α (TGF α), 183–185
 transforming growth factor β (TGF β), 188
Fibrosarcoma, 14, 172, 225
fos oncogenes
 activation of, 21
 growth factors and, 152

hematopoietic malignancies and, 251, 252
fyn oncogene, 121, 122
  transcription and, 123
  tyrosine kinase genes and, 123, 124

gag protein, 13
Gastric cancer
  epidermal growth factor receptor (EGFR) and, 155
  oncogenes in, 213–214
Gene amplification
  c-*myc* oncogene and, 45–46
  N-*myc* oncogene and, 54–55
Giant-cell lung carcinoma, 204
Glioblastoma
  epidermal growth factor receptor (EGFR) and, 154, 155
  oncogenes in, 223
Glioma, 172
  epidermal growth factor receptor (EGFR) and, 154, 155
G_1 phase in cell cycle, 3–4
G protein
  ras oncogene interaction with, 82, 101, 102
  transduction and, 7
Growth factors
  normal cell proliferation and, 4–5
  oncogenes with growth factors similar to, 15–17
  transduction and, 9
GTPase-activating protein (GAP)
  ras oncogene interaction with, 19, 81–86, 90–91, 94–96
G_2 phase in cell cycle, 3, 4
Guanine nucleotide binding, and *ras* oncogenes, 86–88

hck oncogene, 121, 122
  myeloproliferative disorders and, 255
  tyrosine kinase genes and, 123, 124
Head and neck cancers, 221–222
Hematopoietic malignancies
  oncogene activity in, 251–254
  tumor-suppressor genes in, 254
Hepadna viruses, 285
Hepatitis B virus (HBV), 287
Hepatoblastoma, and N-*myc* oncogene, 51
Hepatocellular carcinoma (HCC), 287
Hepatoma, 14, 218
Herpes simplex virus (HSV), 286
Herpes viruses, 11, 285
HER2 gene, 147
H-*ras* oncogene, 74
  bladder cancer and, 220, 221
  breast cancer and, 205–206, 207, 208, 209
  carboxyl methylation of, 89
  cellular differentiation and, 100
  colorectal cancer and, 216
  GTPase-activating protein (GAP) and, 84–85, 91, 95
  inositol phosphates and transformation of, 103
  leukemia and, 247–248, 252
  liver cancer and, 218
  lung cancer and, 210
  melanomas and, 223–224
  oncogenesis and, 14, 19, 100, 104, 105, 106
  primary structure of, 74–77
  renal cancer and, 220
  solid tumors and activation of, 201–204
  three-dimensional structure of protein of, 92–93
  thyroid cancers and, 222
  transduction and, 103–104
hst oncogene
  gastric cancer and, 213
  oncogenesis with, 14
Human cytomegalovirus (HCMV), 286
Human immunodeficiency virus type 1 (HIV-1), 267–268
  epidemiology and clinical characteristics of, 273–274
  Epstein-Barr virus (EBV) infection and, 275–276
  human T-lymphotropic viruses (HTLV-I, HTLV-II) co-infection with, 278
  lymphomas associated with, 273–279
  molecular characterization of, 274–275
  pathogenesis of, 275–279
Human immunodeficiency virus type 2 (HIV-2), 267
Human papilloma viruses (HPVs), 285–286, 287–290
  DNA structure of, 288–289
  pathogenesis of, 287–288
  transcription in infected tissues of, 289
  transforming genes of, 289–290
Human T-cell leukemia virus type I (HTLV-I), 13–14, 267
  adult T-cell leukemia lymphoma (ATLL) and, 267, 268–273
  clinical aspects of infection with, 268
  epidemiology of, 269
  human immunodeficiency virus type 1 (HIV-1) co-infection with, 278
  mechanisms of transformation of, 271–273
  molecular biology of, 270–271
  transmission of, 269–270
Human T-cell leukemia virus type II (HTLV-II), 13, 267, 278
Human T-cell leukemia virus type V (HTLV-V), 267

Immunocytoma, and c-*myc* oncogene, 45
Immunoprecipitation, 35
Infectious mononucleosis, 286
Inositol phosphates
  ras oncogenes and, 102, 103
  transduction and, 6
Insulin

epidermal growth factor receptor (EGFR) and, 151
transduction and, 5
Interferon, and lymphoma cells, 41
Interleukin 1 (IL-1), 273
Interleukin 2 (IL-2), 267
human T-cell leukemia virus type I (HTLV-I) and, 272
Interleukin 3, 254
int-1 oncogene, and growth-factor receptors, 16
Introns, 26

Kaposi's sarcoma, 16, 286
Keratoacanthoma, and *ras* oncogenes, 105
K-*ras* oncogene, 74
bladder cancer and, 220
cervical cancer and, 219
colorectal cancer and, 215, 216
gastric cancer and, 213
inositol phosphates and transformation of, 103
leukemia and, 247–248, 252
liver cancer and, 218
lung cancer and, 210
oncogenesis and, 14, 19, 99, 100, 104, 105, 106, 199, 200
ovarian cancer and, 218
pancreatic cancer and, 217
preleukemia and, 246–247
primary structure of, 74–77
sarcomas and, 225
solid tumors and, 204, 209
thyroid cancers and, 222

Large-cell lung cancer (LCLC), 210–212
lca oncogene, 14
lck oncogene, 121, 122, 130
tyrosine kinase genes and, 123, 124
Leiomyosarcoma, uterine, 218
Leukemias
oncogenes associated with, 14, 241–244, 251
ras oncogenes and, 104, 105
retroviruses and, 267
see also specific leukemias
Library, 31
Liver cancer, 217–218
L-*myc* oncogene, 20, 37, 55–58
breast cancer and, 199
lung cancer and, 210, 211
Lung cancer, 14, 204, 210–212
chromosomal deletion in, 200
DNA analysis of, 210–211
epidermal growth factor receptor (EGFR) and, 155
experimental models of, 210
N-*myc* oncogenes and, 46, 51, 55–58, 199
protein analysis of, 212
ras oncogenes and, 105, 199, 200

retinoblastoma gene in, 310
RNA analysis of, 211–212
Lymphoid cells, and *ras* oncogenes, 99
Lymphomas
bcl-2 oncogene in, 250–251
c-*myc* oncogene and, 41, 47, 48, 249–250
human T-cell leukemia virus type V (HTLV-V) in, 267
ras oncogenes and, 106
retroviruses and, 267
Lymphoproliferative syndrome, with Epstein-Barr virus (EBV), 286, 291
lyn oncogene, 121, 122
tyrosine kinase genes and, 123, 124

Mammary carcinoma
oncogene activation in, 201
transforming growth factor α (TGF α), 181, 184
mcf2 oncogene, 14
mcf3 oncogene, 14
Medulloblastoma, and N-*myc* oncogene, 53
Melanomas, 14, 223–224, 310
Meningiomas
chromosomal deletion in, 200
epidermal growth factor receptor (EGFR) and, 155
oncogenes in, 223
Messenger RNA (mRNA)
c-*myc* oncogene and, 41
molecular biology studies of, 26
Metastatic tumors, and *ras* oncogenes, 106
met oncogene, 225
Mitosis, 3, 4
Molecular biology
concepts of, 25–27
techniques of, 27–36
mos oncogenes, and protein kinases, 18
M phase in cell cycle, 3, 4
Multiple endocrine neoplasia (MEN), 223
Murine erythroleukemia (MEL), and c-*myc* oncogene, 48
Murine mammary tumor virus (MMTV), 205, 206
Murine plasmacytoma (MPC), and c-*myc* oncogene, 44
myb family of oncogenes, 21
myc family of oncogenes, 37–59
activation of, 21
growth factors and, 152
oncogenesis with, 14, 154, 199
see also specific oncogenes
Myelodysplastic syndrome (MDS), 246–247, 255
Myeloproliferative disorders, 255

Nasopharyngeal carcinoma (NPC), 286, 291
Neck cancers, 221–222
neu gene, and epidermal growth factor receptor (EGFR), 145, 147–148

Neuroblastoma, 14, 211, 226–227
  chromosomal deletion in, 200
  N-*myc* oncogene and 53, 54, 55, 199
  ras oncogenes and, 105
Neuroectodermal tumors, 223
Neurofibromas, and chromosomal deletions, 200
Nitrosomethylurea (NMU), and breast cancer, 205
N-*myc* oncogene, 19, 20, 37, 52–55
  brain cancers and, 223
  colorectal cancer and, 215
  expression of, 53–54
  lung cancer and, 210, 211, 212
  neuroblastomas and, 226–227
  oncogenesis and, 54, 154, 199
  Wilms' tumor and, 226
Noncoding sequences, 26
Non-Hodgkin's lymphoma (NHL)
  epidemiology and clinical characteristics of, 273–274
  Epstein-Barr virus (EBV) infection and, 275–276
  human immunodeficiency virus type 1 (HIV-1) and, 273–279
  lymphomas associated with, 273–279
  molecular characterization of, 274–275
  pathogenesis of, 275–279
Northern blot analysis, 34
N-*ras* oncogene, 74
  colorectal cancer and, 215
  gastric cancer and, 213
  GTPase-activating protein (GAP) and, 91, 95
  leukemia and, 247–248, 252
  melanomas and, 223–224
  neuroblastomas and, 226
  oncogenesis with, 14, 19, 209
  preleukemia and, 246–247
  primary structure of, 74–77
  protein palmitylation and, 89
  thyroid cancers and, 222
Nuclear oncogenes, 19–20

Oliodendroglioma, 223
Oncogenes
  cell proliferation and, 10
  classes and functions of, 15–21
  c-*myc* oncogene and, 43–47
  epidermal growth factor receptor (EGFR) and, 147–148, 154–155
  Epstein-Barr virus (EBV) in, 298–299
  human papilloma viruses (HPVs) in, 298–299
  human tumors associated with, 14–15
  L-*myc* oncogene and, 58
  N-*myc* oncogene and, 54
  platelet-derived growth factor (PDGF), and, 171–172
  recessive nature of cancer and, 303–305
  src oncogenes and, 131–134
  transforming growth factor α (TGF α), 180–181, 182, 183–185
  transforming growth factor β (TGF β), 189–190
  see also specific oncogenes
Oncogenesis
  activation of proto-oncogenes in, 20–211
  DNA viruses and, 11
  ras family of oncogenes and, 18–19, 100–101, 104–106
  retroviruses and, 14
  RNA viruses and, 13
  solid tumors and, 199–204
Open reading frame (ORF), c-*myc* oncogene, 38–39
Osteogenic sarcoma, 225
Osteosarcoma, 310
Ovarian carcinoma, 14, 204, 218–219

Palmitate, and *ras* oncogenes, 89–90
Pancreatic cancer, 14, 204
  epidermal growth factor receptor (EGFR) and, 155
  oncogene activity in, 217
Papilloma virus
  Ha-*ras* oncogene and, 201
  see also Human papilloma viruses (HPVs)
Papova viruses, 11, 285
Philadelphia chromosome (Ph^1), 242, 245, 247
Phosphatidyl inositol (PI)
  epidermal growth factor receptor (EGFR) and, 152, 153
  ras oncogenes and, 102–103
Phosphodiesterase, and transduction, 6
Phosphorylation
  epidermal growth factor receptor (EGFR) and, 151
  src oncogenes and, 128–130
Phosphotyrosine
  epidermal growth factor receptor (EGFR) and, 146
  src oncogenes and, 132
Pituitary adenoma, and epidermal growth factor receptor (EGFR), 155
Plasmacytoma, and c-*myc* oncogene, 44
Platelet-derived growth factor (PDGF), 169–173
  brain cancers and, 223
  c-*myc* oncogene and, 48
  c-*src* oncogene and, 130
  epidermal growth factor receptor (EGFR) and, 145
  malignant transformation and, 171–172
  molecular structure and function of, 169–171
  normal cell replication and, 4, 5
  oncogenes with growth factors similar to, 15

transcription and, 9
P-*myc* oncogene, 58
Polyadenylation, 26
Polymerase chain reaction (PCR), 32–34
Polyoma virus
  enhancer sequences of, 9
  ras oncogenes and, 99
  src oncogenes and, 132–133
  transforming growth factor α (TGF α), 183
Poxvirus growth factors, 150
Preleukemia, 246–247
Promoters, 26
Promyelocytic leukemia, 14
  c-*myc* oncogene and, 48
Prostate cancer, 200, 219–220
Protein activity
  c-*mcy* oncogene, 42–43
Protein kinase C (PKC)
  epidermal growth factor receptor (EGFR) and, 151
  transduction and, 6, 9
Protein studies of cells, 34–35
Psoriasis
  epidermal growth factor receptor (EGFR) and, 155
  transforming growth factor α (TGF α), 182

raf oncogenes
  gastric cancer and, 213
  oncogenesis with, 14
  protein kinases in, 18
ras family of oncogenes, 73–106
  activation of, 21
  acute leukemia and, 247–248
  biochemical properties of protein of, 81–98
  cellular differentiation and, 100
  epidermal growth factor receptor (EGFR) and, 153
  experimental carcinogenesis with, 106
  genes related to, 78–80
  lung cancer and, 210
  mechanisms of activation of, 80–81
  members of, 74
  model for function of, 94–96
  oncogenesis and, 14, 18–19, 100–101, 104–106
  preleukemia and, 246–247
  primary structure of, 74–81
  protein structure-function studies of, 92–94
  thyroid cancers and, 222
  transduction interactions and, 7, 101–104
  transformation of cells and, 98–99
  see also specific oncogenes
RAS1 gene, 98, 102
RAS2 gene, 98, 102
Refractory anemia with excess blasts (RAEB), 246
Renal cell carcinoma, 200

c-*myc* oncogene and, 45
transforming growth factor α (TGF α), 181, 182, 184
Restriction endonucleases, in DNA studies, 27
Restriction fragment length polymorphism (RFLP) analysis, 27–28, 304
ret oncogene, 14
Retinoblastoma, 225–226, 310
  chromosomal deletion in, 200, 226
  N-*myc* oncogene and, 51
Retinoblastoma gene
  human cancers and, 310–311
  isolation of, 305–306
  leucine zipper in, 312–314
  oncoproteins and, 314–315
  physiological role of, 316
  structural evidence for, 306–309
Retinoblastoma suppressor gene, 254
Retroviruses
  breast cancer and, 205
  classification of, 267
  c-*myc* oncogene and, 43–44
  leukemias and, 254
  malignancy associated with, 267–279
  oncogenesis and, 14, 21
  ras oncogenes and, 104, 248
  transforming growth factors (TGFs) and, 177
Rhabdomyosarcoma, 14, 225
rho genes, and *ras* oncogenes, 79, 97, 98
R-*myc* oncogene, 58
RNA
  cell culture studies of, 35
  molecular biology studies of, 34–35
  protein studies of, 34–35
  splicing of, 26
  translation and, 25
RNA tumor viruses, 11–14
ros oncogene, and growth-factor receptors, 17
R-*ras* oncogene
  oncogenesis and, 19
  proteins of, 97–98
  structure of, 79

Sarcoma cell lines
  oncogene activation and, 224–225
  platelet-derived growth factor (PDGF) and, 172
  retroviruses and, 248, 267
  src oncogenes and, 131
  transforming growth factor α (TGF α), 180
Sarcoma growth factor (SGF), 149, 177
Screened library, 31
SEC4 gene, and *ras* oncogenes, 97, 98
Seminoma, 219
Serous cystadenocarcinoma, 218
Simian virus 40 (SV40), 11
  enhancer sequences of, 9

nuclear oncogenes in transformation of, 19, 20, 285
platelet-derived growth factor (PDGF) and, 169, 172
ras oncogenes and, 99
retinoblastoma gene and, 315
src oncogenes and, 133
transforming growth factor α (TGF α), 183
Skin carcinomas
oncogene activation in, 223–224
ras oncogenes in, 106, 201
Small-cell lung carcinoma
c-*myc* oncogene and, 46
L-*myc* oncogene and, 55–58
N-*myc* oncogene and, 51
retinoblastoma gene in, 310
Solid tumors, 199–229
cooperation between activated oncogenes in, 204
mechanism of oncogene activation in, 199–201
oncogene activation during carcinogenesis in, 201–204
retinoblastoma gene in, 310
see also specific tumors
Southern hybridization, 27
S phase in cell cycle, 3, 4
Splicing, 26
Squamous tumors
epidermal growth factor receptor (EGFR) and, 154, 155
head and neck, 222
lung cancer, 210–212
skin, 224
transforming growth factor α (TGF α), 181, 182, 184
src family of oncogenes
functions of normal cellular products of, 134–136
general properties of, 122–123
members of, 121–122
oncogenic potential of, 130–134, 255
phosphorylation and, 128–130
primary translation product and, 124–128
tissue distribution of tyrosine kinases and, 123–124
Steroid hormone, and cell proliferation, 4, 9
Stomach cancer, 14, 204; *see also* Gastric cancer
SV40, *see* Simian virus 40 (SV40)

tat protein, 14
T-cell growth factor, 267
T-cell lymphoma, 14
tcl-1 oncogene, 14, 15
tcl-2 oncogene, 14, 15
Teratocarcinoma, 219
c-*myc* oncogene and, 41, 48
N-*myc* oncogene and, 53
Testicular cancer, 219

Tetradecanoyl phorbol-13-acetate (TPA), and transforming growth factor α (TGF α), 182–183
Thyroid cancers, 222
c-*myc* oncogene and, 48
epidermal growth factor receptor (EGFR) and, 155
Thyroid hormone, and cell proliferation, 4, 9, 20
tkl oncogene, 122, 124
T-lymphocytes
c-*myc* oncogene and, 48
src oncogenes and, 135
Transcription, 25
Transformation in cell culture, 35
Transforming growth factor α (TGF α), 177, 178–185
cellular transformation and, 183–185
derivation of, 178–180
synthesis of, 180–183
Transforming growth factor β (TGF β), 177, 185–190
malignant transformation and, 189–190
structural forms of, 185–186
synthesis of, 186–188
Transforming growth factors (TGFs), 177–190
discovery of, 177–178
epidermal growth factor (EGF) and, 143, 144, 177
types of, 177
Translation, 25
trk oncogene, and growth-factor receptors, 17
Tumor-suppressor genes, and hematopoietic malignancies, 254
Tyrosine protein kinases (TPKs)
chronic myelogenous leukemia (CML) and, 243
epidermal growth factor receptor (EGFR) and, 145, 147
groups of, 121
oncoproteins with, 17–18
phosphorylation and, 128–130
platelet-derived growth factor (PDGF) and, 169, 170
src oncogenes and, 123–124
transduction and, 5–6

Uterine cancer, 218

v-*abl* protein, and tyrosine kinase, 18
Vaccinia growth factor, 150
v-*fes* oncogene, 101
v-*fms* oncogene
growth-factor receptors and, 16–17
oncogenesis and, 101
v-*fps* oncogene, 127
v-H-*ras* oncogene, 73, 100, 104
Viral growth factors (VGFs), 150

v-K-*ras* oncogene, 73, 91, 100
v-*mos* oncogene, 101, 104
v-*myb* oncogene, 51, 251
v-*myc* oncogene, 38, 51, 99, 100, 131
v-*raf* oncogene, 104
v-*ras* oncogene, 248
v-*sis* oncogene
  growth-factor receptors and, 15
  oncogenesis and, 101
  platelet-derived growth factor (PDGF)
    and, 169, 171–172
v-*src* oncogene, 101
  oncogenesis and, 130–131, 132
Vulvar cancer, 218

WAGR (Wilm's tumor, Aniridia,
    Genitourinary abnormalities,
    Retardation), 226
Western blot hybridization, 35
Wilms' tumor
  childhood, 226
  N-*myc* oncogene and, 53
  oncogene activation in, 200, 226
Wiskott-Aldrich syndromes (WA), 291

yes-1 oncogene, and gastric cancer, 213
YPT1 protein
  ras oncogene interaction with, 19, 79,
    96–97, 98